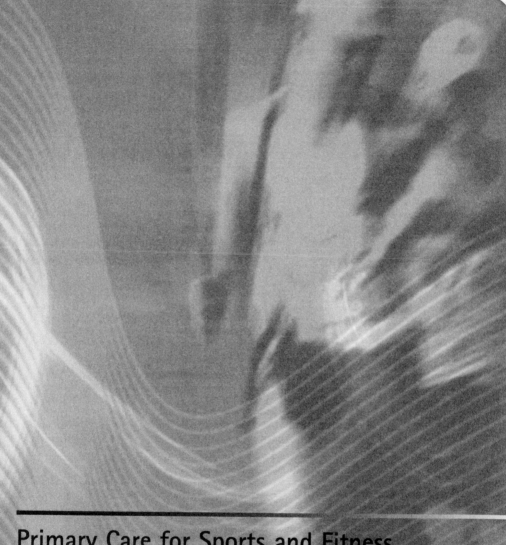

Primary Care for Sports and Fitness
A Lifespan Approach

Brian J. Toy, PhD, ATC
Interim Dean, College of Nursing and Health
 Professions
Associate Professor of Athletic Training,
 Department of Exercise, Health, and Sport
 Sciences
University of Southern Maine

**Phyllis F. Healy, PhD, BC-FNP,
CNL, RN**
Associate Professor of Nursing, School of Nursing
University of Southern Maine

Primary Care
for Sports and Fitness
A Lifespan Approach

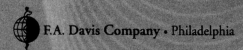 F.A. Davis Company • Philadelphia

F. A. Davis Company
1915 Arch Street
Philadelphia, PA 19103
www.fadavis.com

Printed in the United States of America

Last digit indicates print number: 10 9 8 7 6 5 4 3 2 1

Publisher, Nursing: Joanne Patzek DaCunha, RN, MSN
Developmental Editor: Laura Bonazzoli
Content Development Manager: Darlene Pedersen, RN, MSN
Project Editor: Kristin L. Kern
Manager of Art and Design: Carolyn O'Brien

As new scientific information becomes available through basic and clinical research, recommended treatments and drug therapies undergo changes. The author(s) and publisher have done everything possible to make this book accurate, up to date, and in accord with accepted standards at the time of publication. The author(s), editors, and publisher are not responsible for errors or omissions or for consequences from application of the book, and make no warranty, expressed or implied, in regard to the contents of the book. Any practice described in this book should be applied by the reader in accordance with professional standards of care used in regard to the unique circumstances that may apply in each situation. The reader is advised always to check product information (package inserts) for changes and new information regarding dose and contraindications before administering any drug. Caution is especially urged when using new or infrequently ordered drugs.

Library of Congress Cataloging-in-Publication Data

Toy, Brian J.
  Primary care for sports and fitness : a lifespan approach / by Brian J. Toy, Phyllis F. Healy.
     p. ; cm.
  Includes bibliographical references.
  ISBN-13: 978-0-8036-1492-5
  ISBN-10: 0-8036-1492-6
  1. Sports medicine. 2. Orthopedics. 3. Nurse practitioners. I. Healy, Phyllis F. II. Title.
  [DNLM: 1. Athletic Injuries—Nurses' Instruction. 2. Physical Fitness—Nurses' Instruction. 3. Primary Health Care—Nurses' Instruction. QT 261 T756p 2009]
  RC1210.T69 2009
  617.1'027--dc22

                                                2008041770

This book is dedicated to

– My mom, who watches over our family from afar;

– My dad, who watches over us from above;

– My siblings, who are all accomplished professionals in their chosen careers;

– My daughter, Christine, our princess and Daddy's little girl;

– My son, Aiden, our funny little man;

– My wife, Jacqueline, whose enduring love, support, and understanding allow me to pursue projects like this.

Brian J. Toy

Lovingly dedicated to

– My parents, Vivian (Joe-"Chief") and Cora Foster, smiling from above when once again they realize I do not know what to do when my father is named Vivian!

– My daughter, Megan, and her husband, Ron Raye. Life is so much sweeter because of you both!

Phyllis F. Healy

Acknowledgments

A project of this magnitude cannot be completed without the support of many, many people. In particular, we extend thanks to our contributing authors for helping us produce a quality product. Thanks to Joanne DaCunha and Kristin Kern at F.A. Davis for keeping us on task these past few years and to Laura Bonazzoli who, in the manuscript's early stages, provided excellent insight into the book-writing process. We are grateful to Tracey Fox-Bartels for editing and assuring that the information presented is appropriate for student, and practicing, primary health care providers (and thanks for modeling, Tracey!). Special thanks to Jean Marie Toy, artist extraordinaire, for producing the Patient Teaching Handout figures. We are also indebted to the authors of the numerous F.A. Davis holdings from which we reproduced figures. Thanks to all who reviewed the manuscript. The insight provided was invaluable. To our mentors, past and present, we hope the production of this text pleases you. To our colleagues at the University of Southern Maine, thanks for providing a dynamic place for us to work. To our students, particularly those enrolled in USM's Nurse Practitioner program, this was written with you in mind. We hope you find it useful.

Brian J. Toy, PhD, ATC
Phyllis F. Healy, PhD, BC-FNP, CNL, RN
University of Southern Maine

Contributors

Tracey Fox-Bartels, MSN, FNP, RN
Martin's Point Health Care
Portland, ME

Thomas W. Buford, MS, CSCS
Doctoral Research Assistant, Exercise
    and Biochemical Nutrition Lab
Adjunct Professor, Department of
    Health, Human Performance, and
    Recreation
Baylor University

Tina L. Claiborne, PhD, ATC, CSCS
Assistant Professor and Director of
    Athletic Training Education
Dept. of Exercise Science/Physical
    Education
Adrian College

Karen A. Croteau, EdD, FACSM
Associate Professor of Health Fitness,
    Department of Exercise, Health,
    and Sport Sciences
University of Southern Maine

William F. Simpson, PhD, CES,
    FACSM
Associate Professor and Director,
    Exercise Physiology Laboratory
University of Wisconsin-Superior

Reviewers

Charlotte Covington, MSN, APRN
Family Nurse Practitioner
Associate Professor
Vanderbilt University School of Nursing
Nashville, Tennessee

Sharon Ewing, PhD, FNP, MSN, RN, CS
Clinical Assistant Professor
College of Nursing
University of Arizona
Tucson, Arizona

Linda J. Keilman, MSN, APRN, BC
Assistant Professor
Gerontological Nurse Practitioner
Michigan State University College of
    Nursing
East Lansing, Michigan

Mary Knudtson, DNSc, NP
Professor of Family Medicine
Director of FNP Program
University of California Irvine
Irvine, California

Kathleen Nash, PhD, RN, FNP
Assistant Professor
University of Texas Medical Branch
School of Nursing
Galveston, Texas

Karen Koozer Olson, PhD, FNP
Professor of Nursing
Outreach Programs Coordinator
Texas A&M University
Corpus Christi, Texas

Preface

Primary health care providers are increasingly faced with the responsibility of offering to patients expert advice spanning an array of subject matter related to sports and fitness. Indeed, musculoskeletal injuries are among the most commonly encountered problems in the primary care setting. Recognizing this, in 1998 we proposed that the then Department of Nursing at the University of Southern Maine offer a graduate level course titled *Sports Medicine: Orthopedic Evaluation and Treatment for the Primary Health Care Professional.* The basic premise of this proposal was to offer Nurse Practitioner students, and those practicing in the field, an opportunity to gain more in-depth knowledge in the area of orthopedics than what is typically included in a traditional Nurse Practitioner curriculum. Seeing merit to this proposal, the Department's Graduate Curriculum Committee approved the course offering as a program elective. Over the next few years, course content was modified based on student and faculty feedback and on the ever-changing demands placed on those working in the primary care setting. Thus, though it is impossible for any text to cover all aspects of a subject, the content included in this book is a by-product of 10 years' worth of learning the issues that providers most often encounter in the primary care setting. We hope you find this information helpful.

Brian J. Toy, PhD, ATC
Phyllis F. Healy, PhD, BC-FNP, CNL, RN
University of Southern Maine
April 2008

Contents

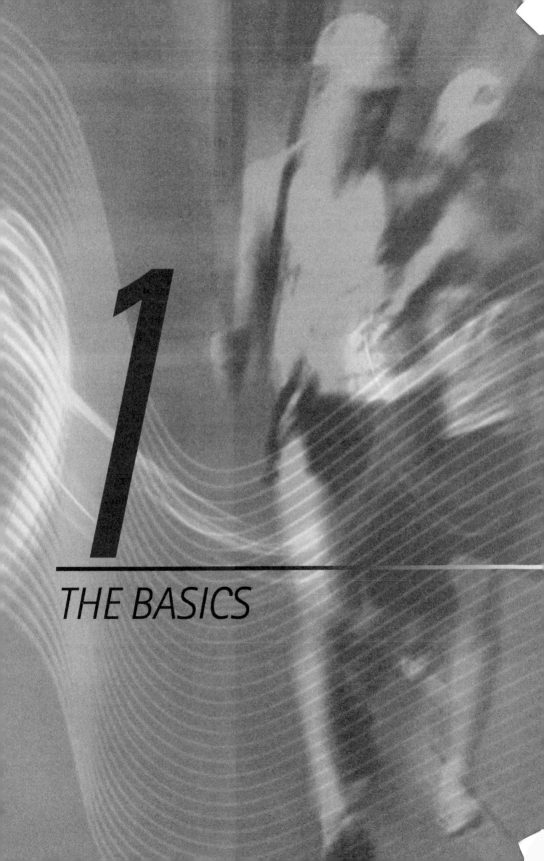

1

THE BASICS

1

Foundations of Musculoskeletal Injury

● Brian J. Toy, PhD, ATC

Before working with people who are interested in participating in sports and fitness activities, primary health care providers must become familiar with body tissues used for exercise. Indeed, understanding what these structures do, recognizing how they are most commonly injured, and knowing what the most common musculoskeletal injuries are, are particularly important when patients report to the primary care setting with a sports-related injury.

Musculoskeletal Definitions

In general, musculoskeletal tissue is divided into two broad classifications: soft and hard. Whereas bone comprises all of the hard tissue within the body, soft tissue includes all things not bone, such as **ligaments** and **tendons**. It is these hard and soft tissues that become injured when the musculoskeletal system is traumatized. In many instances, this means that the joint associated with these tissues is also injured. When working in the primary health care setting, it is important that the health and integrity of hard and soft tissue be assessed during both the pre-participation examination (discussed in Chapter 2) and the orthopedic evaluation process (described in Part II).

Hard Tissue

Bone is comprised of osseous tissue and comes in the following shapes: long, short, flat, and irregular. Sesamoid bones, those which are embedded within a tendon, such as the patella (discussed in Chapter 9), also exist. When the major bones of the body are considered, most long bones are located in the extremities, otherwise known as the *appendicular skeleton*. Exceptions include the short bones of the wrist (carpals) and foot (tarsals) and the flat bones of the pelvis (innominate) and shoulder (scapula). The axial skeleton consists of irregularly shaped bones of the vertebral column and the flat bones of the skull. Regardless of type, when two bones come together, a joint is formed, and the place where this union occurs is referred to as the *joint line*. Though joints can be immovable, otherwise known as *synarthrodial* (e.g., sutures of the skull), or slightly moveable, also referred to as *amphiarthrodial* (e.g., pubic symphysis), it is the diarthrodial, or *synovial*, joints that usually become injured in response to musculoskeletal trauma. The structure and types of diarthrodial joints are discussed later in this chapter.

Major portions of a long bone include the diaphysis, metaphyses, and epiphyses (Fig. 1.1). Whereas compact bone comprises the diaphysis and metaphyses, both compact and spongy bone make up the epiphyses. The diaphysis, or *shaft*, is relatively long and straight and maintains the bone's marrow. This marrow is located in the endosteum-lined medullary cavity, which runs lengthwise within the diaphysis. The metaphyses connect the diaphysis to the proximal and distal epiphyses, which house the bone's secondary ossification centers. The presence of an epiphyseal plate, otherwise known as a *growth plate*, within an epiphysis is a feature exclusive to those bones that have yet to reach full maturity. Once mature, this thin disk of **hyaline cartilage** turns into the epiphyseal line. Except for its proximal and distal ends, each bone is encircled by a fibrous periosteum, a neurovascular-rich structure full of osteoblasts, which aid in new bone formation. A bone's proximal and distal ends are lined by an **articular cartilage**, providing joints with smooth articular surfaces.

In addition to having epiphyseal growth plates, most long bones develop areas that have separate centers of ossification, otherwise known as *apophyses*. These outgrowths

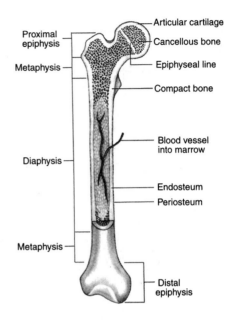

FIGURE 1.1 Portions of a long bone.
From Dillon: *Nursing Health Assessment: A Critical Thinking, Case Studies Approach.* 2003.
Philadelphia: F.A. Davis Company, Fig. 18-2, pg 591, with permission.

are typically located in close proximity to a long bone's epiphyses at its distal or proximal end or both. Commonly termed *tubercles* and *tuberosities*, these apophyseal areas serve as attachment sites for soft tissues such as ligaments and tendons. As discussed later in this chapter, soft tissues subject these apophyses to extreme external forces, such as what happens when a tendon pulls strongly on an apophysis when a muscle contracts.

Soft Tissue

As previously mentioned, soft tissues include all things not bone. Soft tissues most affected by musculoskeletal trauma include **skeletal muscles**, tendons, ligaments, **bursae, nerves, fascia,** and **retinacula**.

Skeletal Muscle and Tendons (Fig. 1.2)

Skeletal muscles consist of contractile elements that, when activated, move diarthrodial joints. For example, when the biceps brachii muscle (described in Chapter 12) is stimulated, it contracts, causing the elbow to flex. Skeletal muscles attach to the bones that they move by way of strong, noncontractile structures called *tendons*. The area where the muscle attaches to the tendon is called the *musculotendinous junction*. Though most muscles have at least one tendon of origin, some, such as the biceps brachii, have more than one. This is because these muscles maintain multiple muscle bellies, requiring that each belly has its own tendon of origin. Like many soft tissues, muscle also has the capability of elongating, or stretching, to a certain degree without being injured, much like a rubber band can stretch within a safe limit without breaking. In contrast, tendons are not flexible, maintaining little, if any, qualities of elasticity.

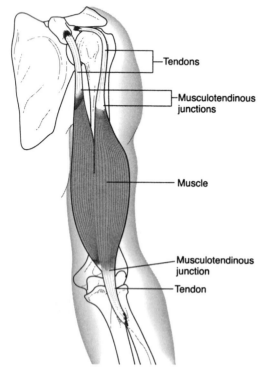

FIGURE 1.2 Parts of a skeletal muscle. From Lippert: *Clinical Kinesiology and Anatomy*, 4th ed. 2006. Philadelphia: F.A. Davis Company, Fig. 10-14, pg 127, with permission.

(PEARL)

Muscles have the capability of stretching, whereas tendons are nonelastic structures.

Diarthrodial Joint Capsule

Though many different types of diarthrodial joints exist, all have the same basic components (Fig. 1.3). That is, they all have a capsule, a ligamentous structure that surrounds the joint, and a synovial membrane, tissue that lines the inner surface of the capsule. The capsule is able to nourish most of the tissues in the region through its vast network of blood vessels. Tissues that cannot benefit from this arrangement are nourished by the joint's synovial fluid, a substance secreted by the synovial membrane. For example, synovial fluid provides the primary nourishment to the joint's interarticular fibrocartilages, such as the menisci of the knee (Fig. 9.4 on page 231). These fibrocartilages attach to the end of one of the joint's bones and serve to keep bones separate from each other. They also stabilize the joint by deepening its socket and cushion the joint by absorbing and dispersing forces applied to it.

As illustrated in Table 1.1, diarthrodial joints are classified by the types of **primary motions** the joint allows. In general, these motions occur actively when a

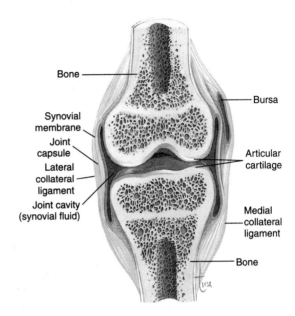

FIGURE 1.3 The structure of a synovial joint.
Adapted from Scanlon: *Essentials of Anatomy and Physiology*, 5th ed. 2007. Philadelphia: F.A. Davis Company, Fig. 6-16, pg 130, with permission.

TABLE 1.1 The different types of diarthrodial joints and the motions they allow

TYPE	MOTIONS	EXAMPLE
Gliding	Side to side	Wrist (intercarpal)
Hinge	Flexion, extension	Knee (tibiofemoral)
Pivot	Rotation (internal and external)	Forearm (proximal and distal radioulnar)
Condyloid	Flexion, extension, abduction, adduction, circumduction, hyperextension (in some instances)	Wrist (radiocarpal)
Ball-and-socket	Flexion, extension, hyperextension, abduction, adduction, circumduction, rotation	Shoulder (glenohumeral)
Saddle	Flexion, extension, hyperextension, abduction, adduction, circumduction, slight rotation	Thumb (carpometacarpal)

person moves the joint himself or herself, or passively, occurring when another person, such a health care provider, moves the joint. In either instance, the amount of motion present for any one movement, such as elbow flexion, is termed the joint's **range of motion** (ROM) for that action. Thus, the terms active ROM (AROM) and passive ROM (PROM) identify the amount of motion a joint has. The motion of **hyperextension** occurs naturally in some joints, such as the shoulder, whereas this is an unnatural movement for other joints, such as the knee. This must be kept in mind when evaluating a patient after a musculoskeletal injury because a joint that hyperextends at the time of injury may or may not be traumatized. Indeed, it is a common misconception among primary health care providers and lay people that "hyperextension" of a joint always leads to injury.

Some joints can naturally hyperextend without being injured, whereas others cannot.

Unlike primary motions, a joint's **accessory motions** are not easily seen or measured. They also cannot occur without the joint's primary motion taking place. However, a joint cannot reach its full AROM or PROM without the presence of these accessory motions. For example, as explained in Chapter 9, the tibia must glide forward, backward, and side to side on the femur for the knee to be able to flex and extend normally. Recognizing that all diarthrodial joints maintain some amount of accessory motion is vital to understanding how a freely moveable joint functions.

Ligaments

Ligaments are tissues that connect bone to bone, making them an important stabilizer of all diarthrodial joints. A ligament is classified as either intrinsic or extrinsic in nature, depending on its relationship to the joint capsule it is associated. Whereas extrinsic ligaments are separate, well-defined structures, intrinsic ligaments are actual thickenings of the capsule. Though not as elastic as muscles, ligaments are supple structures, allowing them to stretch to a certain degree without being injured. Though all diarthrodial joints are supported by a combination of a joint capsule and intrinsic and extrinsic ligaments, well-defined medial (MCL) and lateral (LCL) **collateral ligaments** provide all hinge and condyloid joints with medial and lateral stability (Fig. 1.3).

Medial and lateral collateral ligaments provide hinge and condyloid joints with medial and lateral joint stability and protection.

Bursae

Bursae are synovial fluid–filled sacs located throughout the body (Fig. 1.3). They are responsible for reducing friction between moving tissues, such as between tendon and bone and tendon and tendon. Bursae surround most of the major joints of the body, such as the knee and shoulder, facilitating movement of these structures.

Nerves

Part of the peripheral nervous system, nerves bring information to and from the brain. Whereas afferent nerves provide the brain with sensory information (i.e., pain, touch, etc.), efferent nerves bring directives (i.e., contract a muscle) from the brain to the rest of the body.

Fascia

By and large, all body tissues are covered and interconnected by a dense, fibrous tissue known as *fascia*. Deep fascia supports and protects the hard and soft tissues of the musculoskeletal system. Of note is a special type of fascia, the retinacula, because these bands of tissue are responsible for holding many different tissues in place. For example, the patella retinacula (discussed in Chapter 9) hold the patella in place while it moves within the femoral groove.

Classification and Mechanisms of Musculoskeletal Injury

Musculoskeletal injuries occur in a variety of ways, with various factors increasing a person's risk for developing certain conditions. For example, people with structural abnormalities, such as having a leg length discrepancy (discussed in Chapter 10), or those with flat feet (discussed in Chapter 8), are predisposed to developing a variety of lower extremity and/or low back conditions. These are referred to as *intrinsic risk factors* for causing musculoskeletal injury because they directly relate to body structure. In contrast, extrinsic risk factors are those nonintrinsic things that expose a person to injury, such as employing improper exercise training techniques, using poor footwear, and participating in high-risk activities.[1–3]

In general, musculoskeletal injuries are classified as two types: acute and chronic. An acute musculoskeletal injury is one in which a sudden catastrophe, also known as a *macrotrauma* event, occurs—such as what happens when a person collides with an immovable object or when a tendon suddenly tears. In these instances, the affected tissues are immediately destroyed, and the patient experiences instantaneous pain and disability. This type of condition is usually associated with a specific **mechanism of injury** (MOI), because the person sustaining an acute injury can almost always explain how the injury occurred. In contrast, a chronic, or *overuse*, condition results from repeated microtrauma events, causing the condition to develop over time. In these instances, patients may report moments of pain that dissipate quickly, or they may report an insidious onset of pain that occurs hours or days after the injury occurred. People with an overuse condition usually cannot pinpoint an exact cause of injury, only stating that a particular body part started hurting for no apparent reason. Understanding the differences between acute and chronic injuries and how they occur is important for any primary health care provider charged with assessing musculoskeletal injury.[4,5]

PEARL

Patients with an acute musculoskeletal condition can almost always explain how the injury occurred, whereas people with an overuse condition struggle to pinpoint an exact cause of injury.

Acute Injury

Acute musculoskeletal injuries typically occur when a compressive, tensile, or shearing force is applied to a tissue beyond what the affected tissue can handle (Fig. 1.4). Frequently, this occurs when the body is traumatized from a **valgus**, **varus**, **torsion**, or hyperextension injury mechanism. Gaining an appreciation for the effect these forces and injury mechanisms have on soft and hard tissues enables primary health care providers to assess an injured person better.[6]

Compressive, Tensile, and Shearing Forces

Caused by blunt-force trauma, a compressive, or *axial load*, force, is one that produces a crushing type of injury, such as a **contusion** or **fracture**. For example, whereas the thigh is commonly contused when struck by a hard object, landing on the feet after jumping from a great height may cause one or more bones of the lower extremity to fracture.[7]

A tensile, or *tension*, force, is one that is applied parallel to the affected body tissue(s). Injury results when the tissue is stretched beyond its capacity to lengthen, such as what happens when a muscle or ligament is overstretched. The usual outcome is that the affected tissue tears. In contrast, shearing forces are applied perpendicular to the fibers of affected body tissues. However, like tensile forces, these forces also result in the tearing of the affected structures.[8]

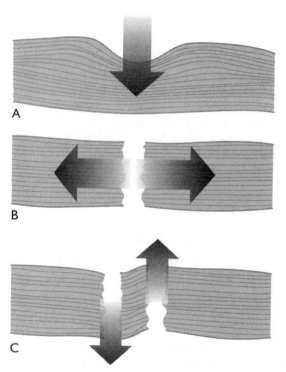

FIGURE 1.4 Forces that injure musculoskeletal tissue: compressive (A), tensile (B), and shearing (C).

Valgus and Varus Injury Mechanisms

A valgus force occurs when a body part, such as the knee, is forced medially, causing the area distal to move away from the midline. When this occurs, the body part's medial structures are at risk of injury. In contrast, a varus force occurs when a body part is forced laterally, causing the area distal to move toward the midline, increasing the chance of injury to lateral structures. When a valgus force is applied to a hinge or condyloid joint, the joint's MCL is at risk of injury, whereas a varus force applied to the same joint increases the chance that the LCL will be traumatized (Fig. 1.5). Typically, these injury mechanisms cause the affected soft tissues to be torn by either a tension or a shearing force.[9]

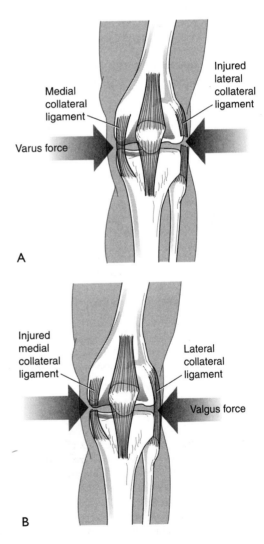

FIGURE 1.5 (A) Varus forces injure lateral structures. (B) Valgus forces injure medial structures.

> Valgus forces applied to the body place the **MCL** of hinge and condyloid joints at risk for injury, whereas varus forces expose the **LCL** to injury.

Hyperextension and Torsion Injury Mechanisms

As its term suggests, a body part, typically a joint, is injured by a hyperextension injury mechanism when it is hyperextended beyond what it is normally capable. This MOI usually results in soft tissue damage from a tensile force. A torsion injury mechanism, otherwise known as a *twisting*, or *rotation*, injury mechanism, occurs when a body part forcefully rotates around a fixed axis. For example, when the foot is firmly planted on the ground, the entire lower extremity must rotate around this fixed point for a person to change direction while walking or running. Doing this places great stress on the ankle, leg, knee, and hip, exposing hard and soft tissues in these regions to shearing-type forces. This injury mechanism offer occurs in conjunction with a valgus, varus, or hyperextension MOI. Indeed, many acute musculoskeletal injuries result from a combination of injury mechanisms.[9]

> A torsion injury mechanism often occurs in conjunction with a valgus, varus, and/or hyperextension MOI.

Chronic Injury

As previously stated, chronic musculoskeletal conditions are often the result of microtrauma. These are the consequences of a person repetitively overloading the body or performing an activity incorrectly and result in conditions such as **stress fractures**, **tendinopathies**, and chronic **bursitis**. Factors that increase the incidence of microtrauma injury include sudden changes to training routine, playing surface, improper footwear; and fatigue. Indeed, exercising or participating in sports when fatigued is a prime cause of all types of musculoskeletal injury.[2,4,5,10–12]

> Exercising or participating in sports when the body is fatigued exposes a person to musculoskeletal injury.

Soft Tissue Conditions

Soft tissue injuries make up the bulk of musculoskeletal conditions seen in the primary care setting. These injuries range from **strains** to **dislocations**, making it vital that primary health care providers understand the basic differences among them.

Muscle Soreness

It is no secret that, at times, exercised muscles become sore. Soreness that begins during and/or immediately after exercise, otherwise known as *acute-onset muscle soreness* (AOMS), develops as a result of factors such as lactic acid production, pain receptor stimulation in the working muscles, and hypoxia due to muscle ischemia. However, when a person stops exercising, pain receptor stimulation ceases, residual lactic acid buildup is removed, and oxygen returns to the muscles. This makes AOMS a fairly transient condition, disappearing an hour or two after exercise. Indeed, contrary to popular belief, the muscle soreness people experience many hours, and sometimes days, after exercise, otherwise known as *delayed-onset muscle soreness* (DOMS), is not due to lactic acid buildup. Rather, DOMS, which typically peaks 24 to 72 hours after exercise, happens when a muscle performs more eccentric contractions (discussed in Chapter 3) during an exercise session than what it is used to. For example, a person who has properly trained to run 5 miles per day at a certain pace usually does not experience muscle soreness as long as he or she runs at the same pace and distance. If, however, the person quickly increases pace and/or running distance, he or she increases the chance of experiencing some degree of DOMS. This soreness only subsides when the muscle fibers damaged during the activity heal.[13,14]

PEARL

Contrary to popular belief, the muscle soreness most people experience several days after exercise is not due to lactic acid buildup in the muscle. Rather, this DOMS is caused when a muscle performs multiple eccentric contractions during an exercise bout.

Tendinopathies

The term *tendinopathies* simply refers to all conditions that involve a tendon. These include **tendinosis**, **tendonitis**, and **paratenonitis**, and though these terms define distinctively different conditions, they are commonly, and incorrectly, used interchangeably in the primary care setting.[15]

Tendinosis

Tendinosis describes a focal area of tendon degeneration that does not exhibit either clinical or histological signs of inflammation. This condition, which develops naturally as a result of aging or tendon overuse, predisposes a person to other tendon injuries, such as a total rupture of a tendon. Tendinosis typically develops when a person places stress on a tendon before the tendon is ready to handle the load. Overloading the tendon in this fashion causes it to degenerate, ultimately leading to injury. A patient can avoid developing tendinosis by employing exercise training techniques that slowly allow tendons to adapt to applied stresses, as discussed in Chapter 3.[4,8,15–17]

Tendonitis

As its suffix indicates, *tendonitis* refers to the inflammation of a tendon. However, when used in the primary care setting, this term refers to a clinical entity and not to a specific inflammatory event. Indeed, it has been shown that the standard inflammatory process (described in Chapter 5) does not occur in people clinically identified with tendonitis. This is because the tendons of these patients are absent of neutrophils, key elements involved in the inflammatory process. In reality, this means that the condition tendonitis has not been shown to exist, making it incorrect for health care providers to use this term to describe conditions of the tendon. Rather, it is more appropriate to use the term *tendinosis*, because this more accurately reflects the degeneration that occurs in most tendon conditions. Furthermore, if the term *tendonitis* is used, parents, patients, coaches, and others interested in the health status of people who participate in sports may not fully appreciate the significance of a tendon injury. For this reason alone, a growing number of health care professionals have stopped using the term *tendonitis*.[4,10,15,18,19]

Because the traditional inflammatory process does not occur when a tendon is injured, people who sustain a tendon injury should be diagnosed as having tendinosis and not tendonitis.

Paratenonitis
Paratenonitis is an umbrella term used to refer to the inflammation and degeneration of the outer layer of a tendon sheath's. This condition, also referred to as **peritendinitis**, **tenosynovitis**, and **tenovaginitis**, typically develops when a tendon comes in close proximity to a fixed structure, such as a bony prominence. It also occurs when a tendon is overused. For example, in the case of **de Quervain's syndrome** (discussed in Chapter 12), tenosynovitis commonly develops in the extrinsic muscles of the thumb as a result of repetitive thumb movement.[15–17,20]

Muscle Contusion and Myositis Ossificans
Simply put, a contusion is a bruise. Though any body tissue can be contused, skeletal muscles are most affected. This acute injury is typically caused by a compressive force resulting from blunt-force trauma. Muscles most at risk of becoming contused include those vulnerable to receiving a direct blow during sporting activities, such as the thigh's quadriceps muscle group (discussed in Chapter 9). Indeed, the requirement that protective equipment be worn by people participating in collision activities, such as football and ice hockey, is to protect the body from being injured in this fashion.[21]

Contusions are graded as mild (first degree), moderate (second degree), and severe (third degree), with severity determined by the amount of motion lost by the joint most affected by the injury. For example, if the ROM of the joint associated with the injured muscle is at least 66% of what is considered normal (determined by comparing the amount of motion either with the contralateral side or with normative data), a mild contusion exists. The affected joint maintains 33% to 66% of normal motion in a moderate contusion, whereas a severe contusion affects more than 66% of the joint's motion.[21]

Though a contusion rarely results in long-term consequences, a severe contusion can lead to **heterotopic ossification** within the injured muscle. Otherwise referred to as *myositis ossificans* (Fig. 9.20 on page 258), this condition also develops when an acute contusion is improperly treated, such as what happens when heat is placed on an injured site before the initial inflammatory process ends (discussed in Chapters 5 and 6). It can also result from a person receiving repeated direct blows to a muscle over an extended period of time, such as what happens when a soccer player gets the muscles on the outside of the shins kicked over and over throughout a playing season. Ultimately, this condition results in the development of a hard, bony mass within the muscle belly, resulting in long-term discomfort and decreases in muscle strength and joint motion.[21]

PEARL

Myositis ossificans can develop from a severe contusion, from improperly treating a contusion, or from a muscle being traumatized by a series of repeated blows over an extended period of time.

Strain

If a muscle or tendon is stretched beyond its ability to lengthen, it will tear, resulting in a strain. This type of acute injury mechanism is typically caused by a tension force, such as what happens when a rubber band is stretched beyond its elastic potential. Referred to as a *pulled muscle* by the lay public, strains also occur when a muscle acts abnormally, such as what happens when it contracts when it is supposed to relax. This usually happens when the working muscles do not coordinate their actions properly, a common result of muscle fatigue. Box 1.1 summarizes those factors believed to increase a person's risk of experiencing a strain. If not treated properly, a patient with an acute muscle strain could eventually be faced with managing a chronic injury.[11,12,22]

Regardless of cause, strains typically occur at the muscle's musculotendinous junction, with muscles spanning two joints, such as the hamstrings (discussed in Chapter 9), maintaining the highest risk of becoming strained. As with contusions, strains are classified as mild (first degree), moderate (second degree), or severe (third degree) injuries. However, in the case of strains, injury severity depends on the amount of tissue damage present, as outlined in Table 1.2. This system is also used to determine the severity of sprains, providing the primary health care provider with a standard method to classify injury to tissues that have been torn.[11,12,14,22,23]

BOX 1.1
FACTORS THAT PREDISPOSE A MUSCLE TO BECOMING STRAINED

Poor muscle strength	Poor coordination of the muscles in the area
Poor flexibility	
Poor posture	History of a previous muscle strain in the area
Improper warm-up	
Fatigue	Strength imbalance of the muscles in the area
Presence of muscle spasms	

TABLE 1.2 Classifying strains and sprains by the amount of tissue damage present

DEGREE OF INJURY	TISSUE DAMAGE
First	Tissue fibers stretched or torn <10%
Second	Tissue fibers torn 10%–50%
Third	Tissue fibers torn >50%

Muscle Spasm

A muscle spasm, otherwise referred to as a *muscle cramp* and known by the lay public as a *charley horse*, is an involuntary contraction of a muscle or group of muscles. Fatigue, dehydration, and electrolyte imbalances within the working muscles are some common causes of muscle spasms. Though not a serious condition, spasms have been identified as a predisposing risk factor for developing other conditions, such as a muscle strain.[24]

Sprain

If a ligament or joint capsule is stretched by external forces beyond its capacity to lengthen, it will tear, resulting in a **sprain**. Typically caused by tension, shearing, and twisting forces, and as shown in Table 1.2, sprains are classified as mild (first degree), moderate (second degree), or severe (third degree), with the injury severity determined by the amount of tissue damaged.[25]

A sprain involves stretching or tearing of a ligament or joint capsule, whereas a strain occurs when a muscle or tendon is stretched or torn.

Dislocation

Though defined as the displacement of any body part, in musculoskeletal medicine, a dislocation, otherwise known as a *luxation*, typically refers to the disarticulation of a joint. This condition can be caused by any injury mechanism if the force applied to the body is great enough to dislodge the joint's bones. When a joint dislocates its capsule, associated ligaments and other surrounding soft tissues are also injured. Indeed, joint injuries that involve multiple third degree ligament sprains typically result in dislocation. Most of the time, a joint that dislocates stays displaced, referred to as an *unreduced dislocation*, until a trained health care provider manipulates, or manually reduces, the joint back into place. Other times, the joint spontaneously reduces, returning to its normal position on its own. In some instances, the bones of an injured joint only partially displace from one another. Referred to as a *subluxation*, this happens in response to a traumatic event, or it can occur spontaneously. Spontaneous subluxations are commonly seen in people who have experienced many previous episodes of multiple dislocations to the point where the capsule is unable to properly hold the joint together. These patients are identified as chronic subluxators.[26–28]

When a joint dislocates, its surrounding capsule and ligaments are almost always severely injured.

Bursitis

Bursitis can be either acute or chronic in nature. Acute bursitis usually occurs when a superficial bursa is injured by a compressive force, resulting from blunt-force trauma, whereas chronic bursitis develops when a deep-lying bursa attempts to prevent friction buildup between adjacent body parts. In either case, bursitis is almost always associated with some degree of swelling, owing to the excessive production of synovial fluid in response to becoming irritated.[29,30]

Neuropathies

Neuropathies refer to diseases and abnormalities of the nervous system. Sensory and motor aspects of a nerve can be affected with any of these conditions. In musculoskeletal medicine, the most common neuropathies encountered include neuralgia, entrapment, neuroma, and neurapraxia.

Neuralgia is defined as any pain that occurs along the path of a nerve. Causes include compression applied directly over a nerve, such as what happens when a pressure wrap is applied in the area of a superficial nerve (discussed in Chapter 6), and the presence of inflammation in the area surrounding a nerve. Entrapment refers to pressure placed on a nerve from surrounding tissues to the point of nerve damage. The results of entrapping a nerve can be transient, such as what happens when a person sits on the sciatic nerve, causing the lower extremity to "fall asleep," or permanent, such as what may happen if a spinal nerve becomes entrapped for an extended period. A neuroma is a mass-like structure that usually develops in an area of a neurovascular bundle. Neuromas commonly develop in the feet (discussed in Chapter 8) as the result of repetitive compressive forces placed on the feet from running and jumping activities. Neurapraxia occurs when a nerve becomes impaired to the point where it cannot conduct electrical impulses. In sports, this typically results from blunt-force trauma directed over the sight of a nerve. Indeed, **transient paresthesia** occurring from the contusion of a superficial nerve is the most common nerve injury seen in those who participate in sports. Fortunately, nerves affected by this injury mechanism almost always recover fully in a relatively short period of time.[8,29,31–33]

Compartment Syndrome

Compartment syndrome is defined as an increase of intracompartmental pressure within a fascial compartment. Though any compartment can be affected, this condition usually occurs in those compartments that naturally have little room within them. When the pressure increase is great enough, the compartment's neurovascular bundles become ischemic, causing a loss of nerve activity and circulation distal to the affected body part.[34,35]

Compartment syndrome can be either an acute or a chronic condition. Acute compartment syndrome (ACS) results from swelling caused by blunt-force trauma, whereas chronic exertional compartment syndrome (CECS) develops from swelling caused by overusing the muscles located in a compartment. In either case, the venous and lymphatic systems' ability to drain fluid from the area is affected (discussed in Chapter 6), ultimately increasing the intracompartmental pressure. In some instances, increases in pressure associated with CECS are caused by muscles hypertrophying to the point where the compartment is unable to accommodate the increased muscle mass.[34,35]

Bone Conditions

Musculoskeletal conditions that involve injuries to bone include fractures and pathologies of the apophyses, epiphyses, and joints.

Fractures

Fractures are the most common hard tissue injury resulting from participation in sports. Otherwise known as *broken bones*, fractures are divided into three different types: simple, compound, and stress. Compound, or *open*, fractures, are ones in which the patient's broken bone penetrates the skin. Patients with a compound fracture are almost always managed by emergency care personnel, rarely seeking treatment in the primary care setting. Thus, the focus here is on simple and stress fractures.

Simple

A simple fracture, also referred to as a *closed fracture,* is a condition in which a broken bone does not penetrate the skin. Caused by a macrotrauma event, simple fractures are classified by how the bone breaks. For example, a longitudinal fracture breaks the bone lengthwise along its shaft, whereas a spiral fracture causes the bone to fracture in a twisting fashion. Fractures of note for those working in the primary care setting are greenstick and avulsion fractures.

Named after how a greenstick splinters when broken, a greenstick fracture is an incomplete fracture of a bone's shaft, leaving part of the cortex and periosteum unharmed. This fracture is unique to children and adolescents, because the bones of younger people are more subtle than those of an adult. This increases the chance that a younger person's bone will not break completely when fractured. In contrast, an avulsion fracture occurs when a muscle-tendon unit exerts a tension force so great that the tendon, and a piece of bone to which it attaches, separate from the rest of the bone. As with greenstick fractures, avulsion fractures happen more frequently to children and adolescents because, in this population, the person's muscle-tendon unit is typically stronger than bone.[36]

Stress

A stress fracture, also called a *fatigue fracture,* is a small defect that occurs when a weakened portion of a bone is subject to repetitive microtrauma. In response, the bone attempts to repair the defect. However, when the stresses placed on the bone outpace the bone's ability to repair the damage, microfracturing continues. If not identified and managed properly, this process continues, ultimately turning a stress fracture into a closed or open fracture.[37]

PEARL

If not managed properly, stress fractures can develop into either a simple or a compound fracture.

Though many factors contribute to their development, as outlined in Box 1.2, stress fractures most often occur when a person makes one or more changes to his or her exercise routine. In the high school and college population, this usually corresponds with a switch of playing seasons (e.g., fall to winter, winter to spring) because these almost always accompany a change in activity, footwear, and surface on which the student athlete participates. It is common for these changes to be made quickly, not allowing the person's body to properly adapt to the new playing conditions. Stress fractures also occur toward the end of the athletic season, after the person has participated in the same activity for an extended period. The lower extremity is most at risk, with stress fractures typically occurring in the feet, leg, and thigh.[38]

Conditions of the Apophysis

In general, the term *apophysitis* is used to describe any inflammation of a bone's apophyses. Most cases of apophysitis are caused by a separation of a muscle-tendon unit from its apophyseal attachment, which, as discussed previously, is usually located

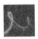

BOX 1.2
FACTORS THAT PREDISPOSE A PERSON TO DEVELOPMENT OF A STRESS FRACTURE

Sudden increase in activity duration, intensity, and/or frequency	Lack of rest between exercise sessions
	Exercising through pain
Change of playing surface	Osteopenia/osteoporosis
Change of activity	Rheumatoid arthritis
Altering footwear	

near or directly on top of an epiphyseal growth plate. **Osgood-Schlatter disease** (discussed in Chapter 9) is a prime example of an apophysitis condition.[39]

Conditions of the Epiphysis

A fracture involving the epiphyseal growth plate is the most common and most serious injury that happens to this portion of the bone. Also known as *physeal fractures*, these conditions are commonly referred to as **Salter-Harris** (S-H) **fractures**, named for two doctors who classified these fractures in a groundbreaking article published in 1963. This system categorizes growth plate fractures based on how the bone is injured (i.e., the MOI) and the relationship the fracture lines have with the epiphysis. Table 1.3 summarizes this classification system. Obviously, S-H fractures should always be ruled out when an adolescent reports bone or joint pain.[40–42]

PEARL

Always suspect a Salter-Harris fracture in adolescents who report
bone or joint pain.

Avascular Necrosis

By definition, avascular necrosis is death of bone tissue due to decreased or total loss of blood supply. Though any tissue can become necrotic, joints are at greatest risk of

TABLE 1.3 Salter-Harris classification for epiphyseal injury

S-H TYPE	DESCRIPTION
I	Metaphysis separated from the epiphysis. Growth plate unaffected.
II (most common)	Growth plate separation and displaced fracture of the metaphysis. Growth plate's potential for future development is unaffected.
III	Fracture through the epiphysis. Growth unaffected as long as proper realignment occurs.
IV	Fracture through the epiphysis and metaphysis. Growth unaffected as long as proper realignment occurs.
V	Compression of epiphysis. Growth disturbance expected.

becoming necrotic after incurring an injury. The aging process also increases the risk of avascular necrosis of the joints. This is particularly true of the hip (discussed in Chapter 10).[43]

Arthritis

The most common forms of arthritis include osteoarthritis (OA), a degenerative joint disease, and rheumatoid arthritis (RA), inflammation of a joint's synovial membrane. A very common condition seen in older adults, OA most commonly affects the knees, hips, feet, spine, and hands. An autoimmune disease, RA is a progressive illness that occurs after the age of 40 and affects females three times more than males.[44]

Gender Differences and Musculoskeletal Injury

Traditional belief holds that there is little difference in the number, type, or severity of musculoskeletal injury rates between males and females who participate in sports and exercise. In 2005, this belief was finally refuted as researchers at the American Academy of Pediatrics National Conference and Exhibition reported that female high school athletes have higher injury rates and risks of injury than males of the same age. Indeed, in recent years, many researchers have established that, in certain instances, females are at a higher risk of becoming injured when compared with their male counterparts participating in the same activity (Box 1.3). Females are also likely to incur certain injuries, such as knee sprains and stress fractures, more often than males. However, males sustain injuries requiring hospitalization in far greater numbers than females. Appreciating these injury pattern differences between the genders is an important component of understanding the complexities involved in evaluating musculoskeletal injury.[1,45-53]

Though females are likely to incur certain injuries, such as knee sprains and stress fractures, males sustain injuries requiring hospitalization in far greater numbers than females.

BOX 1.3
SPORTS IN WHICH FEMALES HAVE A HIGHER INJURY RATE THAN MALES PARTICIPATING IN THE SAME ACTIVITY

Basketball*	Military personnel†
Soccer*	Mountain bike racing‡
Softball (when compared with baseball)*	Martial arts§

*Powell JW, Barber-Foss KD. Sex-related injury patterns among select high school sports. *Am J Sports Med* 2000;28:385.

†Jones BH, Bovee MW, Harris JM, et al. Intrinsic factors for exercise-related injuries among male and female Army trainees. *Am J Sports Med* 1993;21:705.

‡Kronisch RL, Pfeiffer RP, Chow TK, et al. Gender differences in acute mountain bike racing injuries. *Clin J Sport Med* 2002;12:158.

§Pieter W. Martial arts injuries. Med Sport Sci 2005;48:59.

REFERENCES

1. Jones BH, Bovee MW, Harris JM, et al. Intrinsic factors for exercise-related injuries among male and female Army trainees. *Am J Sports Med* 1993;21:705.
2. DiFiori JP. Overuse injuries in children and adolescents. *Phys Sportsmed* 1999;27(1):75.
3. Austermuehle PD. Common knee injuries in primary care. *Nurs Prac* 2001;26(10):26.
4. Leadbetter WB. Cell-matrix response in tendon injury. *Clin Sports Med* 1992;11:533.
5. Merrick MA. Secondary injury after musculoskeletal trauma: a review and update. *J Athl Train* 2002;37:209.
6. Altizer L. Hand and wrist fractures. *Orthop Nurs* 2003;22:232.
7. Hossfeld G, Uehara D. Acute joint injuries of the hand. *Emerg Med Clin North Am* 1993;11:781.
8. Rettig A. Wrist and hand overuse syndromes. *Clin Sports Med* 2001;20:591.
9. Bach BR. Acute knee injuries: when to refer. *Phys Sportsmed* 1997;25(5):39.
10. Almekinders LC, Temple JD. Etiology, diagnosis, and treatment of tendonitis: an analysis of the literature. *Med Sci Sports Exerc* 1998;30:1183.
11. Best TM, Garret WE. Hamstring strains: expediting return to play. *Phys Sportsmed* 1996;24(8):37.
12. Croisier JL. Factors associated with recurrent hamstring injuries. *Sports Med* 2004;34:681.
13. Lenn J, Uhl T, Mattacola C, et al. The effects of fish oil and isoflavones on delayed onset muscle soreness. *Med Sci Sports Exerc* 2002;34:1605.
14. Almekinders LC. Anti-inflammatory treatment of muscular injuries in sport. *Sports Med* 1999;28:383.
15. Maffulli N, Wong J, Almekinders LC. Types and epidemiology of tendinopathy. *Clin Sports Med* 2003;22:675.
16. Selvanetti A, Cipolla M, Puddu G. Overuse tendon injuries: basic science and classification. *Oper Tech Sports Med* 1997;5:110.
17. Rosner JL, Zlatkin MB, Clifford P, et al. Imaging of athletic wrist and hand injuries. *Semin Musculoskelet Radiol* 2004;8:57.
18. Torstensen ET, Bray RC, Wiley JP. Patellar tendinitis: a review of current concepts and treatment. *Clin J Sport Med* 1994;4:77.
19. Scott A, Khan, KM, Roberts CR, et al. What do we mean by the term "inflammation"? A contemporary basic science update for sports medicine. *Br J Sports Med* 2004;38:3720.
20. Almekinders LC. Tendinitis and other chronic tendinopathies. *J Am Acad Orthop Surg* 1998;6:157.
21. Larson CM, Almekinders LC, Daras SG, et al. Evaluating and managing muscle contusions and myositis ossificans. *Phys Sportsmed* 2001;30(2):41.
22. Garrett WE. Muscle strain injuries. *Am J Sports Med* 1996;24:S2.
23. Thorsson O, Lilja B, Nilsson P. Immediate external compression in the management of an acute muscle injury. *Scand J Med Sci Sports* 1997;7:182.
24. U.S. National Library of Medicine. Muscle cramps. *MedlinePlus*. Retrieved from: http://www.nlm.nih.gov/medlineplus/musclecramps.html. Accessed 7/29//08.
25. Safran MR, Benedetti RS, Bartolozzi AR III, et al. Lateral ankle sprains: a comprehensive review, part 1: etiology, pathoanatomy, histopathogenesis, and diagnosis. *Med Sci Sports Exerc* 1999;31(7 suppl):S429.
26. McKinnis LN. *Fundamentals of Musculoskeletal Imaging*, 2nd ed. Philadelphia, PA: FA Davis Co., 2005.
27. Park MC, Blaine TA, Levine WN. Shoulder dislocation in young athletes: current concepts in management. *Phys Sportsmed* 2002;30(12):41.
28. Warme WJ, Arciero RA, Taylor DC. Anterior shoulder instability in sport: current management recommendations. *Sports Med* 1999;28(3):209.
29. Budd GM, Piccioni LH. Identifying and treating common problems in the elbow. *Am J Nurs Pract* 2005;9(2):41.
30. McFarland EG, Mamanee P, Queale WS, et al. Olecranon and prepatellar bursitis: treating acute, chronic, and inflamed. *Phys Sportsmed* 2000;28(3):2000.
31. Parmelee-Peters K, Eathorne SW. The wrist: common injuries and management. *Prim Care* 2005;32:35.
32. Hockenbury RT. Forefoot problems in athletes. *Med Sci Sports Exerc* 1999;31(7 suppl):S448.
33. Simons SM. Foot injuries of the recreational athlete. *Phys Sportsmed* 1999;27(1):57.

34. Schon LC, Baxter DE, Clanton TO. Chronic exercise-induced leg pain in active people: more than just shin splints. *Phys Sportsmed* 1992;20(1):100.

35. Swain R. Lower extremity compartment syndrome: when to suspect acute or chronic pressure buildup. *Postgrad Med* 1999;105(3):159.

36. England SP, Sundberg S. Management of common pediatric fractures. *Pediatr Clin North Am* 1996;43:991.

37. Knapp TP, Garrett WE Jr. Stress fractures: general concepts. *Clin Sports Med* 1997;16:339.

38. Perron AD, Brady WJ, Keats TA. Management of common stress fractures: when to apply conservative therapy, when to take an aggressive approach. *Postgrad Med* 2002;111(2):95.

39. Adirim TA, Cheng TL. Overview of injuries in the young athlete. *Sports Med* 2003;33:75.

40. Salter RB, Harris WR. Injuries involving the epiphyseal plate. *J Bone Joint Surg* 1963;45A:587.

41. Huurman WW. Injuries to the hand and wrist. *Adolescent Med* 1998;9:611.

42. Le TB, Hentz VR. Hand and wrist injuries in young athletes. *Hand Clin* 2000;16:597.

43. Boettcher EG, Bonfiglio M, Hamilton HH, et al. Non-traumatic necrosis of the femoral head. *J Bone Joint Surg Am* 2007;52A:312.

44. U.S. Department of Health and Human Services. *Arthritis and Exercise*. Bethesda, MD: National Institute of Arthritis and Musculoskeletal and Skin Diseases, 2001.

45. Lansee RR, Strauss RH, Leizman DJ, et al. Injury and disability in matched men's and women's intercollegiate sports. *Am J Public Health* 1990;80:1459.

46. Whiteside PA. Men's and women's injuries in comparable sports. *Phys Sportsmed* 1980;8:130.

47. Little L. Female athletes have higher injury rates. *Medscape Medical News*. Retrieved from: http://doctor.medscape.com/viewarticle/514418. Accessed 1/27/08.

48. Powell JW, Barber-Foss KD. Sex-related injury patterns among select high school sports. *Am J Sports Med* 2000;28:385.

49. Kronisch RL, Pfeiffer RP, Chow TK, et al. Gender differences in acute mountain bike racing injuries. *Clin J Sport Med* 2002;12:158.

50. Pieter W. Martial arts injuries. *Med Sport Sci* 2005;48:59.

51. Leech E. Preparing a female collegiate athlete for anterior cruciate ligament reconstruction and rehabilitation. *Orthop Nurs* 2003;22(3):169.

52. Protzman RR, Griffs CG. Stress fractures in men and women undergoing military training. *J Bone Joint Surg Am* 1977;59:825.

53. Dempsey RL, Layde PM, Laud PW, et al. Incidence of sports and recreation related injuries resulting in hospitalization in Wisconsin in 2000. *Inj Prev* 2005;11:91.

SUGGESTED READINGS

Hart ES, Albright MB, Rebello GN, et al. Broken bones. Common pediatric fractures: part I. *Orthop Nurs* 2006;25(4):251.

Hawkins D, Metheny J. Overuse injuries in youth sports: biomechanical considerations. *Med Sci Sports Exerc* 2001;33:1701.

Khan KM, Cook JL, Taunton JE, et al. Overuse tendinosis, not tendonitis. *Phys Sportsmed* 2000;28(5):38.

WEB LINKS

http://www.pueblo.gsa.gov/cic_text/health/sports/injuries. Accessed 7/29/08.
   U.S. Department of Health and Human Services Web site dedicated to sports injuries. Reviews what sports injuries are, explains the difference between acute and chronic injuries, and identifies who is at greatest risk for sports injuries.

http://www.niams.nih.gov/Health_Info/Sprains_Strains/default.asp. Accessed 7/29/08.
   National Institute of Arthritis and Musculoskeletal and Skin Diseases Web site dedicated to answering questions about strains and sprains.

http://www.arthroscopy.com/sp22000.htm. Accessed 7/29/08.
   Provides an in-depth description of growth plate injuries, including diagnosis, treatment, and rehabilitation.

2

The Pre-Participation Examination

● **Brian J. Toy, PhD, ATC**

The medical examination used to clear a person for participation in athletics has traditionally been referred to as the "preseason physical" examination. However, with more and more Americans participating in sports and performing regular exercise, health care providers are increasingly referring to this examination as a **pre-participation examination** (PPE). This broader term is more reflective of the patient population requesting the examination.

In content and sequence, the PPE does not differ greatly from the standard health assessment process. However, the goals and objectives of the PPE, the patient population seeking it, the state laws requiring middle and high school students to complete it, and the legal implications all make performing a PPE a unique experience for many primary health care providers.

Goals and Objectives

The goal of the PPE is not to disqualify people from participating in physical activity. Indeed, across the United States, the percentage of people precluded from participating in interscholastic athletics for medical reasons is extremely low, less than 2.0% of all those examined. Rather, the primary goal of a PPE is to ensure the health and safety of the patient.[1-5]

PEARL

The primary goal of the PPE is to ensure the health and safety of a person who wants to participate in sports or exercise.

To meet this goal, several objectives must be pursued. These include[4,6,7]

• screening for conditions which may be life threatening or disabling or may predispose to injury or illness,
• identifying patients at greatest risk of morbidity or mortality,
• detecting conditions that may limit performance,
• developing baseline data for future comparison,
• evaluating physical fitness,
• fulfilling administrative, insurance, and legal requirements,
• implementing injury prevention programs,
• bringing immunizations up-to-date.

Because the PPE for many adolescents provides the primary, and sometimes only, contact between the person and the health care system, the screening process for this age group also provides an opportunity to provide counseling and to perform a general health maintenance examination. At this time, general wellness topics, such as the use of tobacco products, alcohol, and recreational drugs, can be discussed.[4,6,7]

Professionals Approved to Perform a PPE

In general, the PPE can be completed by any health care provider approved by the state to perform such a screening. Historically, such approval was granted only to medical and osteopathic physicians. However, evolving state practice acts of other health care professions, including Nurse Practitioners, Doctors of Chiropractic Medicine, Physician Assistants, and Naturopathic Clinicians, have, in certain instances, granted the authority to perform PPEs to these providers.[7,8]

To ensure compliance with state law, review state practice acts before performing a PPE.

Timing and Frequency

For various reasons, the timing and frequency of PPEs for student athletes can be challenging. For members of the general population, the PPE is often scheduled when, and as often as, the patient or the patient's primary care provider requests it.

Timing for Interscholastic and Intercollegiate Athletes

Ideally, the PPE should be performed a minimum of 6 weeks before a person wants to begin participating in sports. Following this guideline provides sufficient time to refer the patient for any needed follow-up by other health care providers and to initiate any treatment and rehabilitation plans before the activity's start date. However, it is typical for patients and schools to schedule the PPE within days of the activity's first scheduled session. This is not problematic if no health care concerns are found. However, problems do arise when patients require referral for treatment before participation. In such cases, the person should be disqualified pending further evaluation.[4]

A comprehensive PPE should be administered 6 weeks before an interscholastic or intercollegiate athletic start date.

From a practical standpoint, PPE screenings for interscholastic and intercollegiate athletes should be scheduled at least one athletic season before the initiation of the athlete's participation start date. Thus, the PPE for students who want to participate in a winter sport should occur soon after the start of the academic year. Athletes desiring to participate in a spring sport should complete the PPE no later than the initiation of the winter sports season. Students who want to participate in fall sports should complete a PPE during the spring of the preceding academic year. If students are screened in the spring, processes need to be implemented to ensure that students can report health care concerns that arise over the summer months before beginning fall sports practice. Because there is a natural disconnect between academic years, it is usually the fall student athlete who seeks PPE within a few days of an activity's start date.[4]

To reduce the need for disqualifications based on poor timing of the PPE, primary health care providers need to develop a close working relationship with people in the community who are responsible for securing PPEs for student athletes. This usually includes employees of interscholastic and intercollegiate programs, such as certified athletic trainers, coaches, athletics directors, principals, and designated team physicians. Providers need to communicate with these people so that a reasonable working time frame for PPE implementation can be developed. Parents must be included in the process, either directly or through school-sponsored associations such as parent-teacher organizations. Collaboration is particularly important if large numbers of students need to be screened by a certain date.[4,5,7,9]

Frequency for Interscholastic and Intercollegiate Athletes

For legal and other reasons, many interscholastic and intercollegiate athletic programs require student athletes to successfully complete a comprehensive PPE once each year. However, most published guidelines do not recommend a full PPE annually. Instead, they recommend a comprehensive PPE for all students entering middle school, high school, or college and for students transferring from one institution to another. For returning students who already passed an initial, comprehensive examination and want to participate in sports in the current year, the completion of an abridged PPE is recommended. In addition to obtaining height, weight, blood pressure (BP), and pulse rate (PR) measurements, the abridged screening includes updating the patient's medical history. The history update provides an opportunity for conditions the patient may have acquired since completing the initial screening or since the last update to be evaluated and allows for any illnesses or injuries previously identified to be reevaluated. It is also recommended that a full cardiovascular evaluation occur every 2 years for high school participants.[4,7,9–12]

PEARL

A comprehensive PPE should be completed by all students entering middle school, high school, or college and for those transferring from one institution to another.

Timing and Frequency for Nonathletic Populations

Though published recommendations exist regarding the timing and frequency of medical clearance for student athletes, consensus related to screening timing and frequency for other populations engaging in sports or general exercise programs does not exist. Nevertheless, all people who engage in physical activity and/or participate in sports should follow the student athlete PPE guidelines. Specifically, patients should receive a comprehensive PPE whenever they plan to initiate a new sport or exercise program, or when they want to initiate activity at a higher level, e.g., advancing from recreational ice-skating to participating on a community ice hockey team.

Portions of the PPE

As noted earlier, a key objective of the PPE is to identify patients at greatest risk of morbidity or mortality resulting from participating in sports or exercise. Unfortunately, scientific data on the effectiveness of PPEs in meeting this objective are lacking. Thus, clearing a person to participate in sports is primarily based on clinical findings and a risk estimate as it applies to each patient. For example, though it may be safe to clear a person with an identified cardiac abnormality to participate in the sport of archery, it may be unwise to clear the same patient to play football.[13]

Introduction

State regulations differ regarding the medical information required to clear middle and high school athletes for participation. It is for this reason the National Federation of State High School Associations (NFHS) has not standardized the interscholastic PPE. Similarly, the National Collegiate Athletic Association (NCAA) outlines areas of emphasis, but does not specify required portions, of a college examination. This lack of standardization has resulted in a PPE process that maintains inequities between and among school districts, colleges, and universities. Thus, when performing a PPE for interscholastic athletes, establish which portions of the PPE are required by state statute, and determine which specific forms need to be completed. For college athletes, obtain copies of forms, and discuss PPE requirements with university officials.[10,14,15]

Before performing a PPE, determine what the state requires for an interscholastic student athlete to be cleared for participation.

History

As with any standard health assessment, the majority of problems affecting a patient can be identified by obtaining a thorough medical history. Thus, through this portion of the PPE, most conditions that preclude participation are identified. In the case of minors, parents or legal guardians must be involved in completing the history portion of the health questionnaire.[4]

Most conditions that exclude a person from participation or require referral are identified in the history portion of the PPE.

When obtaining a health history from female patients, include the information listed in Box 2.1. These questions help identify the presence of conditions, such as a menstrual irregularity or an eating disorder, that might cause the examination to be adapted. For example, the incidence of exercise-induced **secondary amenorrhea** is significant in this population, typically occurring in females who participate in long-duration, aerobic-based activities such as distance running. Adolescent girls and women identified with this condition may have disordered eating or a gynecological or metabolic condition. Thus, these patients require education regarding the **female athlete triad** (discussed in Chapter 4) and the interrelationship of secondary amenorrhea, decreased bone density, and the development of stress fractures.[4,7,16,17]

Even with menstruating females, include questions related to eating habits and eating disorders because disordered eating is prevalent among female athletes. The highest prevalence is among athletes participating in activities that place an emphasis on aesthetic value or leanness for optimal performance, such as gymnastics, cheerleading, and figure skating. In contrast, the excessive blood loss accompanying **menorrhagia** contributes to iron deficiency anemia, especially if the patient does not eat meat, poultry, or fish. These foods are high in heme iron, which is much more readily absorbed by the body than plant sources of iron. In patients with menorrhagia, a blood test to screen for iron deficiency anemia may be warranted.[16,18]

BOX 2.1
FEMALE-SPECIFIC HEALTH HISTORY QUESTIONS

Reproductive
- Age at menarche
- Date of most recent menstrual period
- Flow of menstrual period (heavy, moderate, mild)
- Average length of time between menstrual periods
- Average length of menstrual period
- Number of menstrual periods experienced within the past 12 months
- Hormonal birth control being used
- History of pregnancy
- Current pregnancy

Nutritional status
- Confirmed history of an eating disorder
- Weight at PPE compared with weight 1 year ago
- Personal feeling about present weight
- History of excessive dieting
- Average number of meals consumed in a day
- Nutrition source of the average meal (fats, carbohydrates, protein)
- Body fat percentage*
- 24-Hour food recall*

*Performed if nutritional and/or eating disorder status is questioned.
PPE = pre-participation examination.

Adapted from: Johnson MD. Tailoring the preparticipation exam to female athletes. *Phys Sportsmed* 1992;20(7):61; AAFP, AAP, ACSM, et al. *Preparticipation Physical Evaluation*, 3rd ed. Minneapolis, MN: The Physician and Sports Medicine: A Division of the McGraw-Hill Companies, 2005; Tanner SM. Preparticipation examination targeted for the female athlete. *Clin Sports Med* 1994;13(2):337.

Physical Examination

Though portions of the physical examination are standard regardless of the activity the person desires to partake, participation in certain activities requires that this portion of the examination be focused on different body regions and systems. For example, the musculoskeletal system of long-distance runners should be assessed for overuse conditions, whereas the skin of people who wrestle must be evaluated for contagious dermatological diseases.

Height and Weight

Height and weight are measured as part of every PPE and yearly follow-up. A consistent record of height and weight allows the person's general health status to be monitored. Furthermore, these data may be helpful in identifying factors contributing to other medical problems. For example, increases in body weight may be related to the presence of hypertension and exacerbate low back discomfort.[4]

Blood Pressure

As with height and weight, BP is obtained as part of every PPE and yearly review. Regardless of age, seated ranges of systolic and diastolic BPs should be between 100 and 140 mm Hg and between 60 and 90 mm Hg, respectively. When determining hypertension status, use the recommendations of *The Seventh Report of the Joint National Committee on Prevention, Detection, Evaluation, and Treatment of High Blood Pressure*.[4,9,11,19]

Though increases in BP can be attributed to many factors, an initial high reading need not be alarming. Involvement in pre-examination physical activity, ingestion of stimulants such as caffeine, and the anxiety created by the PPE process itself, commonly referred to as *white coat syndrome*, may artificially inflate BP measurements. In addition, people involved in physical activities that require static muscular contraction (e.g., weight lifting) may present with BPs at the upper limits of the normal ranges. The use of an improper cuff size can also affect recording accuracy. If an initial reading of 140/90 mm Hg or higher is obtained, repeat the reading after the patient has been allowed to sit quietly and undisturbed for 5 minutes. If necessary, secure a third measurement after the patient lies down and rests for an additional 10 minutes. To ensure accuracy, a BP that remains elevated above 135/85 should be monitored over a period of several days.[4,6,9,19]

Once high BP has been confirmed, refer the patient to a cardiologist. The participation status for a hypertensive individual varies depending on the severity of the condition. To determine the effect that subsequent treatment programs have in controlling hypertension, BP readings should be obtained every 2 months for these patients.[20]

Pulse Rate

Obtaining a patient's resting PR is also part of every PPE and yearly review. This is usually taken at the radial artery with the patient seated. Recognize that PRs taken at this site can vary between 60 and 100 beats/min across the life span. In addition, because the heart of a person who is physically fit works very efficiently, it is common for a well-conditioned individual, regardless of age, to maintain a resting PR in the 40- to 60-beats/min range. Thus, consider a low PR finding for an active person to be within normal limits unless pathology related to a low PR has been identified. Note that a patient with **anorexia nervosa** (discussed in Chapter 4) may have a very low resting PR (e.g., 30 to 40 beats/min), whereas an elevated PR may be associated with anemia. Both of these conditions are more commonly seen in females.[16]

Eyes and Visual Acuity

When assessing eye function, confirm that the pupils are equal, round, and reactive to light and accommodation (PERRLA). In the absence of other symptoms, such as those associated with a head injury, refer abnormal pupil findings to an ophthalmologist. Evaluate visual acuity with a Snellen eye chart. Refer findings that exceed 20/40 in either eye for correction. Though poor vision can impair a person's athletic performance, checking for proper vision can also help to prevent injuries because visual acuity helps the athlete to avoid bodily contact with other participants, field equipment, and airborne objects.[4,5,7,9]

In addition to documenting visual acuity, confirm that the retina in each eye is intact. A detached retina may preclude the person from participation in strenuous and collision activities. Participation with sight in only one eye may be fine for certain activities (e.g., cross-country running) but inadvisable for other activities (e.g., ice hockey). Patients insisting on participating in activities that may place the remaining good eye in danger should understand the risks of participation, wear adequate eye protection, and sign a release of liability as presented in Patient Teaching Handout (PTH) 2.1.[13]

Ears, Nose, Mouth, and Throat

The general health of the ears, nose, mouth, and throat are assessed as during any typical health assessment. With athletes who participate in swimming and other water sports, evaluate for irritation or infection of the external and middle ears (discussed in Chapter 13). Check the external portion of the wrestler's ear for excess fluid buildup, which occurs as a result of repetitive rubbing of the ears of these athletes against wrestling mats (discussed in Chapter 13). Perform a brief oral mucosa screen for patients with a history of oral tobacco use.[4,7]

Cardiovascular

The cardiovascular screening is arguably the most significant portion of the PPE. Its main objective is to identify those at risk for experiencing **sudden cardiac death** (SCD). Unfortunately, in sports, SCD typically occurs in people who, within the previous year, presented with few or no symptoms and were medically cleared to participate. Even when combined with a thorough cardiac history, a cardiovascular physical examination offers no guarantee that a potentially fatal underlying pathology will be detected.[1,11,21]

PEARL

Obtaining a comprehensive health history and completing a thorough cardiovascular evaluation are the best ways to identify people most at risk for sudden cardiac death.

The most common cause of SCD in young athletes is **hypertrophic cardiomyopathy** (HCM). Indicators for HCM include family history of SCD, chest pain of unknown origin, exercise-induced syncope, exertional dyspnea, coronary artery abnormalities, and myocarditis. Because **Marfan's syndrome**, which manifests clinically, is a prime risk factor for SCD, the PPE should include an evaluation for this syndrome.[11,13,21-23] Box 2.2 outlines the physical characteristics of a person with Marfan's syndrome.

PEARL

Hypertrophic cardiomyopathy is the most common cause of exercise-induced sudden cardiac death in people younger than 35 years.

 BOX 2.2
PHYSICAL CHARACTERISTICS OF MARFAN'S SYNDROME

Tall, thin stature	Hyperextensible joints
Long, thin fingers	Retinal detachment
Lens abnormalities (dislocated; myopia; ectopic)	Height >95th percentile
	Arm span greater than height
Anterior thoracic deformity (pectus excavatum)	Mitral valve prolapse
	Steinberg's thumb sign (opposed thumb
High, narrow hard palate	reaches past ulna border of hand)

Adapted from: Ades PA. Preventing sudden death. *Phys Sportsmed* 1992;20(9):75; Missri JC, Sweet DD. Marfan syndrome: a review. *Cardiovasc Rev Rep* 1982;3:1648; McKeag DB. Preparticipation screening of the potential athlete. *Clin Sports Med* 1989;8:373.

To detect people most at risk for SCD, perform the cardiovascular examination in a quiet setting and, at a minimum, include essentials of the cardiovascular pre-participation screening as identified by the American Heart Association (AHA). These elements consist of[11]

- seated brachial BP,
- precordial auscultation in the standing and supine positions,
- assessment of the femoral pulses, and
- evaluation for Marfan's syndrome.

Identification of any cardiovascular abnormality mandates referral to a cardiologist. A complete cardiovascular workup, which includes any combination of a 12-lead electrocardiogram, stress echocardiogram, and graded exercise stress test (GXT), determines the extent of the abnormality. Excellent resources exist to help interpret the results of such a workup and provide guidance in determining whether it is safe for a person to participate. These resources include the AHA recommendations regarding sports participation for young patients with genetic cardiovascular diseases and the 36th Bethesda Conference recommendations for determining competition eligibility for athletes with cardiovascular abnormalities.[8,24]

Pulmonary

Usually performed in conjunction with the cardiac screening, auscultation of the lungs should reveal clear breath sounds accompanied by symmetric diaphragm excursion. Difficulty breathing or coughing spells during exercise may indicate the presence of **exercise-induced bronchospasm** (discussed in Chapter 3), which can be the result of asthma, environmental allergies, seasonal rhinitis, or smoking. Patients with wheezing, crackles, rhonchi, rubs, or rales should be referred for further lung function testing.[4]

Gastrointestinal

Before examining the gastrointestinal system, review the patient's diet and eating habits to determine whether the patient's energy and nutrient intake appropriately supports the desired physical activity and to screen for the presence of disordered eating (discussed in Chapter 4). Auscultate the abdomen, and then palpate for masses. Any finding of acute **organomegaly** should temporarily preclude participation until the condition is further investigated, because an enlargement of certain organs may be associated with pathology. For example, enlargement of the spleen suggests mononucleosis (discussed in Chapter 14). Eventual clearance for participation with an enlarged organ depends on many factors, including the cause of the condition and the activity the person desires to pursue.[7]

Genitourinary

Evaluate males for the presence of an inguinal hernia (discussed in Chapter 14); an undescended, absent, or atrophied testicle; or a testicular mass. For females, review menstrual history, incidence of pelvic inflammatory disease, and status of the ovaries. A traditional genitourinary examination for the female is usually not a standard portion of the PPE. For sexually active patients, review the use of birth control and safe sex practices. If indicated, evaluate for the presence of sexually transmitted disease, and provide counseling for prevention.[4,7]

Any person desiring to participate in sports with one functional kidney or testicle should be individually assessed, apprised of the risks, and provided with extra equipment to protect the involved area. If the remaining organ is diseased, is abnormally positioned, or has previously been injured, seriously consider disqualification, particularly if the person desires to participate in collision or contact activities. Secure a release of liability (PTH 2.1) if the patient insists on participating with one functional kidney or testicle.[7,13,25]

Neurological
During the neurological portion of the PPE, assess for a history of seizures and incidence of previous head injury. If a patient reports untreated episodes of seizures or lingering symptoms of a head injury, exclude the patient from participation until further investigation is completed. Other neurological testing includes evaluation of cranial nerves, reflexes, balance, and coordination.[4]

Musculoskeletal
An ideal PPE includes comprehensive strength, range of motion (ROM), and ligament laxity testing for all of the body's freely moveable joints. Because of time constraints, this is usually not possible. Thus, this portion of the evaluation is usually limited to the body's major joints. Evaluate both strength and ROM as outlined in Table 2.1, because these tests are sensitive for detecting major orthopedic abnormalities. Any asymmetrical findings, or findings that cause pain or undue discomfort, should be further investigated by performing a more thorough evaluation of the involved body part. If needed, refer patients to an orthopedist for evaluation.[4,5,9]

Dermatological
Observe the patient's skin for signs of infection and any other suspicious lesions. Patients being treated for contagious skin conditions should be excluded from activities that require body contact between participants until the lesion is no longer communicable. Noncontagious lesions usually do not warrant exclusion but should be treated appropriately.[7,13]

Variations for Specific Populations

Variations of the PPE for people not participating in interscholastic or intercollegiate sports are rarely discussed or written about. As a result, performing the PPE for patients in the general population who want to participate in community sports or vigorous exercise, especially if they have not engaged in regular physical activity for several years, can be challenging. In contrast, the process of screening athletes with special needs is the subject of a fair amount of professional literature. Several studies of special-needs athletes have been conducted in response to initiatives such as the Special Olympics and the Paralympics and the passage of federal laws such as the Americans with Disabilities Act (ADA).[4,26–28]

Life Span
Though finding accepted screening guidelines for nonstudent patients can be challenging, to the extent possible, tailor the examination to the population being assessed. Thus, have these patients complete a standard health assessment, taking into account factors such as age, cardiovascular health, current physical condition, and type of activity being pursued. Use a self-administered health history survey, such as the Physical

TABLE 2.1 Pre-participation examination musculoskeletal examination

PATIENT SITTING	PATIENT STANDING
Elbow ROM and strength: Patient performs flexion and extension actively and against resistance.	Posture and shoulder asymmetry: Examiner observes back, front, and side of patient.
Forearm ROM and strength: Patient performs supination and pronation actively and against resistance.	Active cervical spine ROM: Patient extends (looks up), flexes (chin to chest), lateral flexes (ear to shoulder), and rotates (chin to shoulder).
Wrist ROM and strength: Patient performs flexion and extension actively and against resistance.	Active back extension: Patient looks to the ceiling (with knees straight).
Hand ROM and strength: Patient performs active flexion/extension (clench and open fist) and abduction/adduction (spread fingers apart and close) actively and against resistance.	Scoliosis check: Examiner visualizes spine posteriorly while patient touches toes (with knees straight).
Quadriceps strength and symmetry: Patient contracts/relaxes quads from a seated position.	Shoulder strength: Examiner provides resistive scapula elevation (shoulder shrug) and abduction.
Knee ROM and strength: Patient performs flexion and extension actively and against resistance.	Active shoulder ROM–Apley's scratch test series: Patient touches opposite acromioclavicular joint, superior angle of scapula, and inferior angle of scapula.
Lumbar spine and hamstring flexibility: Patient sits and touches toes with knees straight.	Leg and foot strength: Patient stands on toes and stands on heels.
	Gait analysis: Patient walks toward/away from examiner.
	Hip, knee, and ankle function: Patient duckwalks away from examiner (four steps).

ROM = range of motion.

Adapted from: AAFP, AAP, ACSM, et al. *Preparticipation Physical Evaluation,* 3rd ed. Minneapolis, MN: The Physician and Sports Medicine: A Division of the McGraw-Hill Companies, 2005; McKeag DB. Preparticipation screening of the potential athlete. *Clin Sports Med* 1989;8:373; Sanders B, Nemeth WC. Preparticipation physical examination. *J Orthop Sports Phys Ther* 1996;23:149.

Activity Readiness Questionnaire (Fig. 2.1), for people desiring to participate in a program of regular exercise. This tool, which consists of seven questions, identifies patients who should complete a comprehensive PPE before initiating an exercise program.[9,29]

Children and Adolescents

Current evidence supports the participation of children and adolescents in most athletic activities. However, these patients should be evaluated for conditions that may expose them to increased risk of injury. Specifically, determine whether the patient is

Physical Activity Readiness
Questionnaire - PAR-Q
(revised 2002)

PAR-Q & YOU

(A Questionnaire for People Aged 15 to 69)

Regular physical activity is fun and healthy, and increasingly more people are starting to become more active every day. Being more active is very safe for most people. However, some people should check with their doctor before they start becoming much more physically active.

If you are planning to become much more physically active than you are now, start by answering the seven questions in the box below. If you are between the ages of 15 and 69, the PAR-Q will tell you if you should check with your doctor before you start. If you are over 69 years of age, and you are not used to being very active, check with your doctor.

Common sense is your best guide when you answer these questions. Please read the questions carefully and answer each one honestly: check YES or NO.

YES	NO	
☐	☐	1. Has your doctor ever said that you have a heart condition <u>and</u> that you should only do physical activity recommended by a doctor?
☐	☐	2. Do you feel pain in your chest when you do physical activity?
☐	☐	3. In the past month, have you had chest pain when you were not doing physical activity?
☐	☐	4. Do you lose your balance because of dizziness or do you ever lose consciousness?
☐	☐	5. Do you have a bone or joint problem (for example, back, knee or hip) that could be made worse by a change in your physical activity?
☐	☐	6. Is your doctor currently prescribing drugs (for example, water pills) for your blood pressure or heart condition?
☐	☐	7. Do you know of <u>any other reason</u> why you should not do physical activity?

If you answered

YES to one or more questions

Talk with your doctor by phone or in person BEFORE you start becoming much more physically active or BEFORE you have a fitness appraisal. Tell your doctor about the PAR-Q and which questions you answered YES.

- You may be able to do any activity you want — as long as you start slowly and build up gradually. Or, you may need to restrict your activities to those which are safe for you. Talk with your doctor about the kinds of activities you wish to participate in and follow his/her advice.
- Find out which community programs are safe and helpful for you.

NO to all questions

If you answered NO honestly to all PAR-Q questions, you can be reasonably sure that you can:
- start becoming much more physically active – begin slowly and build up gradually. This is the safest and easiest way to go.
- take part in a fitness appraisal – this is an excellent way to determine your basic fitness so that you can plan the best way for you to live actively. It is also highly recommended that you have your blood pressure evaluated. If your reading is over 144/94, talk with your doctor before you start becoming much more physically active.

DELAY BECOMING MUCH MORE ACTIVE:
- if you are not feeling well because of a temporary illness such as a cold or a fever – wait until you feel better; or
- if you are or may be pregnant – talk to your doctor before you start becoming more active.

PLEASE NOTE: If your health changes so that you then answer YES to any of the above questions, tell your fitness or health professional. Ask whether you should change your physical activity plan.

Informed Use of the PAR-Q: The Canadian Society for Exercise Physiology, Health Canada, and their agents assume no liability for persons who undertake physical activity, and if in doubt after completing this questionnaire, consult your doctor prior to physical activity.

No changes permitted. You are encouraged to photocopy the PAR-Q but only if you use the entire form.

NOTE: If the PAR-Q is being given to a person before he or she participates in a physical activity program or a fitness appraisal, this section may be used for legal or administrative purposes.

"I have read, understood and completed this questionnaire. Any questions I had were answered to my full satisfaction."

NAME _____

SIGNATURE _____   DATE _____

SIGNATURE OF PARENT _____   WITNESS _____
or GUARDIAN (for participants under the age of majority)

Note: This physical activity clearance is valid for a maximum of 12 months from the date it is completed and becomes invalid if your condition changes so that you would answer YES to any of the seven questions.

© Canadian Society for Exercise Physiology   Supported by: Health Canada / Santé Canada

FIGURE 2.1 PAR-Q & YOU questionnaire used to evaluate the health status of patients aged 15 to 69 desiring to start an exercise program.
Canadian Society for Exercise Physiology. 185 Somerset St. West, Suite 202, Ottawa, Ontario, Canada K2P 0J2 (with permission).

cognitively and physically mature enough to pursue the desired activity. For example, it may be wise to counsel a tall, lean, male middle school student with weak neck muscles (which predisposes the patient to cervical spine injury) away from the sport of football and into the sport of cross-country running. Once more fully developed, it may be safer for this student to participate in football or other riskier activities.[9,13]

Middle and Older Adults

The most common cause of SCD in people older than 35 years is coronary artery disease (CAD). Thus, focus the PPE for these adults on the detection of previously undiagnosed CAD. In general, healthy people with no known underlying pathology can begin a moderate exercise program (discussed in Chapter 3) without first administering a GXT. However, as exercise intensity and age increase, the need for a GXT increases. Obtain extensive personal and family histories and order a maximal GXT for patients desiring to engage in vigorous competitive events, such as masters athlete competitions, as well as for people who maintain a moderate to high CAD risk profile. Follow the recommendations published by prominent health care organizations such as the AHA and the American College of Sports Medicine when deciding on the need to obtain a GXT in the adult and elderly populations[11,13,30] (Table 2.2).

TABLE 2.2 Age-related treadmill graded exercise stress test screening guidelines

POPULATION (YEARS OF AGE)	EXERCISE STRESS TESTING—NO	EXERCISE STRESS TESTING—YES
Adult (30–65)	Moderate (40%–60% Vo_2max) exercise routine; asymptomatic, irrespective of CAD risk factors, age, or gender* Vigorous (>60% $Vo_{2\ max}$) exercise routine; asymptomatic, fewer than 2 CAD risk factors for* • men aged <45 • women aged <55	Vigorous (>60% Vo_2max) exercise routine for* • men aged >45 • women aged >55 • those with 1 or more CAD risk factors • those with known coronary, pulmonary, or metabolic disease 2 or more CAD risk factors (other than age or gender) or 1 markedly abnormal CAD risk factor for† • men aged >40 • women aged >50
Elderly/older adult (>65)		CAD risk factors with and without symptoms* Sedentary individuals*

CAD = coronary artery disease; Vo_2max = maximal oxygen consumption in 1 minute.

*American College of Sports Medicine. *Guidelines for Exercise Testing and Prescription*, 7th ed. Philadelphia, PA: Lippincott Williams & Wilkins, 2006.

†Maron BJ, Thompson PD, Puffer JC, et al. Cardiovascular preparticipation screening of competitive athletes: a statement for health professionals from the Sudden Death Committee (clinical cardiology) and Congenital Cardiac Defects Committee (cardiovascular disease in the young), American Heart Association. *Circulation* 1996;94:850.

Coronary artery disease is the most common cause of exercise-induced sudden cardiac death in people older than 35 years.

Years of inactivity increase the risk for middle and older adults to experience musculoskeletal injury as they attempt to become more active. Indeed, people who exercise only periodically are more likely to experience acute musculoskeletal injury than those who exercise regularly. Thus, for these patients, it is essential to review the mechanism of any previous injury and provide advice on injury prevention and physical conditioning techniques. Implement treatment and rehabilitation programs for any identified injury.

In many instances, older patients decide to initiate a fitness program in response to a recently diagnosed disease or injury. For example, a 70-year-old female diagnosed with osteoporosis may wish to begin a strength-training program, whereas a 73-year-old male with hypertension may decide to enroll in an aerobics class for older adults. Thus, comprise the PPE for the elderly patient to the medically necessary portions of a comprehensive screening, bearing in mind the effects an exercise program may have on the medical condition.[9,31]

Individuals with Special Needs

The PPE for people with special needs does not differ much from the PPE offered to any other patient. Overall, the examination should carefully screen for selective findings common to this population, such as visual, cardiovascular, neurologic, dermatologic, and musculoskeletal impairments. Recognize that organizations such as the Special Olympics require that all athletes be examined by a physician or appropriately trained provider before participating in a sanctioned Special Olympics contest. Through its Healthy Athletes initiative, the Special Olympics developed the MedFest screening program to facilitate a standard PPE for its participants. The medical portion of this screening includes height, weight, BP, cardiovascular, abdominal, and musculoskeletal assessments. Needed follow-up medical care is part of the screening process for all participants.[4,26]

Become familiar with the required content of the Special Olympics PPE for people with special needs.

Disqualification and Legal Considerations

Legal problems related to the PPE primarily occur when a health care provider does not disqualify someone who should have been disqualified, or does disqualify someone who then insists on a legal right to participate. In certain instances, mandates help to guide the primary health care provider with regard to the legal boundaries related to clearing a person to participate in or disqualifying a person from participating in organized sports.

Factors Affecting a Patient's Ability to Participate

When making a final decision on a person's ability to participate, consider these factors:

- the demands of the sport in which the individual desires to participate (Table 2.3),
- the potential for the identified condition to place the participant or others at risk,
- whether the patient can safely participate during the initiation and continuation of a proper course of treatment, and
- the probability that participating in contact sports or other high-risk activities (Table 2.4) may exacerbate the condition.

TABLE 2.3 Classification of sports by strenuousness

HIGH TO MODERATE INTENSITY		
HIGH TO MODERATE DYNAMIC AND STATIC DEMANDS	HIGH TO MODERATE DYNAMIC AND LOW STATIC DEMANDS	HIGH TO MODERATE STATIC AND LOW DYNAMIC DEMANDS
Boxing*	Badminton	Archery
Crew or rowing	Baseball	Auto racing
Cross-country skiing	Basketball	Diving
Cycling	Field hockey	Horseback riding (jumping)
Downhill skiing	Lacrosse	Field events (throwing)
Fencing	Orienteering	Gymnastics
Football	Race walking	Karate or judo
Ice hockey	Racquetball	Motorcycling
Rugby	Soccer	Rodeo
Running (sprint)	Squash	Sailing
Speed skating	Swimming	Ski jumping
Water polo	Table tennis	Water-skiing
Wrestling	Tennis	Weight lifting
	Volleyball	

LOW INTENSITY (LOW DYNAMIC AND LOW STATIC DEMANDS)
Bowling
Cricket
Curling
Golf
Riflery

*Participation not recommended by the American Academy of Pediatrics.

American Academy of Pediatrics Committee on Sports Medicine and Physical Fitness. Medical conditions affecting sports participation. *Pediatrics* 2001;107(5):1205 (with permission).

TABLE 2.4 Classification of sports by contact

CONTACT OR COLLISION	LIMITED CONTACT	NONCONTACT
Basketball	Baseball	Archery
Boxing*	Bicycling	Badminton
Diving	Cheerleading	Bodybuilding
Field hockey	Canoeing or kayaking	Bowling
Football	(white water)	Canoeing or kayaking
• Tackle	Fencing	(flat water)
Ice hockey†	Field events	Crew or rowing
Lacrosse	• High jump	Curling
Martial arts	• Pole vault	Dancing§
Rodeo	Floor hockey	• Ballet
Rugby	Football	• Modern
Ski jumping	• Flag	• Jazz
Soccer	Gymnastics	Field events
Team handball	Handball	• Discus
Water polo	Horseback riding	• Javelin
Wrestling	Racquetball	• Shot put
	Skating	Golf
	• Ice	Orienteering‖
	• In-line	Power lifting
	• Roller	Race walking
	Skiing	Riflery
	• Cross-country	Rope jumping
	• Downhill	Running
	• Water	Sailing
	Skateboarding	Scuba diving
	Snowboarding‡	Swimming
	Softball	Table tennis
	Squash	Tennis
	Ultimate frisbee	Track
	Volleyball	Weight lifting
	Windsurfing or surfing	

*Participation not recommended by the American Academy of Pediatrics.

†The American Academy of Pediatrics recommends limiting the amount of body checking allowed for hockey players aged 15 years and younger to reduce injuries.

‡Snowboarding has been added since previous statement was published.

§Dancing has been further classified into ballet, modern, and jazz since previous statement was published.

‖A race (contest) in which competitors use a map and compass to find their way through unfamiliar territory.

American Academy of Pediatrics Committee on Sports Medicine and Physical Fitness. Medical conditions affecting sports participation. *Pediatrics* 2001;107(5):1205 (with permission).

Ultimately, the following questions should be answered when determining a patient's participation status[4]:

• Does an identified problem place the patient at increased risk for injury or illness?
• Is another participant at risk for injury or illness because of the problem?

• Can the patient participate with treatment?
• Can limited participation be allowed while treatment is being completed?
• What activities, if any, can the patient participate in safely?

The American Academy of Pediatrics Committee on Sports Medicine and Fitness has outlined disqualification guidelines for common medical conditions (Table 2.5). These guidelines divide clearance decisions into three classifications: cleared, cleared with qualifications, and not cleared. Table 2.5 also provides an explanation for each medical condition assigned one of these classifications. Use these guidelines when determining which findings necessitate referral and which preclude participation.[13]

TABLE 2.5 Medical conditions and sports participation*

CONDITION	MAY PARTICIPATE
Atlantoaxial instability (instability of the joint between cervical vertebrae 1 and 2) *Explanation*: Athlete needs evaluation to assess risk of spinal cord injury during sports participation.	Qualified yes
Bleeding disorder *Explanation*: Athlete needs evaluation.	Qualified yes
Cardiovascular disease	
Carditis (inflammation of the heart) *Explanation:* Carditis may result in sudden death with exertion.	No
Hypertension (high blood pressure) *Explanation*: Those with significant essential (unexplained) hypertension should avoid weight and power lifting, bodybuilding, and strength training. Those with secondary hypertension (hypertension caused by a previously identified disease) or severe essential hypertension need evaluation. The National High Blood Pressure Education Working Group defined significant and severe hypertension.	Qualified yes
Congenital heart disease (structural heart defects at birth) *Explanation*: Those with mild forms may participate fully; those with moderate or severe forms or who have undergone surgery need evaluation. The 26th Bethesda Conference defined mild, moderate, and severe disease for common cardiac lesions.	Qualified yes
Dysrhythmia (irregular heart rhythm) *Explanation*: Those with symptoms (chest pain, syncope, dizziness, shortness of breath, or other symptoms of possible dysrhythmia) or evidence of mitral regurgitation (leaking) on physical examination need evaluation. All others may participate fully.	Qualified yes

(table continues on page 42)

TABLE 2.5 Medical conditions and sports participation* (continued)

CONDITION	MAY PARTICIPATE
Heart murmur *Explanation*: If the murmur is innocent (does not indicate heart disease), full participation is permitted. Otherwise, the athlete needs evaluation (see congenital heart disease and mitral valve prolapse).	Qualified yes
Cerebral palsy *Explanation*: Athlete needs evaluation.	Qualified yes
Diabetes mellitus *Explanation*: All sports can be played with proper attention to diet, blood glucose concentration, hydration, and insulin therapy. Blood glucose concentration should be monitored every 30 minutes during continuous exercise and 15 minutes after completion of exercise.	Yes
Diarrhea *Explanation*: Unless disease is mild, no participation is permitted, because diarrhea may increase the risk of dehydration and heat illness. See fever.	Qualified no

Eating disorders
  Anorexia nervosa
  Bulimia nervosa
   Explanation: Patients with these disorders need medical and psychiatric assessment before participation.
	Qualified yes

Eyes
  Functionally one-eyed athlete
  Loss of an eye
  Detached retina
  Previous eye surgery or serious eye injury
   Explanation: A functionally one-eyed athlete has a best-corrected visual acuity of less than 20/40 in the eye with worse acuity. These athletes would have significant disability if the better eye were seriously injured, as would those with loss of an eye. Some athletes who previously have undergone eye surgery or had a serious eye injury may have an increased risk of injury because of the weakened eye tissue. Availability of eye guards approved by the American Society for Testing and Material and other protective equipment may allow participation in most sports, but this must be judged on an individual basis.
	Qualified yes

CONDITION	MAY PARTICIPATE
Fever	No
Explanation: Fever can increase cardiopulmonary effort, reduce maximum exercise capacity, make heat illness more likely, and increase orthostatic hypertension during exercise. Fever may rarely accompany myocarditis or other infections that may make exercise dangerous.	
Heat illness, history of	Qualified yes
Explanation: Because of the increased likelihood of recurrence, the athlete needs individual assessment to determine the presence of pre-disposing conditions and to arrange a prevention strategy.	
Hepatitis	Yes
Explanation: Because of the apparent minimal risk to others, all sports may be played that the athlete's state of health allows. In all athletes, skin lesions should be covered properly, and athletic personnel should use universal precautions when handling blood or body fluids with visible blood.	
Human immunodeficiency virus infection	Yes
Explanation: Because of the apparent minimal risk to others, all sports may be played that the athlete's state of health allows. In all athletes, skin lesions should be covered properly, and athletic personnel should use universal precautions when handling blood or body fluids with visible blood.	
Kidney, absence of	Qualified yes
Explanation: Athlete needs individual assessment for contact, collision, and limited-contact sports.	
Liver, enlarged	Qualified yes
Explanation: If the liver is acutely enlarged, participation should be avoided because of risk of rupture. If the liver is chronically enlarged, individual assessment is needed before collision, contact, or limited-contact sports are played.	
Malignant neoplasm	Qualified yes
Explanation: Athlete needs individual assessment.	
Musculoskeletal disorders	Qualified yes
Explanation: Athlete needs individual assessment.	

(table continues on page 44)

TABLE 2.5 Medical conditions and sports participation* (continued)

CONDITION	MAY PARTICIPATE
Neurological disorders	
History of serious head or spine trauma, severe or repeated concussions, or craniotomy	Qualified yes
Explanation: Athlete needs individual assessment for collision, contact, or limited-contact sports and also for noncontact sports if deficits in judgment or cognition are present. Research supports a conservative approach to management of concussion.	
Seizure disorder, well-controlled	Yes
Explanation: Risk of seizure during participation is minimal.	
Seizure disorder, poorly controlled	Qualified yes
Explanation: Athlete needs individual assessment for collision, contact, or limited-contact sports. The following noncontact sports should be avoided: archery, riflery, swimming, weight or power lifting, strength training, or sports involving heights. In these sports, occurrence of a seizure may pose a risk to self or others.	
Obesity	Qualified yes
Explanation: Because of the risk of heat illness, obese persons need careful acclimatization and hydration.	
Organ transplant recipient	Qualified yes
Explanation: Athlete needs individual assessment.	
Ovary, absence of one	Yes
Explanation: Risk of severe injury to the remaining ovary is minimal.	
Respiratory conditions	
Pulmonary compromise, including cystic fibrosis	Qualified yes
Explanation: Athlete needs individual assessment, but generally, all sports may be played if oxygenation remains satisfactory during a graded exercise test. Patients with cystic fibrosis need acclimatization and good hydration to reduce the risk of heat illness.	
Asthma	Yes
Explanation: With proper medication and education, only athletes with the most severe asthma will need to modify their participation.	
Acute upper respiratory infection	Qualified yes
Explanation: Upper respiratory obstruction may affect pulmonary function. Athlete needs individual assessment for all but mild disease. See fever.	

CONDITION	MAY PARTICIPATE
Sickle cell disease	Qualified yes
Explanation: Athlete needs individual assessment. In general, if status of the illness permits, all but high-exertion, collision, and contact sports may be played. Overheating, dehydration, and chilling must be avoided.	
Sickle cell trait	Yes
Explanation: It is unlikely that persons with sickle cell trait have an increased risk of sudden death or other medical problems during athletic participation, except under the most extreme conditions of heat, humidity, and possibly increased altitude. These persons, like all athletes, should be carefully conditioned, acclimatized, and hydrated to reduce any possible risk.	
Skin disorders (boils, herpes simplex, impetigo, scabies, molluscum contagiosum)	Qualified yes
Explanation: While the patient is contagious, participation in gymnastics with mats; martial arts; wrestling; or other collision, contact, or limited-contact sports is not allowed.	
Spleen, enlarged	Qualified yes
Explanation: A patient with an acutely enlarged spleen should avoid all sports because of risk of rupture. A patient with a chronically enlarged spleen needs individual assessment before playing collision, contact, or limited-contact sports.	
Testicle, undescended or absence of one	Yes
Explanation: Certain sports may require a protective cup.	

*This table is designed for use by medical and nonmedical personnel.

"Needs evaluation" means that a physician with appropriate knowledge and experience should assess the safety of a given sport for an athlete with the listed medical condition. Unless otherwise noted, this is because of variability of the severity of the disease, the risk of the injury for the specific sports listed in Table 2.4, or both.

American Academy of Pediatrics Committee on Sports Medicine and Physical Fitness: Medical conditions affecting sports participation. *Pediatrics* 2001;107:1205 (with permission).

PEARL

Before clearing a person for participation, refer patients with abnormal findings to the proper physician entity.

When faced with the decision of whether to approve for participation or disqualify a patient who presents with an injury or illness outside medically accepted guidelines, it is generally recommended that this decision be deferred to a physician. Usually, a primary care physician makes the decision upon consultation with specialists. In some instances, a physician may disqualify a patient for a transient condition but allow participation once the situation has been brought within medically accepted limits. Alternatively, the presence of a particular injury or illness may preclude a person from participating in some activities but not others. Certainly, most people are able to participate in some form of physical activity, sport, or exercise program.[4]

A physician should make the final participation determination for people who present with remarkable PPE findings.

Legal Considerations
Medically clearing a person to participate in physically intensive and potentially dangerous activities can be a daunting task for any health care provider. The consequences of allowing a high-risk individual to partake in such activities could prove fatal. However, clearing an athlete does not automatically make the provider legally liable for injury or death due to an undisclosed medical condition such as a cardiovascular abnormality. Liability would most likely occur only if deviations from accepted medical practice had occurred during the PPE, and only if it can be shown that the use of established diagnostic criteria and methods would have disclosed a medical abnormality.[11]

Mandates
Traditionally, the PPE process has been governed by external mandates. For example, almost all state high school associations governing interscholastic athletics require a medical evaluation before a student can participate at the middle or high school levels. Other organizations, such as the NCAA, publish guidelines for member institutions to follow with regard to the administration of such examinations. These mandates may be viewed as burdensome because they typically have to be completed in a short time frame, such as at the beginning of an athletic season or at the start of a school year. However, most medical, legislative, and school administrative personnel agree that offering participants a PPE meets the moral and ethical responsibilities of maintaining the person's health and safety needs.[10,11,14,32]

Legislation
Though interscholastic and intercollegiate administrative personnel usually grant health care professionals the authority to medically disqualify a patient from participation, patients who feel that they are able to compete may claim a legal right to do so. Indeed, legal decisions have permitted student athletes to participate despite known medical risks and despite a medical disqualification being made. Furthermore, health care providers routinely follow differing medical clearance recommendations, because definitive guidelines are lacking. Thus, it is not uncommon for a second medical opinion to lead to a disagreement about whether a person should be cleared to participate. Nonetheless, in no instance should a person be cleared to participate if sound medical reasoning for allowing participation is lacking. In addition to the moral and ethical quandary such a decision could cause, taking such an action could be libelous.[33-36]

In no instance should a person be cleared to participate in sports
or exercise if sound medical reasoning for allowing
participation is lacking.

Since enactment of the 1973 Rehabilitation Act and the 1990 ADA, the health
care provider's authority to exclude people from participation in sports has been
increasingly challenged. These federal statutes, which prohibit unfair discrimination
against individuals who have physical abnormalities or impairments, have given physically impaired athletes the legal means by which to challenge medical sports participation decisions. Though schools can require athletes to demonstrate certain physical
qualifications, established by medical personnel, in order to compete, they cannot
exclude athletes who can satisfy all of the sports requirements in spite of physical
impairment. For example, it has been ruled illegal to exclude a person who has a missing or nonfunctioning paired organ (e.g., eye, kidney) from participating in high school
and college contact and collision sports. Regardless, reasonable physical qualifications
for participation in institutionally sponsored athletic events can be established and can
be used to disqualify individuals from participating.[28,33–35]

Seemingly contradictory judicial decisions regarding impaired patients' rights
have also challenged the authority of health care providers to disqualify individuals
from athletic participation. For example, though some court decisions have upheld
the right to medically exclude people, other decisions have sided with those who
have claimed a legal right to play. Thus, in certain situations, it may be determined
that the best legal option is to recommend, versus exclude, nonparticipation in
sporting activities because of a preexisting medical condition. By approaching each
PPE patient individually, incorporating the best medical information available, and
developing a positive rapport with the patient (including parents or legal guardians
in the case of minors), the patient can gain an appreciation for, and better understanding of, the PPE process and reasons for a disqualification recommendation. In
cases where the patient's parents or legal guardians insist on allowing participation
against medical advice, secure a signed release of liability (PTH 2.1) indicating that
all have been advised about and understand the potential dangers of participation.
However, the effectiveness of these waivers in protecting providers from lawsuits is
questionable and can vary among states.[13,28,35]

Secure a signed release of liability for patients who want to
participate against medical advice.

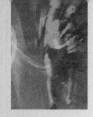

CASE STUDY
Pre-Participation Examination*

SCENARIO
In October, a 19-year-old male college student presents for his first college PPE before beginning ice hockey practice as part of the college team.

PERTINENT HISTORY
Medications: Denies regular use. Uses over-the-counter ibuprofen prn (about 400 mg once per week) for various musculoskeletal discomforts. Denies use of supplements. Takes a daily multivitamin.

Family History: Denies family history of sudden death before age 50, any history of Marfan's syndrome, hypertrophic cardiomyopathy, or other heart disease.

PERSONAL HEALTH HISTORY
Tobacco Use: Denies a history of smoking or oral tobacco use.

Alcohol Intake: None during the week but usually drinks the equivalent of 3 or 4 beers after completion of the weekly Saturday night ice hockey game. Reports less alcohol consumption in the off-season.

Caffeinated Beverages: Drinks a minimum of 1 caffeinated regular soda per day.

Diet: Maintains an excessive caloric intake as he prepares for his first college ice hockey season. Claims that the position he plays (defense) necessitates that he "bulk up" to compete at the college level. Diet is well rounded, with an emphasis on protein intake.

Exercise: Two hours of ice-skating per day, 6 days a week. In an attempt to increase muscle mass, he weight trains 3 to 4 days per week. Weight training sessions last 30 to 40 minutes.

Past Medical History: Unremarkable until age 17, when he sustained a left lower flank injury after being slammed into a goalpost at high speed. Initial evaluation by the athletic trainer revealed localized, radiating pain and immobility with increasing severity that made performing a physical examination extremely difficult. Hematuria was discovered, and the patient was immediately transported to the hospital. Magnetic resonance imaging was ordered and revealed the presence of only one kidney, a congenital abnormality he was unaware of until that time. A conservative treatment plan of rest and no participation in contact or collision sports was followed. He has not played ice hockey or any other competitive sport since the injury occurred. However, as previously noted, he has been exercising vigorously in preparation for the upcoming season. The patient claims his primary care physician in his home town thinks he can continue his ice hockey career as long as he wears extra padding to protect his kidney.

PERTINENT PHYSICAL EXAMINATION
Blood pressure: 120/78 mm Hg. Heart rate: 56 bpm. Respiratory rate: 16 breaths/min. Height: 73 inches. Weight: 210 pounds.

Appearance: Muscular, medium build.

*Because of space limitations, these cases are not meant to be comprehensive but are used as exemplar cases for the point being illustrated.

Abdominal and Genitourinary Examinations: No tenderness to palpation in left lower flank or elsewhere. Though not required in a standard PPE, a urinalysis stick examination reveals no presence of hematuria.

RED FLAGS FOR THE PRIMARY HEALTH CARE PROVIDER TO CONSIDER

From the patient's history, it is highly questionable whether this athlete should be allowed to continue his participation in a sport that places his remaining, already damaged kidney at risk. Even with added protection, the consequences of reinjury include the potential of prolonged dialysis and kidney transplantation.

RECOMMENDED PLAN

- Delay approval for athletic participation pending further evaluation and consultation.
- Contact primary care physician to obtain copies of the patient's complete medical history.
- Engage the athlete and the college's athletic administrative personnel in conversation regarding participation risks.
- If athlete is cleared to participate, have him sign a release of liability with copies housed in your office and in the patient's medical file at the college.

REFERENCES

1. Magnes SA, Henderson JM, Hunter SC. What conditions limit sports participation? Experience with 10540 athletes. *Phys Sportsmed* 1992;20(5):143.
2. Fuller CM, McNulty CM, Spring DA, et al. Prospective screening of 5615 high school athletes for risk of sudden cardiac death. *Med Sci Sports Exerc* 1997;29:1131.
3. Smith J, Laskowski ER. The preparticipation physical examination: Mayo Clinic experience with 2739 examinations. *Mayo Clin Proc* 1998;73:419.
4. American Academy of Family Physicians (AAFP), American Academy of Pediatrics (AAP), American College of Sports Medicine (ACSM), et al. *Preparticipation Physical Evaluation*, 3rd ed. Minneapolis, MN: The Physician and Sports Medicine: A Division of the McGraw-Hill Companies, 2005.
5. Sanders B, Nemeth WC. Preparticipation physical examination. *J Orthop Sports Phys Ther* 1996;23:149.
6. Armsey TD, Hosey RG. Medical aspects of sports: epidemiology of injuries, preparticipation physical examination, and drugs in sports. *Clin Sports Med* 2004;23:255.
7. Gemberling C. Preparticipation sports evaluation: an overview. *Nurse Pract Forum* 1996;7(3):125.
8. Maron BJ, Zipes DP. 36th Bethesda Conference: eligibility recommendations for competitive athletes with cardiovascular abnormalities. *J Am Coll Cardiol* 2005;45:1313.
9. McKeag DB. Preparticipation screening of the potential athlete. *Clin Sports Med* 1989;8:373.
10. National Collegiate Athletics Association. *Sports Medicine Handbook, 2006-2007*. Indianapolis, IN. Retrieved from: http://www.ncaa.org/library/sports_sciences/sports_med_handbook/2006-07/2006-07_sports_medicine_handbook.pdf. Accessed 1/25/08.
11. Maron BJ, Thompson PD, Puffer JC, et al. Cardiovascular preparticipation screening of competitive athletes: a statement for health professionals from the Sudden Death Committee (clinical cardiology) and Congenital Cardiac Defects Committee (cardiovascular disease in the young), American Heart Association. *Circulation* 1996;94:850.
12. Maron BJ, Thompson PD, Puffer JC, et al. Cardiovascular preparticipation screening of competitive athletes: addendum. American Heart Association. *Circulation* 1998;97:2294.
13. American Academy of Pediatrics Committee on Sports Medicine and Fitness. Medical conditions affecting sports participation. *Pediatrics* 2001;107:1205.
14. National Federation of State High School Associations. Sports medicine: NFHS encourages pre-participation physical evaluations. Press release. Nov. 4, 1998.
15. Schnirring L. News Briefs: High school association declines national PPE form. *Phys Sportsmed* 1999;27(1):25.
16. Johnson MD. Tailoring the preparticipation exam to female athletes. *Phys Sportsmed* 1992;20(7):61.
17. Kadel NJ, Teitz CC, Kronmal RA. Stress fractures in ballet dancers. *Am J Sports Med* 1992;20:445.
18. Baker WF. Iron deficiency in pregnancy, obstetrics and gynecology. *Clin North Am* 2000;14:1061.
19. JNC 7 Express. The Seventh Report of the Joint National Committee on Prevention, Detection, Evaluation and Treatment of High Blood Pressure. U.S. Department of Health and Human Services. National Institutes of Health Publication No. 03-5233, 2003. Retrieved from: http://www.nhlbi.nih.gov/guidelines/hypertension/express.pdf. Accessed 7/29/08.
20. Maron BJ, Araújo CGS, Thompson PD, et al. AHA science advisory: recommendations for preparticipation screening and the assessment of cardiovascular disease in masters athletes. An advisory for healthcare professionals from the working groups of the World Heart Federation, the International Federation of Sports Medicine, and the American Heart Association Committee on Exercise, Cardiac Rehabilitation, and Prevention. *Circulation* 2001;103:327.
21. Van Camp S, Bloor CM, Mueller FO, et al. Nontraumatic sports death in high school and college athletes. *Med Sci Sports Exerc* 1995;27:641.
22. Ades PA. Preventing sudden death. *Phys Sportsmed* 1992;20(9):75.
23. Missri JC, Sweet DD. Marfan syndrome: a review. *Cardiovasc Rev Rep* 1982;3:1648.

24. Maron BJ, Chaitman BR, Ackerman MJ, et al. Recommendations for physical activity and recreational sports participation for young patients with genetic cardiovascular diseases. *Circulation* 2004;109(22):2807.
25. Sharp DS, Ross JH, Kay R. Attitudes of pediatric urologists regarding sports participation by children with a solitary kidney. *J Urol* 2002;168:1811.
26. Special Olympics. Healthy athletes: MedFest. Retrieved from: http://www.specialolympics.org. Accessed 7/29//08.
27. American Academy of Pediatrics Committee on Sports Medicine. Atlantoaxial instability in Down syndrome. *Pediatrics* 1984;74(1):152.
28. Nichols AW. Sports medicine and the Americans with Disabilities Act. *Clin J Sport Med* 1996;6(3):190.
29. Canadian Society for Exercise Physiology. Physical Activity Readiness Questionnaire: PAR-Q and You. Retrieved from: http://www.csep.ca/main.cfm?cid=574&nid=5110. Accessed 7/29/08.
30. American College of Sports Medicine. *Guidelines for Exercise Testing and Prescription*, 7th ed. Philadelphia, PA: Lippincott Williams & Wilkins, 2006.
31. Kligman EW, Hewitt MJ, Crowell DL. Recommending exercise to healthy older adults: the preparticipation evaluation and exercise prescription. *Phys Sportsmed* 1999;27(11):42.
32. Glover DW, Maron BJ. Profile of preparticipation cardiovascular screening for high school athletes. *JAMA* 1998;279(22):1817.
33. Mitten JD. When is disqualification from sports justified? Medical judgment vs. patients' rights. *Phys Sportsmed* 1996;24(10):75.
34. Mitten MJ. Team physician and competitive athletics: allocating legal responsibility for athletic injuries. *University of Pittsburgh Law Review* 1993;55:129.
35. *Grube v Bethlehem Area School District*, 550 F Supp 418 (ED Pa 1982).
36. *Wright v Columbia University*, 520 F2d 789 (ED Pa 1981).

SUGGESTED READINGS

Herringer J. Cautiously delegate medical histories, physical exams. *Nurs Manage* 2003;34(2):20.
Maheady DC. Special Olympics physicals: a winning opportunity for nurse practitioner students. *Clin Excell Nurse Pract* 1998;2(2):112.
Miller SK. Professional practice: Does NP scope of practice include physical exams for work and sports? *Patient Care Nurse Pract* 2001;4(6):84.

WEB LINKS

www.aap.org. Accessed 7/29/08.
   Web site of the American Academy of Pediatrics. An all encompassing site dedicated to children's health. Sections are available for health care providers and parents alike.

www.ameicanheart.org. Accessed 7/29/08.
   Provides information to all things associated with heart disease. Links for local information are also available.

www.acsm.org. Accessed 7/29/08.
   Web site of the American College of Sports Medicine. Provides an array of information on health, exercise, and disease prevention for clinicians, educators, fitness professionals, and the public. Includes specific links related to pre-participation screening for both athletes and the general population.

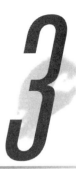

3

Physical Fitness

● **Karen A. Croteau, EdD, FACSM; Edited by Brian J. Toy, PhD, ATC** hysical activity, a core component of a healthy lifestyle, has been identified by Healthy People 2010 as one of the 10 leading health indicators in the United States. Documented benefits of regular moderate physical activity include preventing chronic diseases, disability, and premature death and improving quality of life. Despite knowing the many benefits of being physically active, most people are not active on a regular basis, and levels of physical activity remain low among all segments of the population. Indeed, almost 40% of all adults in the United States engage in no leisure-time physical activity whatsoever. This can somewhat be attributed to advances in technology, allowing people to vastly curtail the amount of exercise they get on a daily basis. Therefore, it is essential that primary health care providers educate patients about the virtues of physical activity.[1-4]

Physical Activity, Exercise, and Physical Fitness

Though all are important components of health, the terms *physical activity, exercise,* and *physical fitness* have different meanings. Because these terms are sometimes used interchangeably, primary health care providers need to be able to distinguish among the three when working with patients.

Physical Activity

Physical activity is defined as any bodily movement that requires the use of muscle contractions, expends energy, and produces progressive health benefits. The 1996 Surgeon General's Report (SGR) on Physical Activity and Health concludes that all people, regardless of age, can reap substantial health benefits by performing at least 30 minutes of moderately intense physical activity on most, if not all, days of the week. The SGR report also states that people can experience similar benefits whether the 30-minute recommendation is done continuously or cumulatively in two to three bouts of 10 to 15 minutes. Recent guidelines published by the American College of Sports Medicine (ACSM) and the American Heart Association (AHA) have added to these recommendations, stating that adults between the ages of 16 to 65 should participate in 30 minutes of moderately intense physical activity 5 days each week or 20 minutes of vigorous physical activity 3 days each week. Globally, these recommendations dispute the notion that a person must partake in long bouts of somewhat intense exercise, such as jogging or bicycle riding, to produce health benefits. Indeed, performing many different types of everyday activities, such as walking to and from work or school, taking the stairs instead of the elevator, and performing various household chores, suffice as physical activity. Fortunately, these activities are easier for most people to perform, particularly those who normally lead a sedentary lifestyle. This makes the concept of engaging in physical activity much less intimidating to the general public.[2,5,6]

For most people, health benefits can be achieved by regularly participating in 30 minutes of moderately intense physical activity on at least 5 days a week.

Exercise

Exercise is a type of physical activity that requires planned, structured, and repetitive bodily movement with a purpose of improving or maintaining one or more components of physical fitness. Examples of exercise include structured walking programs, running, cycling, swimming, strength training, and various group exercise classes. Although participation in physical activity, as explained above, does provide health benefits, greater benefits can be attained by participating in longer and/or more vigorous bouts of exercise.[2,5]

Physical Fitness

Physical fitness is a multidimensional concept defined as a set of attributes that people possess or achieve that relate to the ability to perform physical activity. Composed of the physical aspects of well-being that contribute to an optimal quality of life, physical fitness is divided into health-related and skill-related components. The discussion here is limited to the health-related components, because these are the most relevant to primary health care providers.

The components of health-related physical fitness include[5]

- **cardiorespiratory endurance**, also known as *aerobic fitness*,
- **muscular strength**,
- **muscular endurance**,
- **flexibility**, and
- **body composition**.

Health Benefits of Physical Activity and Exercise

Because of the high rates of sedentariness and physical inactivity among the U.S. population, exercising regularly can substantially help the average person become healthier. The SGR lists a number of health-related benefits associated with physical activity. Recent research findings have expanded this list. In all, these benefits include the physiological adaptations that the body makes in response to becoming physically fit, a reduction of disease risk, maintenance of **functional fitness**, improvement of psychological well-being, and increases in longevity and quality of life.[2,6,7]

Physiological Adaptations

Physiological adaptations include changes that affect the structure of the body in response to an exercise stimulus and are specific to the type of activity performed. These adaptations include improvements in cardiorespiratory endurance, muscular strength and endurance, and flexibility.[8]

PEARL

Physiological adaptations resulting from partaking in physical activity and/or exercise include improvements in cardiorespiratory endurance, muscular strength and endurance, and flexibility.

Cardiorespiratory Endurance

Cardiorespiratory endurance is arguably the most important component of health-related physical fitness. Specific adaptations the body makes in response to cardiorespiratory endurance exercise include increased[9,10]

- vital capacity of the lungs, permitting more oxygen to enter the body;
- cardiac output, enabling the heart to pump more blood within 1 minute;
- stroke volume (SV), allowing the heart to pump more blood with each beat;
- red blood cell count, enhancing the oxygen-carrying capacity of blood;
- capillary density of both heart and skeletal muscles, allowing for greater gas exchange;
- number and size of mitochondria in working muscles, resulting in the production of more energy;
- fat-burning enzymes in working muscles, permitting more fat to be used as fuel; and
- amount of oxygen the body utilizes in 1 minute (Vo_2max).

Cardiorespiratory endurance exercise also decreases[9,10]

- resting heart rate (RHR) by increasing SV,
- submaximal oxygen consumption by using less oxygen at lower intensity levels, and
- exercise recovery time.

Muscular Strength and Endurance

Increases in muscular strength and endurance are accomplished through resistance exercise training. Specific adaptations to performing these exercises include[8]

- better muscle tone;
- increase in quantity of contractile proteins;
- muscle **hypertrophy**;
- preservation of, or increase in, **lean body mass** (LBM);
- improved posture and physical appearance;
- increased **resting metabolic rate** (RMR);
- enhanced ability to perform activities of daily living (ADLs);
- enhanced performance in occupational, recreational, and athletic activities; and
- musculoskeletal injury prevention.

Flexibility

Regularly performing flexibility or stretching exercises affects all soft tissues in the area being stretched. These include muscles, tendons, ligaments, joint capsules, and fascia (all discussed in Chapter 1). Specific adaptations the body makes in response to stretching include[8]

- increased muscular flexibility;
- increased joint range of motion (ROM);
- improved posture and physical appearance;
- decreased symptoms of low back pain;
- prevention and minimization of delayed-onset muscle soreness (DOMS) (discussed in Chapter 1);
- reduction of stress and muscle tension;
- promotion of relaxation; and
- enhanced performance in occupational, recreational, and athletic activities.

Though it is widely believed that performing stretching exercises before and/or after engaging in physical activity prevents muscular injury, this relationship has yet to be established. Indeed, some believe that stretching before activity actually increases a person's risk of straining a muscle. Clearly, more research is needed in this area.[11,12]

Reduction of Disease Risk

Results of numerous studies indicate an association between physical activity and reduced risk of chronic diseases such as coronary artery disease (CAD) and stroke, both prevalent diseases of the cardiovascular system. CAD risk factors impacted by regular physical activity include reduced resting systolic and diastolic blood pressures (BPs), increased high-density lipoprotein levels, reduced triglyceride levels, reduced total and intra-abdominal body fat, improved glucose tolerance and insulin sensitivity, and reduced adhesiveness and aggregation of blood platelets. Regular physical activity and/or exercise is also associated with lower rates of type 2 diabetes, chronic back pain, osteoporotic fractures, colon and breast cancer, and gallbladder disease.[2,7,9,13,14]

Maintenance of Functional Fitness

Functional fitness can be improved and maintained through regular physical activity, helping various populations, such as older adults, to perform ADLs. This allows many elderly people to live independently. Functional fitness also increases a person's ability to perform occupational, recreational, and sport activities, allowing all segments of the population to participate in these endeavors.[2,15,16]

Improvement of Psychological Well-Being

In addition to the numerous physical benefits associated with participating in physical activity and exercise, psychological benefits also exist. These include a reduction of anxiety and depression and improvements in mood and emotional well-being. Being physically active also relieves tension, raises energy levels, and helps a person cope with stress.[2]

Increase in Longevity and Quality of Life

It is well documented that people who are physically active throughout life also benefit from increases in both quantity (longevity) and quality of life. Indeed, people with higher levels of physical fitness have lower death rates from all causes of death, also known as *all-cause mortality*.[2,17]

Exercise Variables

When developing an exercise program for a patient, certain variables must be appropriately manipulated for desired cardiorespiratory, resistance, and flexibility body adaptations to occur. These variables include exercise frequency, intensity, time (duration), and type (mode) and are commonly referred to by the acronym FITT[9]:

- F = frequency
- I = intensity
- T = time
- T = type

Frequency and Intensity

Frequency refers to the number of exercise sessions a person performs per week (e.g., three times), whereas *intensity* refers to how hard a person exercises. For cardiorespiratory endurance, exercise intensity is reported either as a percentage of a person's maximal heart rate (HRmax), measured in beats per minute, or as a percentage of the individual's Vo_2max, measured in liters per minute or milliliters per kilogram of body weight per minute. Though determining a person's Vo_2max provides the most accurate means of measuring aerobic exercise intensity, the methods used to arrive at this information can be challenging to use, particularly when working with the general public. Thus, most primary health care providers determine a patient's proper cardiorespiratory endurance exercise intensity using the HRmax method. This easy-to-use technique is described later in this chapter.

Frequency refers to the number of exercise sessions a person performs per week, whereas intensity refers to how hard a person exercises.

For resistance exercise, intensity is measured as a percentage of a person's maximal lifting capacity for one repetition (1-RM), with a repetition defined as lifting and lowering a weight one time. Flexibility intensity is measured by the ROM associated with a particular joint and directly relates to how far a person can stretch a particular body part.

Time (Duration) and Type (Mode)

Exercise duration refers to how long a specific exercise session lasts. Cardiorespiratory endurance exercise duration is measured in time, such as walking or jogging for 30 minutes, whereas resistance exercise duration is expressed as repetitions, otherwise known as *reps*, and sets, with a set defined as a group of reps. Resistance training duration is communicated by identifying the number of sets performed followed by the number of reps (e.g., three sets of 10 reps). Stretching duration refers to both the length of time it takes to perform an individual stretch and the number of reps performed. For example, it is common to tell a patient to perform three reps of the same stretch while instructing him or her to hold each stretch for 15 seconds.

The mode of exercise refers to the type of exercise performed. For example, jogging is a mode of exercise, as are weight lifting, biking, and playing tennis. However, when discussing resistance training, exercise mode also refers to the type of muscular contraction used to perform the exercise. This should be explained to patients who desire to use resistance training as part of an exercise regimen.

Two basic types of muscle contraction exist: isometric and isotonic. In an isometric contraction, the fibers of a muscle contract without changing the muscle's length and without moving the joint(s) on which the muscle acts. This usually occurs when a muscle contracts against an unyielding object, such as what happens when a person pushes against a brick wall. In contrast, an isotonic contraction occurs when the muscle fibers and joint(s) on which the muscle acts produce movement. Two types of isotonic contractions exist: concentric and eccentric. Whereas muscle fibers shorten during a concentric contraction, such as what happens when a person contracts the biceps brachii to lift a glass from a table, they lengthen during an eccentric contraction, such as what happens when the biceps brachii contracts while returning a glass to the table. Because an eccentric contraction produces more force than a concentric contraction, it is much harder on a muscle to perform this type of contraction. Indeed, recall from Chapter 1 that performing many eccentric contractions during exercise is the prime cause of DOMS experienced by most people after long and/or intense bouts of exercise.[8]

People who become physically active for health benefits, and not to become competitive in a specific sport, may want to vary their mode of exercise from time to time. Otherwise referred to as *cross-training*, this approach to implementing an exercise program helps some people to stay motivated and decreases the chance for overuse muscle injury by periodically altering the areas of the body being stressed during activity.

Principles of Training

To improve the health-related components of physical fitness, the principles of progressive overload, specificity, reversibility, recuperation, and individual differences must be considered when designing and implementing an exercise program.[8]

Progressive Overload

The progressive overload principle states that to improve physical fitness, a training stimulus greater than what a person is accustomed must be provided, and applied, in a gradual manner. This means that the frequency, intensity, and duration of a person's exercise session should be periodically increased in an incremental fashion. For example, to increase cardiorespiratory endurance, the amount of time spent exercising, the number of exercise days, and/or the intensity of each exercise session must be increased. When applying the progressive overload principle to strength training, it is necessary to increase the number of reps performed and/or the amount of weight lifted. By repeatedly applying this principle, muscles and body systems adapt with improved efficiency and capacity.[8]

To improve physical fitness, a training stimulus greater than what a person is accustomed to must be provided.

Specificity

The specificity principle states that to receive specific results from an exercise program, the program must target a specific energy system and/or muscle group. For example, a person needs to run, versus performing another activity, such as biking, to improve running performance. Obviously, following this principle is more important to people who want to become better at a specific sport than it is for those who want to gain the general health benefits of exercise.[8]

Reversibility

Also referred to as the *use-and-disuse*, *de-training*, and *use-it-or-lose-it* principle, the reversibility principle states that any positive benefits gained as a result of exercising are lost when a person becomes sedentary. Generally, people who have high levels of physical fitness have longer "grace" periods of fitness maintenance, whereas those with lower levels of fitness tend to lose the effects of exercise more quickly.[8]

Recuperation

The recuperation principle states that the body's energy systems and muscles need adequate time to recover and adapt between exercise sessions. For example, a recuperation period of 1 to 2 days per week is recommended for people participating in cardiorespiratory endurance exercise, whereas muscular strength training requires a longer recovery period between exercise sessions. Specific recovery periods for each component of health-related fitness are discussed later in the chapter.[8]

The body's energy systems and muscles need adequate time to recover and adapt between exercise sessions.

Individual Differences

The individual differences principle refers to the fact that people vary in terms of initial fitness levels and in the body's ability to respond to exercise training. Indeed, genetic makeup is the prime factor in determining both the response a person experiences with training and the maximal level of physical fitness the person can attain. This means that, regardless of a person's dedication to an exercise program, it is impossible for someone without the proper genetic composition to achieve fitness and/or skill levels beyond what the body can obtain. For example, some people's cardiorespiratory and musculoskeletal systems allow them to exercise close to their HRmax or VO_2max for extended periods, influencing their ability to perform well in activities such as long-distance running. This genetic predisposition to excel in certain activities is the prime reason why so few people have the ability to become involved in things such as professional sports and Olympic-level competitions.[8]

Genetic makeup is the prime factor in determining both the response a person experiences with training and the maximal level of physical fitness that he or she can attain.

Body Composition

Body composition refers to the amount of fat, versus the amount of LBM, that the body maintains and is expressed as a relative percentage of body fat (BFP). In general, a healthy BFP for males younger than 35 years is 8% to 22%, whereas this range for men 35 and older is 10% to 25%. For females younger than 35 years, a healthy range is 20% to 35%, whereas this range for females 35 and older is 23% to 38%. Precise measures of body fat can be made through techniques such as **dual-energy x-ray absorptiometry (DEXA) scanning** and **hydrostatic weighing**. Although these tests are both highly reliable, they are equipment intensive, are expensive, and require highly trained personnel to administer. Thus, most primary health care providers estimate a person's body composition by using methods such as bioelectrical impedance (BIA), skinfold measurements (SMs), body mass index (BMI), and waist circumference (WC).[8,9]

Bioelectrical Impedance

Measuring body composition through BIA consists of passing a weak electrical current from one body limb to another. In the clinical setting, this is done through the use of a handheld or analyzer/scale BIA unit, devices that can be purchased easily. This method of estimating BFP is based on the premise that an electrical current moves more easily through muscle because of its high water content and is impeded by fat because of its low water content. Because a person's hydration status has a great impact on the accuracy of this test, the BIA unit's directions must be closely followed if this method of determining a patient's BFP is used in the clinical setting.[8]

Skinfold Measurements

Using SMs to estimate BFP remains a common way for primary health care providers to determine a patient's body composition. The use of these measurements is grounded in the belief that at least one-third of the body's fat is located under the skin. Thus, by measuring the amount of subcutaneous fat in several key body areas, a patient's total BFP can be estimated. Though this method is very effective, the precision with which a provider is able to accurately determine a patient's BFP is directly affected by the person's ability to properly use a skinfold caliper. Simply put, the correct use of a skinfold caliper, like any psychomotor skill, takes practice. It is for this reason that this method should only be used if the person taking the measurements has been properly trained or has extensive experience in using a skinfold caliper. Refer to any standard fitness evaluation textbook for common skinfold body sites and related charts when using SMs to determine a patient's BFP.[8,9]

Body Mass Index

Expressed as a number calculated from a patient's weight and height, the BMI method of determining a patient's body composition has gained widespread popularity among primary health care providers. This technique is easy to administer and is useful in identifying patients at risk for premature illness and death. The following formula is used to determine a person's BMI[18]:

$$\text{weight (lb)}/[\text{height (in.)}]^2 \times 703$$

For example, the BMI for a 40-year-old male who weighs 190 pounds and stands 69 inches is determined as follows:

$$\text{BMI} = 190/[69]^2 \times 703$$

$$= 190/4761 \times 703$$

$$= 0.0399 \times 703$$

$$= 28.1$$

Refer to Table 3.1 to interpret this data. As this table reveals, the patient in this example is classified as overweight, as any adult with a BMI between 25 and 29.9 would be. An adult with a BMI at or above 30 is classified as obese.[18]

TABLE 3.1 Interpretation of BMI for adults	
BMI	**WEIGHT STATUS**
Below 18.5	Underweight
18.5–24.9	Normal weight
25.0–29.9	Overweight
30.0 and above	Obese

BMI = body mass index.

Centers for Disease Control, Department of Health and Human Services. Body Mass Index Home. Retrieved from: http://www.cdc.gov/nccdphp/dnpa/healthyweight/assessing/bmi/adult_BMI/about_adult_BMI.htm#Interpreted. Accessed 7/29/08.

Because BMI changes substantially as children and teens age, determining a person's BMI for patients aged between 2 to 20 is gender and age specific. Thus, the term *BMI for age* is used to refer to BMI measurements for this population. Refer to the Centers for Disease Control and Prevention BMI Web site to calculate and interpret BMI measurements for children and teens.[18,19]

Although a person's BMI establishes whether they are overweight or obese, it does not differentiate between how much body fat or LBM a person has. Nevertheless, it is a reliable indicator of body fatness, because the correlation between a patient's BMI and actual BFP is high. However, variations in age, gender, and physical fitness status affect this relationship as follows[18]:

- at the same BMI, women tend to have more body fat than men do;
- at the same BMI, older people tend to have more body fat than younger adults do; and
- highly trained athletes may have a high BMI because of increased muscularity rather than increased body fatness.

PEARL

A person's **BMI** is a reliable indicator of body fatness because the correlation between **BMI** and actual **BFP** is high.

Waist Circumference

Whereas BMI provides a general indication of a patient's body fatness, the WC shows the distribution of a person's body fat. It is this distribution that has been recognized as an important predictor of chronic illnesses such as hypertension, type 2 diabetes, lipid disorders, and CAD related to obesity. This makes obtaining a patient's WC a vital part of any assessment technique for people desiring to become physically active. A person's WC is established by measuring the circumference of the patient's waist between the navel and xiphoid process. Females with a WC >35 inches and males with a WC >40 inches have an increased risk of developing a chronic illness due to obesity.[9]

Exercise Programming

As discussed in Chapter 2, before starting an exercise program and/or becoming involved in competitive athletics, a person should complete either a comprehensive pre-participation examination (PPE) or a Physical Activity Readiness Questionnaire (PAR-Q). After it is determined that a patient is healthy enough to exercise, individualized exercise programs can be developed by incorporating the following components:

- warm-up period,
- flexibility exercises,
- cardiorespiratory endurance exercise,
- muscular strength and endurance exercises, and
- cool-down period.

Although an ideal exercise program includes all of these elements, the actual program is dependent on the patient's goals. For example, a person desiring to run a marathon race should concentrate on cardiorespiratory endurance exercise, with less emphasis placed on resistance training. Also, although highly effective exercise programs can be developed, it is just as important to apply behavior modification principles to assist the patient to adhere to the program. These principles are covered later in this chapter. Finally, after they have initiated an exercise program, the fitness status of the patient must be reassessed periodically. This allows an opportunity to provide the patient with positive feedback and encouragement, for improvements to be noted and for program modifications to be made.

Warm-Up

Before initiating any exercise session, it is important to advise patients to prepare the body for activity. Do this by explaining to the patient how to properly warm up the body. This includes telling people to warm up before stretching, because many people believe they should stretch to warm up. Emphasize to patients that it is proper to "warm up to stretch, not stretch to warm up."

Advise patients to warm up the body before performing flexibility exercises and other forms of exercise.

The purpose of the warm-up is to prepare the body for the physiological demands of exercise. Specifically, warming up increases[9]

- blood flow to the heart and active muscles;
- oxygen consumption and release to active muscles;
- temperature of active muscles; and
- elasticity of muscles, tendons, and ligaments.

A proper warm-up consists of both general and specific aspects. Whereas a general warm-up includes the completion of full body movements, such as walking briskly or jogging, the specific warm-up prepares the body to perform the skills it needs to complete the exercise session. For example, before performing a resistance exercise, instruct patients to complete a few repetitions of the planned exercise with a weight much lighter than what the person uses to complete the exercise. For a cardiorespiratory workout, have patients perform the same activity at a lower intensity, such as biking more slowly than usual. Though the duration of the warm-up session depends on the person's fitness level and the intensity and duration of the pending workout, advise patients to spend 5 to 15 minutes preparing the body for exercise.

Advise patients to spend 5 to 15 minutes warming up before initiating exercise.

Flexibility Exercise

Though there are many ways to increase flexibility of the body's soft tissues, the most common, and safest, is through performing static stretching exercises. This involves placing a body part, such as the thigh, in a position so the soft tissues in the area are stretched without the body part moving.

Guidelines for Implementing Flexibility Exercise

To obtain the maximal benefits of a stretch, the soft tissues in the area must be in a relaxed state. This is particularly true when trying to stretch muscles because it is difficult to increase the flexibility of a muscle when it is contracting. For example, it is easier to stretch the hamstrings (discussed in Chapter 9) when seated than when standing, because in the standing position the hamstrings must contract to keep the body erect. Also, performing flexibility exercises is an individual matter and should not be viewed as a competition between people, because trying to "outstretch" another person could result in serious injury.

Flexibility exercise is an individual matter and should not be viewed as a competition between people.

When teaching patients how to perform flexibility exercises, instruct them to stretch to a point of mild tension or slight discomfort, not to a point of pain. When patients reach this point, tell them to "hold" the stretch for 15 to 30 seconds. Initially, have patients perform two repetitions of each stretch prescribed at least 3 days per week. Have them progress to the point where they are performing four repetitions of each stretch on most days of the week. They should also perform these stretches after every exercise session and before each vigorous exercise session. Flexibility exercise guidelines are summarized in Table 3.2. Stretching exercises for each major muscle group are presented in Patient Teaching Handout (PTH) 3.1.

Cardiorespiratory Endurance Exercise

Recall that the definition of cardiorespiratory endurance is the ability of the body to deliver and utilize oxygen during prolonged exercise. Though the many benefits of this form of exercise were previously discussed, it bears repeating that aerobic exercise is particularly important in preventing CAD. Thus, with few exceptions, cardiorespiratory endurance exercise is the cornerstone of any exercise program.

TABLE 3.2 Flexibility exercise guidelines	
Frequency	2–3 d/wk (minimal) 5–7 d/wk (ideal) Before and after activity
Intensity	Stretch to point of mild tension or slight discomfort, but not to point of pain
Time (duration)	15–30 seconds, 2–4 reps/stretch
Type (mode)	Static stretching of all major muscle groups
Progression	Gradually increase duration and frequency

PEARL

Cardiorespiratory endurance exercise is the cornerstone of any exercise program.

Guidelines for Implementing Cardiorespiratory Endurance Exercise

As previously mentioned, the ACSM recommends that people perform physical activity of moderate intensity at least 5 days per week or vigorous activity at least 3 days per week. Thus, advise patients interested in exercising for general fitness to perform aerobic exercise 3 to 5 days per week. Realize the number of days recommended is directly dependent on the intensity level of the planned exercise sessions. For example, participation in activities requiring lower intensity levels, such as walking, require more participation days than those activities of higher intensity, such as jogging, so sufficient aerobic fitness gains can be achieved. For most people, the additional health benefits realized by performing higher-intensity aerobic exercise more than 5 days per week do not outweigh the risk of incurring musculoskeletal injury commonly seen when exercising this frequently. Therefore, reserve recommending participation in high-intensity exercises more than 5 days per week for competitive athletes.

PEARL

Advise patients seeking health benefits of exercise to participate in aerobic activities 3 to 5 days per week.

Establishing and monitoring cardiorespiratory exercise intensity levels is of prime importance when developing a cardiorespiratory endurance exercise program, because these levels must be sufficient to produce desired physiologic effects. However, they cannot be so intense that the person is unable to continue the activity for any length of time. Determining the proper intensity level involves establishing the person's training, or target, heart rate range (THRR). The THRR represents the range where the person's heart rate (HR) can fluctuate during exercise while still providing aerobic benefits. For most people, this range is equivalent to 70% to 94% of HRmax or 50% to 85% of **heart rate reserve** (HRR). Use the formula provided in Box 3.1 to determine a person's HRmax, HRR, and THRR. When prescribing an exercise program for the novice exerciser, be sure to start with a low-intensity THRR (e.g., 60% to 70% of HRmax), progressing to a higher intensity once the person develops some level of aerobic fitness. So they can monitor exercise session intensity, teach patients how to measure their HR at the radial artery in the wrist, multiplying the number of beats occurring in 15 seconds by 4 to obtain the number of beats per minute.

As with exercise frequency, how long an exercise session lasts is inversely proportional to intensity level. That is, the greater the exercise intensity is, the shorter the exercise session is. This is because it is difficult to exercise for an extended period at a high intensity level. To ensure that patients get all of the benefits of cardiorespiratory endurance exercise, advise patients to perform between 20 and 60 minutes of activity in their THRR per exercise session. This can be accomplished by performing intermittent bouts of activity throughout the day as suggested by the SGR or by completing one continuous bout of exercise. Sedentary people and patients with low aerobic fitness levels who are just beginning an exercise program may benefit by starting with intermittent bouts of exercise, gradually progressing until they can keep their HR in their THRR for 20 minutes of continuous exercise.

BOX 3.1
How to determine THRR using RHR, HRmax, and HRR

Example: Jane, a 40-year-old woman of average fitness level, wants to begin a cardiorespiratory endurance exercise program. Determine Jane's

• resting heart rate (RHR).

$$RHR = 60 \text{ bpm}$$

• maximal heart rate (HRmax) by subtracting her age from 220.

$$220 - 40 = 180 \text{ bpm}$$

• heart rate reserve (HRR) by subtracting her RHR from her HRmax.

$$180 - 60 = 120 \text{ bpm}$$

• target heart rate range (THRR) by multiplying her HRR by the desired intensity ranges. Add her RHR to these numbers:

$$120 \text{ bpm} \times 50\% = 60 + 60 \text{ (RHR)} = 120 \text{ bpm}$$

$$120 \text{ bpm} \times 60\% = 72 + 60 \text{ (RHR)} = 132 \text{ bpm}$$

$$THRR = 120\text{--}132 \text{ bpm}$$

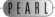

For each exercise session, advise patients to perform 20 to 60 minutes of either continuous or intermittent cardiorespiratory endurance exercise in their THRR.

The type of exercise required to develop cardiorespiratory endurance should employ large muscle groups in activities that are rhythmic and continuous. Examples include walking, running, hiking, cycling, swimming, rowing, dancing, skating, and cross-country skiing. Exercise performed on stationary machines, such as stair-climbers and elliptical trainers, are also examples of aerobic exercise. Some sports, such as basketball, soccer, and tennis, have the potential to develop aerobic fitness as long as the activity is performed with the appropriate intensity and duration. Factors to consider when helping a patient to select an aerobic activity include the person's health status, fitness level, ultimate goals, and, most importantly, interest level. Strongly advise patients to choose an aerobic activity they find enjoyable, because this greatly influences whether they will adhere to an exercise program. Consider suggesting walking for novice exercisers, because it is familiar and accessible, and it is easy for patients to self-regulate exercise intensity with this activity.

Strongly advise patients to choose an aerobic activity they find enjoyable, because this greatly influences whether they will adhere to an exercise program.

After determining the frequency, intensity, duration, and mode of exercise the person plans to pursue, periodically increase the duration, frequency, and intensity of the exercise sessions. Base the decision to increase these parameters on the patient's health status, tolerance to the current level of training, and desire to change the exercise program. Indeed, the key to designing an appropriate aerobic exercise program is for the patient to progress to a point where the exercise sessions meet his or her goals, such as obtaining a certain fitness level or reducing BFP. Realize that increasing exercise variables before the patient is ready may affect the patient's adherence to the program. Cardiorespiratory endurance exercise guidelines are summarized in Table 3.3.

Muscular Strength and Endurance Exercise

Maintaining good muscular strength and endurance is important for enhanced posture, reduced chance of musculoskeletal injury, prevention of osteoporosis, and improvement or maintenance of functional fitness. For older adults, muscular strength is more important than all other aspects of physical fitness, because the ability to perform ADLs, necessary to remain independent as people age, depends on sufficient strength levels. Participants in recreational and competitive sports also need adequate levels of muscular strength and endurance to perform chosen activities.

TABLE 3.3 Cardiorespiratory endurance exercise guidelines

Frequency	3–5 d/wk
Intensity (THRR)	50%–85% HRR
Time (duration)	20–60 minutes (continuous or intermittent)
Type (mode)	Dynamic, large muscle group activity (e.g., walking, jogging, cycling, swimming, soccer, aerobics)
Progression	Gradually increase duration, frequency, and intensity

HRR = heart rate reserve; THRR = target heart rate range.

For older adults, muscular strength is more important than all other aspects of physical fitness, because the ability of a person to perform ADLs depends on sufficient strength levels.

Guidelines for Implementing Resistance Exercise

Resistance exercise recommendations are dependent on whether the patient has a goal of increasing muscular strength, increasing muscular endurance, or maintaining general fitness. In general, advise patients desiring to increase muscular strength to perform these exercises with a resistance close to 100% of their 1-RM. Also, instruct people interested in enhancing muscle strength to decrease the number of reps performed. Recommend less weight and more reps for patients who want to increase muscle endurance and for people who want to maintain general fitness.

Regardless of the goal, advise patients to resistance train 2 to 3 nonconsecutive days per week, because this allows muscles adequate recovery period between workouts. Usually, more recovery time is needed for people trying to increase strength as compared with those trying to increase muscle endurance and those interested in maintaining general fitness. Once the resistance training program has been implemented, periodically apply the overload principle to ensure that patients continually experience desired effects. Do this by increasing the resistance, the number of sets, or the number of reps the person performs. Follow the guidelines summarized in Table 3.4 when prescribing such exercises for patients. Use the list of general resistance training guidelines provided in Box 3.2 when advising patients who are interested in starting a resistance training program.

Advise people interested in gaining muscle strength to resistance train 2 to 3 nonconsecutive days per week

TABLE 3.4 Muscular strength and endurance training guidelines

	TRAINING GOAL		
	GENERAL FITNESS	MUSCULAR STRENGTH	MUSCULAR ENDURANCE
Frequency	2–3 d/wk	2–3 d/wk	3–5 d/wk
Intensity	60%–75% 1-RM	80%–100% 1-RM	40%–60% 1-RM
Repetitions	8–12	6–8 or less	10–30
Sets	1–3	2–6	3–6
Rest between sets	1–2 minutes	2–5 minutes	2 minutes
Type (mode)	1–2 exercises for each muscle group	>2 exercises for each muscle group	>1 exercise for each muscle group
Progression	Increase repetitions, intensity, and sets	Increase repetitions, intensity, and, sets	Increase repetitions, intensity, and sets

1-RM = maximal lifting capacity for one repetition.

BOX 3.2
SPECIFIC GUIDELINES FOR MUSCULAR STRENGTH AND ENDURANCE EXERCISE

- Select at least one exercise per major muscle group (legs, thighs, chest, upper back, shoulders, biceps, triceps, abdominals, lower back).
- Begin with the larger muscle groups first, and then work the smaller muscle groups.
- Lift in a slow and controlled manner.
- Perform exercises through the joint's safest range of motion.
- Use a spotter (for safety and motivation) when performing free weight exercises.
- Maintain a training log indicating weight, number of reps, and number of sets for each exercise.
- Do not hold your breath when lifting. Breathe out during the lift; breathe in when lowering the weight.
- Always precede a resistance training session with a warm-up and follow with a cool-down.
- Discontinue training if you feel light-headed or experience any unusual discomfort or pain.

Most people use free weights, such as dumbbells and barbells, and/or commercial weight machines to perform resistance training exercises. Although using these devices is certainly appropriate, not every patient has access to such equipment. Fortunately, any number of household items, such as soup cans placed in a bag, can be used to provide the resistance necessary to perform strength training exercises. Refer to PTH 3.2 for examples of basic strengthening exercises that can be performed at home.

Cool-Down

When developing an exercise program, emphasize to patients the importance of the cool-down portion of the exercise session. The purpose of the cool-down is to gradually return all body systems, such as HR, BP, and metabolism, to normal. In addition, a properly performed cool-down removes metabolic wastes (e.g., lactic acid) from working muscles. This ensures adequate circulation and prevents blood from pooling in the extremities. Cooling down also prevents, or delays, the development of DOMS and reduces the potential for postexercise cardiac rhythm disturbances.[8]

Emphasize the importance of the cool-down portion of the exercise session
to patients.

The cool-down differs from the warm-up in that a cardiovascular activity is generally performed after all forms of exercise. Accordingly, to cool down after the completion of an aerobic activity, patients should gradually reduce the intensity of the activity they just completed. Recommend that people performing resistance training cool-down by performing an aerobic exercise of their choosing. As with the warm-up, advise patients to spend 5 to 15 minutes cooling down after exercise. Instruct patients to check their HR during the cool-down session, because a gradual return of the HR to its resting level is a sign that the body is cooling off properly. The more physically fit a person is, the more quickly his or her HR will return to RHR level. Instruct the person to perform stretching exercises before the HR returns to its resting state.

Behavior Modification Principles

Adopting a healthy behavior, or stopping an unhealthy one, can be challenging. Indeed, despite knowing the many benefits of physical activity and formal exercise, 50% of all people quit within the first 3 to 6 months of beginning an exercise program. Therefore, it is important for primary health care providers to know about the many factors that influence exercise behavior. It is also essential to understand the importance of employing behavior modification principles to increase the likelihood that a patient stays compliant with an exercise program.[20]

Stages of "Readiness to Change" Model

Changing a behavior is a process that takes time, and successful behavior change requires readiness on the part of the participant. The stages of "readiness to change" state that a person progresses through different stages when it comes to behavior change and that there are underlying processes operating at each stage. This holds true for people involved in physical activity and exercise. Therefore, it is important to identify a person's stage of readiness for change before techniques to address specific processes can be selected. These stages of behavior change include[21,22]

- precontemplation: no intention of changing a behavior in the immediate future;
- contemplation: thinking about changing a behavior in the next 6 months;
- preparation: seriously considering changing a behavior in the next month;
- action: actively doing things to change a behavior;
- maintenance: sticking with a behavior for up to 5 years; and
- termination/adoption: sticking with a behavior for more than 5 years with no fear of relapse.

Box 3.3 provides a work sheet that can be used to identify which stage of change a patient is in. To do this, have the patient check off the statement that most accurately describes his or her current exercise behavior. Each statement corresponds to a stage of change, with the first statement corresponding to precontemplation and the final statement corresponding to termination/adoption. Once the stage a patient is in is determined, use the techniques outlined in Table 3.5 to enhance exercise behavior and to prevent relapses, which are defined as discontinuing a healthy behavior or returning to an unhealthy behavior.[10]

Goal Setting

Setting realistic goals is essential in initiating and maintaining behavior change. When helping patients set goals, use the acronym SMART, which states that goals should be[10]

BOX 3.3
SAMPLE WORK SHEET FOR DETERMINING STAGE OF READINESS TO CHANGE WITH EXERCISE

Stage of Change
Please indicate which statement most accurately describes your current exercise behavior.
____ I do not currently exercise, and I do not intend to exercise in the foreseeable future (precontemplation).
____ I do not currently exercise, but I want to start an exercise program in the next 6 months (contemplation).
____ I do not currently exercise, but I intend to start an exercise program within the next month (preparation).
____ I currently exercise on a regular basis, but I have only done so within the past 6 months (action).
____ I currently exercise on a regular basis, and I have done so for >6 months but >5 years (maintenance).
____ I currently exercise on a regular basis, and I have done so for >5 years (termination/adoption).

Adapted from Hoeger WK, Hoeger SA. *Principles and Labs for Fitness and Wellness*. Belmont, CA: Thomson Wadsworth, 2008; American College of Sports Medicine. *ACSM's Guidelines for Exercise Testing and Prescription*, 7th ed. Philadelphia, PA: Lippincott Williams & Wilkins, 2006; Lox CL, Martin Ginis KA, Petruzzello SJ. *The Psychology of Exercise*. Scottsdale, AZ: Holcomb Hathaway, 2006.

TABLE 3.5 Techniques for enhancing exercise participation based on stage-of-change

STAGE	TECHNIQUE
Precontemplation	Discuss benefits of exercise as it relates to the patient's health. Provide written materials about the importance of exercise. Share other patient success stories.
Contemplation	Review pros and cons of exercise. Discuss barriers to exercise and how to overcome. Provide a list of local exercise programs and facilities. Have the patient undergo a fitness evaluation.
Preparation	Assist the patient in setting short-term, realistic goals. Review importance of scheduling exercise. Provide the patient with an exercise prescription. Review strategies for increasing daily lifestyle physical activity. Recommend purchase of a pedometer to track daily physical activity.
Action	Recommend use of an exercise log, calendar, or progress chart. Encourage use of a workout buddy or exercising in a group. Discuss the importance of finding enjoyable activities. Conduct a follow-up fitness evaluation. Assist the patient in setting new goals. Recognize patient accomplishments. Encourage use of personal rewards for meeting goals.
Maintenance	Emphasize use of a variety of exercises. Review the importance of strength and flexibility training. Discuss potential relapse situations and how to overcome. Reinforce the importance of regular exercise.

Adapted from Hoeger WK, Hoeger SA. *Principles and Labs for Fitness and Wellness.* Belmont, CA: Thomson Wadsworth, 2008; American College of Sports Medicine. *ACSM's Guidelines for Exercise Testing and Prescription,* 7th ed. Philadelphia, PA: Lippincott Williams & Wilkins, 2006; Lox CL, Martin Ginis KA, Petruzzello SJ. *The Psychology of Exercise.* Scottsdale, AZ: Holcomb Hathaway, 2006.

- Specific: State the exact goal you wish to achieve (e.g., walk for 30 minutes for 5 days per week). Write it down, and tell someone else.
- Measurable: State the exact amount of improvement you wish to make in a way that can be measured (e.g., lose an average of 1 pound of weight per week).
- Acceptable: Goals must be your own, to motivate and challenge you.
- Realistic: Your goals should be challenging yet achievable. Break down a long-term goal into short-term goals to keep you motivated.
- Time-specific: Give yourself a deadline to reach your short-term and long-term goals.

It is also important to have patients reassess goals periodically to determine whether they have met their original goals. If so, it may be time for the patient to set new goals. If the original goal has not been met, assess whether it is still a SMART goal for the patient. If not, advise the person to set new goals.

Overcoming Barriers

There are numerous reasons why people do not participate in regular physical activity. Otherwise referred to as *barriers*, some reasons are within a person's control, whereas others are external in nature. Table 3.6 identifies typical reasons why people do not exercise and offers some suggestions for overcoming these barriers.

TABLE 3.6 Common reasons why people do not exercise and suggested strategies to overcome these barriers

BARRIER TO EXERCISE	STRATEGIES TO OVERCOME BARRIER
Lack of time	Schedule physical activity into your day and make it a priority. Plan ahead for busy times.
Too tired/not enough energy	Focus on the benefit of increased energy after physical activity. Plan on a shorter workout (once you start, you may keep going).
Lack of motivation	List the pros and cons of being more physically active. Focus on the benefits you hope to achieve. Use short-term goals that can be realistically met. Reward yourself. Ready your workout clothes the night before your exercise day.
Lack of enjoyment/boredom	Participate in a variety of activities until you find one that you enjoy. Cross-train, exercise to music, and/or join a class with an enthusiastic leader.
Lack of social support	Find a workout partner. Join a fitness facility or exercise class.
Lack of knowledge	Read materials on physical activity. Question your primary health care provider. Join a local fitness facility that employs a personal trainer.
Physical limitations	Work with a health care provider to determine which activities can be done given your physical limitation (e.g., swimming is a good alternative to running for those who have lower extremity injuries).
Bad weather	Check for available indoor activities and facilities. Purchase home exercise equipment.

Fitness for Special Populations

Though the general principles of exercise prescription described in this chapter apply to all people, they may have to be modified when working with certain populations. Although it is impossible to include every population for which this is necessary, this section provides information related to those special populations that primary health care providers typically encounter. Though it is wise for all who desire to become physically active to be medically cleared before starting an exercise program, insist that people who classify as a special-population patient complete a PPE before exercising.

Obese and Overweight

It should come as no surprise that excess consumption of food and reduced rates of physical activity are the primary causes of the weight gain epidemic currently occurring in the United States. With all population groups in this country experiencing increases in obesity rates, it is important to tell patients that too much body fat and/or body weight is associated with a variety of conditions, including hypertension, hyperlipidemia, type 2 diabetes, CAD, and stroke. For an overweight or obese person to experience significant weight loss, he or she must partake in at least 60 minutes of physical activity per day. This translates to an energy expenditure of at least 2000 kcal per week for both short-term weight loss and long-term maintenance goals. It is important that overweight and obese people participate in both cardiorespiratory endurance exercise and resistance training, because these activities burn calories, decrease body fat, increase LBM, and increase RMR.[9,10]

Elderly

Regular participation in physical activity affords a variety of benefits to older adults. For example, while helping to reduce the risk factors for CAD and stroke, aerobic exercise provides a variety of psychological benefits. Most importantly, elderly people who are physically active are able to perform ADLs and maintain independent living longer than those who are inactive. Recall, however, that older adults, as advised in Chapter 2, may need to complete a stress test before beginning an exercise program.

It is recommended that elderly exercisers avoid participating in high-impact activities, such as running and high-impact aerobic dance, because of the excess stresses they place on joints. Thus, older patients should participate in low-impact and nonimpact activities, such as walking, swimming, cycling, and water aerobics, because these decrease the chance of causing musculoskeletal injury. In addition, encourage older adults to participate in balance training programs, because doing so helps prevent falls in this population.[9,23]

With some modifications, elderly patients with preexisting conditions such as osteoarthritis (OA), rheumatoid arthritis (RA) (both discussed in Chapter 1), and **osteoporosis** can also safely participate in regular exercise. Indeed, exercise is an important part of the total management plan for those with OA and RA, because participation in physical activity leads to improved joint function and decreases pain. Similarly, regular exercise helps to increase bone density of patients with osteoporosis. Use the information provided in Table 3.7 when providing exercise advice for patients with OA, RA, and osteoporosis.[9,24–26]

TABLE 3.7 Suggested exercise parameters for those with osteoarthritis, rheumatoid arthritis, and osteoporosis

OSTEOARTHRITIS AND RHEUMATOID ARTHRITIS	OSTEOPOROSIS
Perform short bouts (e.g., 10 minutes) of aerobic exercise at low intensities.	Select a weight-bearing, low-impact activity, such as walking.
Participate in activities that can be performed in warm water (e.g., water aerobics).	Perform muscular strength and endurance activities at least twice a week.
Participate in a variety of activities (i.e., cross-train).	Perform daily flexibility, functional, and balance exercises.
Include daily stretches and functional activities (e.g., climbing stairs).	Exercise with an upright posture.
Avoid exercise during periods of symptom exacerbation or flare-up.	Avoid forward bending and twisting.
Avoid exercising in the morning (RA patients).	Exercise in a safe environment with minimal floor obstacles.

RA = rheumatoid arthritis.

Children and Adolescents

It is unfortunate that the subsequent health problems currently seen from inactivity in the U.S. adult population, such as obesity, have also become common in children and adolescents. Establishing regular physical activity patterns in these populations helps provide immediate health benefits (e.g., weight loss, weight maintenance, stress reduction), prevents the development of future chronic conditions, and prepares children and adolescents for participation in recreational and sports activities later in life.

When providing exercise advice for these populations, keep in mind that children and adolescents are not simply small adults. This means that there are some unique considerations that must be taken into account when developing an exercise program for them. These include ensuring that they[27]

- accumulate at least 60 minutes or more of age-appropriate physical activity on most days of the week;
- use a variety of age-appropriate activities that work all muscle groups;
- include weight-bearing activities;
- are properly supervised, especially when performing resistance exercises;
- perform exercises using body weight as resistance (e.g., push-ups);
- avoid intense or maximal training; and
- are discouraged from extended periods of inactivity (2 hours or more).

Pregnant Women

In general, participation in regular physical activity of moderate intensity is safe for people who are pregnant. However, because many physiologic changes occur with pregnancy, such as increases in joint laxity, expectant mothers should be educated about the potential adverse effects of participating in physical activity. These include increases in sacroiliac and hip joint pain, maternal blood volume, RHR, cardiac output, and insulin resistance. Pregnancy also leads to reduced lung volume of the expectant mother. Primary exercise safety concerns for this population center on preventing increases in core temperature, ensuring oxygen availability, and preventing uterine contractions. Nevertheless, as long as exercise is performed in a safe fashion, the benefits of being physically active when pregnant far outweigh the risks. These benefits include decreases in low back pain, stress, anxiety, depression, digestion trouble, and constipation. Expectant mothers who exercise also have more energy to complete ADLs and are more likely to experience a controlled weight gain throughout their pregnancy. When compared with patients who remain inactive, people who exercise during pregnancy recover from labor more quickly, have smaller postpartum bellies, and experience a faster return to prepregnancy weight.[28,29]

As long as exercise is performed in a safe fashion, the benefits of being physically active when pregnant far outweigh the risks.

Though it is safe for expectant mothers to exercise, people who want to either start or continue to be physically active during pregnancy should[29]

- participate in light-intensity, low-impact activities, such as walking, aquatics, and cycling;
- avoid exercising in the supine position after the first trimester;
- not overstretch already lax joints; and
- avoid contact activities and those which present a high risk of falling.

Diabetics

Regardless of the type of diabetes a patient has, all diabetics should become physically active, because doing so helps control the disease and enhances the person's quality of life. Indeed, when combined with proper diet and medication, exercise is a cornerstone of diabetes management. The goal of developing an exercise program for this population is to ensure that the patient is able to maintain metabolic control while avoiding hypoglycemia (blood glucose levels <65 mg/dL) during and after exercise. Achieving this can be challenging, especially for type 1 diabetics because of the complexities involved with regulating blood glucose levels in these patients.[30–32]

PEARL

A main goal in the development of an exercise prescription for a diabetic is for the person to maintain metabolic control while avoiding hypoglycemia during and after exercise.

Be aware that different forms of exercise have varying effects on blood glucose response. For example, blood glucose levels rise minimally in response to anaerobic exercise, such as low-level weight training. Thus, participating in these activities makes it easier for the diabetic to maintain proper blood glucose levels. In contrast, participating in aerobic exercise, such as running or bicycling, greatly affects blood glucose levels. This is because these activities rely on fats and carbohydrates (CHOs) (discussed in Chapter 4) to produce the blood glucose needed to fuel these activities. In addition, when the intensity of an aerobic exercise increases, the body becomes more reliant on CHO stores, further affecting blood glucose levels. Thus, it should come as no surprise that certain variables, such as exercise type, duration, and intensity, must be considered when developing an exercise program for the diabetic patient. The patient's current fitness level must also be taken into account, because diabetics who are less fit initially experience greater fluctuations in blood glucose levels when beginning an exercise program.[30-32]

When developing an exercise program for the type 1 diabetic, use the information provided in Box 3.4 as a guide. For this population, modifying diet and insulin intake before, during, and after exercise is a trial-and-error process for each new activity in which the diabetic participates. Be sure to refer the patient to a specialist if he or she has trouble regulating blood glucose levels.[30-32]

In addition to helping patients manage type 2 diabetes, exercise also plays a major role in preventing this disease from developing, because, for many people, this condition is precipitated by inactivity. Thus, as long as type 2 diabetics have been cleared for exercise through the PPE process, they should participate in aerobic activities of long duration (e.g., 1 hour in length) because this facilitates fat loss. Fortunately, type 2 diabetics do not have to monitor blood sugar levels during exercise, though they should do so before and after activity.[30,31]

BOX 3.4
GENERAL EXERCISE GUIDELINES FOR THE TYPE 1 DIABETIC

- Perform more repetitions and more exercise sets, with lower weight, when resistance training.
- Exercise in the morning, when circulating insulin levels are low.
- Modify food intake and/or insulin dosage before activity.
- Consume extra rapidly absorbed CHOs as necessary during and after exercise.
- Learn your own glycemic response to different exercise conditions.
- Identify when changes in insulin or food intake are needed.
- Monitor blood sugar levels before, during, and after exercise.
- Maintain quick access to simple CHOs to treat hypoglycemia, should it occur.
- Avoid prolonged periods of exercising at near-maximal intensity.
- Avoid activities (e.g., heavy weightlifting) that require performing repeated Valsalva maneuvers.
- Check insulin levels often during the exercise session. Use this information to balance future insulin dosage and CHO intake before, during, and after exercise.

CHO = carbohydrate.

Asthmatics

In general, airway obstruction during exercise is caused by one of three conditions: chronic asthma, exercise-induced asthma (EIA), or exercise-induced bronchospasm (EIB). Because the differences between EIA and EIB have yet to be fully explained, these terms are frequently used interchangeably. The term EIA is used here to explain airway obstruction triggered by exercise.[33,34]

For years, there was a perception that people with chronic asthma were less capable of exercising as compared with their healthy counterparts. Typically, this made asthmatics less physically active than nonasthmatics. This difference was explained, in part, by reports stating that in childhood some asthmatics felt they could not keep up with other children during play. Ultimately, this reduced level of physical activity among asthmatic children led to reduced aerobic fitness levels in this population.[35,36]

Today, we know that asthmatics, particularly children and adolescents, can maintain physical activity levels comparable with those of nonasthmatics. Indeed, exercise is an important part of a comprehensive asthma management plan because asthmatics who are aerobically conditioned can exercise without breathing as hard. Asthmatics who are physically fit also experience decreases in both the number and the severity of asthmatic events. Thus, not only is it unnecessary to disqualify chronic asthmatics from participating in exercise and sporting activities, but these patients should be encouraged to become physically active.[35-37]

PEARL

Asthmatics should be encouraged to become physically active because exercise is an important part of a comprehensive asthma management plan.

Unlike chronic asthma, EIA is a reversible airway obstruction that occurs during or after exertion. Though its exact pathophysiology is still unknown, EIA occurs in both chronic asthmatics and otherwise healthy people. Causes of this condition include cooling of the bronchial mucosa, such as what occurs when a person exercises in cold, dry air, and the introduction of chemical irritants, such as pollutants, into the airway. Regardless, people with EIA do not experience the bronchodilation normally associated with physical activity. Rather, they experience bronchoconstriction 5 to 8 minutes after the initiation of an exercise bout, with maximal constriction occurring within 15 minutes. This process is responsible for causing the feeling of breathlessness commonly associated with EIA. Other symptoms of EIA include chest tightness, coughing (which may be the patient's only symptom), excessive sputum production, wheezing, chest or abdominal pain, nausea and vomiting, headache, and fatigue. Once the person with EIA stops exercising, pulmonary function typically returns to its original level within 30 to 60 minutes, though symptoms may be most severe within 15 minutes of exercise termination. Activities such as running and bicycling, which require the exerciser to incrementally increase the rate and depth of breathing, cause EIA more than activities such as tennis and racquetball, where sustained increases in the depth and rate of breathing rate are less likely to occur. Use the information provided in Box 3.5 as a guide when developing an exercise program for the asthmatic.[35-37]

BOX 3.5
GENERAL EXERCISE GUIDELINES FOR THE ASTHMATIC

- Choose activities that require exercise in a humid environment (e.g., indoor swimming).
- Avoid exercising in cold, dry air and when pollen count or air pollution is high.
- Cover the mouth and nose with a scarf or surgical mask to help warm and humidify the air when exercising in the cold is unavoidable.
- Perform nasal breathing exercises before activity because these warm and humidify air passages.
- For those who live in urban areas, refrain from exercising outside during rush hour.
- Choose activities that demand short bursts of energy, rather than activities that require periods of extended exercise.
- Refrain from exercise during times of viral infection.
- Perform an extended cool-down period because this may lessen EIA symptom severity.

EIA = exercise-induced asthma.

People With Coronary Artery Disease

Sadly, CAD continues to be the leading cause of morbidity and mortality in the United States. High-fat diets, a sedentary population, cigarette smoking, increasing obesity rates, and high stress levels contribute to these outcomes. Fortunately, most premature deaths caused by CAD are preventable when an exercise program is implemented along with the proper use of medication, behavior modification, and diet. Indeed, exercise is the cornerstone of a treatment plan for reversing the effects of CAD. It does this by[2,9,30,38,39]

- reversing the buildup of plaque in the arteries,
- improving the heart's oxygen supply,
- raising the amount of high-density lipoproteins in circulating blood,
- lowering BP,
- aiding in weight loss,
- reducing triglyceride levels,
- reducing total and intra-abdominal body fat,
- improving glucose tolerance and insulin sensitivity, and
- reducing adhesiveness and aggregation of blood platelets.

The primary goal of prescribing an exercise program for patients with CAD is to improve the person's functional capacity and exercise tolerance. Considerations to take into account when developing an exercise program for these patients include setting short-term, attainable goals for exercise tolerance and weight loss and suggesting that they participate in aerobic activities that require the use of large muscle groups, such as walking, cycling, swimming, and rowing. Advise patients to exercise at a moderate intensity (60% of HRmax) without triggering symptoms. Instruct patients to start with a few minutes of exercise a day (e.g., 10 minutes), gradually working toward the ultimate exercise goal of 30 minutes of moderate activity on most days of the week. Be sure to refer people who have had coronary artery bypass surgery, angioplasty, or myocardial infarction to a specialist, because these patients are better served by participating in a formal cardiac rehabilitation program.[38,39]

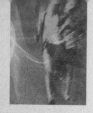

CASE STUDY
Physical Fitness

SCENARIO
A 36-year-old female comes to your practice desiring to start a physical fitness program. She currently walks and bikes occasionally in the neighborhood with her children. Once a week, the family goes to the local pool for family swim.

PERTINENT HISTORY
Medications: None.

Family History: Father died at age 62 of a heart attack. Mother is still alive, though experiencing congestive heart failure.

PERSONAL HEALTH HISTORY
Tobacco Use: Does not currently smoke, though she smoked 1 pack of cigarettes per day between the ages of 16 and 30.

Recreational Drugs: Denies use.

Alcohol Intake: 1 to 2 drinks per week.

Caffeinated Beverages: 2 to 3 cups of caffeinated coffee per day.

Diet: Eats a bowl of cereal with a glass of orange juice for breakfast, a turkey or tuna sandwich with cheese for lunch, morning and afternoon snacks of a banana or an energy bar, and chicken or fish with vegetables and bread for dinner. Has an occasional bowl of ice cream or popcorn in the evening. Drinks plain water for fluids.

Exercise: Was involved in athletics in high school and recreational sports in college. Her amount of physical activity slowly decreased as her family obligations increased. Currently not engaged in any formal exercise, but does currently walk, and occasionally swims and bikes.

Past Medical History: Generally healthy. No surgeries or major injuries. Mild to moderate spring and late summer hay fever. Three live births: two in her 20s and one in her early 30s.

PERTINENT PHYSICAL EXAMINATION*
Heart rate: 60 bpm. Blood pressure: 138/78 mm Hg. Height: 65 inches. Weight: 157 pounds. Body mass index (BMI): 26.5. Waist circumference (WC): 41 in.

RED FLAGS FOR THE PRIMARY HEALTH CARE PROFESSIONAL TO CONSIDER
• Family history of cardiac disease.
• WC >40 in.
• BMI indicates overweight status (26.5).

*Focused examination limited to key points for this case.

RECOMMENDED PLAN

- Cardiorespiratory endurance
Frequency: 3 nonconsecutive days/week
Intensity: HRmax = 220 − age = 185
  HRR = HRmax − RH = 185 − 60 = 125
  THR1 = (HRR × 50%) + RHR = (125 × 50%) + 60 = 62.5 + 60 = 122.5
  THR2 = (HRR × 60%) + RHR = (125 × 60%) + 60 = 75 + 60 = 135
  THRR = 122−135 bpm
Time: 20 minutes continuous
Type: walking

Progress: to 30 minutes, 4 days/week, 60% to 70% HR

- Muscular strength and endurance
Frequency: 3 nonconsecutive days/week
Intensity: approximately 60% of 1-RM
Time:
  Reps: 8
  Sets: 1
Type: exercises outlined in PTH 3.2

Progress: increase reps each session; increase weight load once 12 reps is reached

- Flexibility
Frequency: after every workout
Intensity: stretch to the point of slight discomfort
Time: 2 reps at 15 seconds for each stretch
Type: static stretches as outlined in PTH 3.1

Progress: increase to 3 reps and up to 20 to 30 seconds per stretch after 4 weeks

REFERENCES

1. U.S. Department of Health and Human Services. *Healthy People 2010: Understanding and Improving Health.* Washington, DC: U.S. Department of Health and Human Services, 2000.
2. U.S. Department of Health and Human Services. *Physical Activity and Health: A Report of the Surgeon General.* Washington DC: U.S. Government Printing Office, 1996.
3. Centers for Disease Control, Merck Institute of Aging and Health. *The State of Aging and Health in America Report.* Washington, DC: Merck Company Foundation, 2004.
4. Schoenborn CA, Barnes PM. *Leisure-Time Physical Activity Among Adults: United States, 1977-98. Advanced Data From Vital and Health Statistics,* No. 325. Hyattsville, MD: National Center for Health Statistics,. 2002.
5. President's Council on Physical Fitness. Definitions: health, fitness, and physical activity. *Research Digest.* 2000. Retrieved from: http://www.fitness.gov/pcpfs_research_digs.htm. Accessed 7/29/08.
6. Haskell WL, Lee I, Pate RR, et al. Physical activity and public health: updated recommendation for adults from the American College of Sports Medicine and the American Heart Association. *Med Sci Sports Exerc* 2007;39:1423.
7. Bean JF, Vora A, Frontera WR. Benefits of exercise for community-dwelling older adults. *Arch Phys Med Rehabil* 2004;85:S31.
8. American College of Sports Medicine. *ACSM's Resource Manual for Guidelines for Exercise Testing and Prescription,* 5th ed. Philadelphia, PA: Lippincott Williams & Wilkins, 2005.
9. American College of Sports Medicine. *ACSM's Guidelines for Exercise Testing and Prescription,* 7th ed. Philadelphia, PA; Lippincott Williams & Wilkins, 2006.
10. Hoeger WK, Hoeger SA. *Principles and Labs for Fitness and Wellness.* Belmont, CA: Thomson Wadsworth, 2008.
11. Thacker SB, Gilchrist J, Stroup DF, et al. The impact of stretching on sports injury risk: a systematic review of the literature. *Med Sci Sports Exerc* 2004;36:371.
12. Herbert RD, Gabriel M. Effects of stretching before and after exercising on muscle soreness and risk of injury: systematic review. *BMJ* 2002;325:468.
13. Blair S, Kohl HI, Paffenbarger RJ, et al. Physical fitness and all-cause mortality: a prospective study of healthy men and women. *JAMA* 1989;262:2395.
14. Talbot LA, Morrell CH, Metter EJ, et al. Comparison of cardiorespiratory fitness versus leisure time physical activity as predictors of coronary events in men aged <65 years and >65 years. *Am J Cardiol* 2002;89:1187.
15. Clark DO. The effect of walking on lower body disability among older Blacks and Whites. *Am J Pub Health* 1996;86:57.
16. Verfaillie DF, Nichols JF, Turkel E, et al. Effects of resistance, balance, and gait training on reduction of risk factors leading to falls in elders. *J Aging Phys Act* 1997;5:213.
17. Kesaniemi YK, Danforth E, Jensen, MD, et al. Dose-response issues concerning physical activity and health: an evidence-based symposium. *Med Sci Sports Exerc* 2001;33:S351.
18. Centers for Disease Control, Department of Health and Human Services. Body Mass Index Home. Retrieved from: http://www.cdc.gov/nccdphp/dnpa/bmi/index.htm. Accessed 7/29/08.
19. Pietrobelli A, Faith MS, Allison DB, et al. Body mass index as a measure of adiposity among children and adolescents: a validation study. *J Pediatrics* 1998;132:204.
20. Dishman RK. Increasing and maintaining exercise and physical activity. *Behav Ther* 1991;22:345.
21. Prochaska J, DiClemente C. Transtheoretical therapy, toward a more integrative model of change. *Psych Theory Res Prac* 1982;19:276.
22. Dunn AL, Marcus BH, Kampert JB, et al. Comparison of lifestyle and structured interventions to increase physical activity and cardiorespiratory fitness: a randomized trial. *JAMA* 1999;281:327.
23. The National Blueprint: Increasing Physical Activity Among Adults Aged 50 and Older. 2002. Retrieved from: http://www.agingblueprint.org. Accessed 7/29/08.
24. U.S. Department of Health and Human Services. *Arthritis and Exercise.* Bethesda, MD: National Institute of Arthritis and Musculoskeletal and Skin Diseases, 2001.
25. National Osteoporosis Foundation. *America's Bone Health: The State of Osteoporosis and Low Bone Mass in Our Nation.* Washington, DC: National Osteoporosis Foundation, 2002.

26. U.S. Department of Health and Human Services. *Bone Health and Osteoporosis: A Report of the Surgeon General.* Rockville, MD: Public Health Service, 2004.
27. National Association for Sport and Physical Education. *Physical Activity for Children: A Statement of Guidelines for Children Ages 5-12.* Reston, VA: American Alliance for Health, Physical Education, Recreation, and Dance, 2004.
28. ACOG Committee. Opinion No. 267: Exercise during pregnancy and the postpartum period. *Obstet Gynecol* 2002;99:171.
29. American College of Sports Medicine. *ACSM Roundtable Consensus Statement: Impact of Physical Activity During Pregnancy and Postpartum on Chronic Disease Risk.* 2006.
30. Colberg SR, Swain D. Exercise and diabetes control: a winning combination. *Phys Sportsmed* 2000;28(4):63.
31. Draznin MB. Type 1 diabetes and sports participation. *Phys Sportsmed* 2000;28(12):49.
32. American Diabetes Association. Clinical practice recommendations 2000: diabetes mellitus and exercise. *Diabetes Care* 2000;23(suppl 1):S50.
33. Hermansen CL. Exercise-induced bronchospasm vs. exercise-induced asthma [letter]. *Am Fam Physician* 2004;69:808.
34. Sinha T, David AK. Exercise-induced bronchospasm vs. exercise-induced asthma [letter reply]. *Am Fam Physician* 2004;69:808.
35. Welsh L, Roberts R, Kemp J. Fitness and physical activity in children with asthma. *Sports Med* 2004;34:861.
36. Leski M. Exercise-induced asthma. *South Med J* 2004;97:859.
37. Lacroix VJ. Exercise-induced asthma. *Phys Sportsmed* 1999;27(12):75.
38. Cox MH. Exercise for coronary artery disease: a cornerstone of comprehensive treatment. *Phys Sportsmed* 1997;25(12):27.
39. Cox MH. Exercise for mild coronary artery disease. *Phys Sportsmed* 1997;25(12):35.

SUGGESTED READINGS

Manson JE, Skerrett PJ, Greenland P, et al. The escalating pandemics of obesity and sedentary lifestyle: a call to action for clinicians. *Arch Intern Med* 2004;164(3):249.

McInnis KJ, Franklin BA, Rippe JM. Counseling for physical activity in overweight and obese patients. *Am Fam Physician* 2003;67:1249.

Richardson CR, Schwenk TL. Helping sedentary patients become more active: a practical guide for the primary care physician. *J Clin Out Manage* 2007;14(3):161.

WEB LINKS

www.acefitness.org. Accessed 7/29/08.
  Web site of the American Council on Exercise. Provides health and fitness information for both fitness professionals and the general public. Outlines opportunities for people working in the fitness industry and health care settings to become certified fitness professionals.

www.nsca-lift.org. Accessed 7/29/08.
  Web site of the National Strength and Conditioning Association. Provides practical applications of strength and conditioning techniques based on research findings. Offers information regarding personal trainer certification opportunities to aspiring fitness professionals.

http://www.fitness.gov. Accessed 7/29/08.
  Sponsored by the U.S. Department of Health and Human Services, this is the health, physical activity, fitness, and sports information Web site of the President's Council on Physical Fitness. Provides the general public with information on how to start a physical fitness program.

4

Nutrition for the Primary Health Care Provider

William F. Simpson, PhD, FACSM, Brian J. Toy, PhD, ATC, Thomas W. Buford, MS, CSCS and Tracey Fox-Bartels, MSN, FNP, RN

Proper nutrition is an essential element of maintaining optimal health and body composition, as well as in achieving maximal athletic performance. While natural variability between people makes it impossible to create one diet to recommend to all, examining scientific principles makes it easier for persons to eat a diet that ensures optimal health or maximizes athletic potential. Unfortunately, the popular media is saturated with misinformation, leading to confusion and poor nutritional choices made by much of the public. This confusion plays a large role in the increasing prevalence of obesity within the United States. Thus, the aim of this chapter is to provide a framework within which accurate nutrition information can be supplied to patients. However, this framework must not be confused with a one-size-fits-all recipe, because each person responds differently to a given diet. Ultimately, a patient must adjust these recommendations if his or her body does not respond as expected. Primary health care providers must educate patients and provide stopgap solutions.

Basic Nutrition

Simply put, nutrition is the science of examining the consumption of **nutrients** through the diet. These nutrients are subdivided into two classifications: **macronutrients** and **micronutrients.**[1,2]

Macronutrients

Macronutrients consist of the three nutrients that are required in large quantities in the diet: carbohydrates (CHOs), proteins (PROs), and fats. These nutrients provide the energy required to maintain the body's functions as well as uphold cellular structure and homeostasis. Whether in energy production or in cellular structure, these nutrients play a vital role in the overall health of an individual.

Carbohydrates

Carbohydrates are naturally occurring compounds composed of carbon, hydrogen, and oxygen. When ingested, they provide the body with approximately 4 kcal/g of energy. Three major classes of CHOs exist: monosaccharides, oligosaccharides, and polysaccharides. The single sugar monosaccharides include glucose, otherwise known as *dextrose*; fructose; and galactose. Oligosaccharides are chains of sugars that contain between 2 and 10 monosaccharides each. The most common, the disaccharides, those sugars composed of two monosaccharides, include lactose, maltose, and sucrose. Polysaccharides are complex CHOs that contain many chains of monosaccharides. Starches and fibers are the primary types of dietary polysaccharides, whereas glycogen, a polysaccharide found in animals, is the storage form of glucose in the body. It is found primarily in the liver and skeletal muscle.[1,2]

When compared, simple CHOs are primarily more calorie dense, yet less nutrient dense, than complex CHOs. This makes the consumption of monosaccharides a major problem in the sedentary population because of the ease with which these simple sugars convert to fat when ingested. Because they are absorbed more slowly and provide greater nutrient value than do monosaccharides, polysaccharides are promoted as the healthier food source. Indeed, starch, the storage form of CHOs in plants, is a viable energy source because it digests slowly and provides energy for longer periods than do simple CHOs. In contrast, fiber, which comes in soluble and insoluble forms, is indigestible, making it a poor supplier of energy. However, fiber plays many useful roles in digestion. **Soluble fiber** maximizes nutrient uptake time by slowing the rate at which food travels through the small intestine. In contrast, **insoluble fiber**, commonly referred to as *cellulose*, removes toxins from the body and adds bulk to fecal matter. To maintain proper health, most people should consume 6 to 8 g CHO/kg body weight per day, and adults should ingest 20 to 30 g fiber per day. Table 4.1 summarizes the types and common names of CHOs and lists typical food sources for each class of CHO.[1-4]

PEARL

The bulk of a person's carbohydrate intake should be in the form of polysaccharides, and most people should consume 6 to 8 g **CHO/kg** body weight per day.

TABLE 4.1 Types of carbohydrates and their common food sources

CARBOHYDRATE	COMMON NAME	FOOD SOURCES
Monosaccharides		
Glucose	Dextrose	Fruits, sweeteners
Fructose	Fruit sugar	Fruits, honey
Galactose		Milk products
Oligosaccharides and disaccharides		
Sucrose (glucose + fructose)	Table sugar	Sugar cane, beet sugar, high-fructose corn syrup, honey, maple syrup, brown sugar
Lactose (glucose + galactose)	Milk sugar	Milk and milk products
Maltose (glucose + glucose)	Malt sugar	Germinating seeds, beer, cereal
Polysaccharides		
Starch	Dextrin	Potatoes, corn, wheat, rye, and legumes
Fiber	Hemicellulose	
• Soluble	Pectin	Fruits, legumes, oats, rye, barley, wheat, rice, bran
• Insoluble	Gums	
	Cellulose	
	Mucilage	Vegetables, wheat, bran, oats, legumes, beans, fruits, vegetables
	Psyllium	
	Lignin	

Regardless of how they enter the body, all CHOs are converted into glucose. Once glucose enters the bloodstream, it is either immediately used for energy or stored in the liver and skeletal muscles as glycogen. It is in this form that glucose is saved for use at a later time because glycogen is the primary substance the body breaks down into glucose to meet daily energy demands. However, once liver and skeletal muscle glycogen stores are maximized, glucose remaining in the blood is converted and stored as fat. Other than endurance athletes who perform aerobic training for longer than 1 to 2 hours each day, most people generally maintain maximal glycogen storage within the liver and skeletal muscle.[1,3,4]

As previously mentioned, polysaccharides should make up the bulk of a person's CHO intake because, when compared with monosaccharides, they have the ability to provide the body with needed nutrients and are less likely to becomes stored as fat. However, advising exactly which foods a patient should eat can be challenging. One way to do this is to determine the glycemic index (GI) of a food. This index is a system of classifying CHOs based on how quickly a food raises blood insulin levels. In general, foods with a GI at, above, or near 100, otherwise refereed to as *high-GI* foods, such as sugared soft drinks, cause a steep, quick rise in insulin production. In contrast, foods with a GI below 55, also known as *low-GI* foods, such as oat bran, cause a more gradual, sustained insulin spike. A diet consisting of low-GI foods has been shown to protect against the development of obesity and colon cancer and contributes to higher blood high-density lipoprotein (HDL) concentrations.[1,3–8]

PEARL

Foods with a high glycemic index raise blood insulin levels quickly.

Though the GI index provides excellent guidance with regard to the effect a food has on insulin levels, too often people examine GI charts and conclude that all foods with a high GI should be avoided. This is because the GI system only classifies foods based on how much they contribute to a person's blood sugar level and not on the amount of CHO they contain. Taking into account both a food's GI index and the amount of CHO it contains is a more accurate way to determine the healthiest foods. This can be accomplished by determining a food's glycemic load (GL). A food's GL is determined by multiplying its GI by the grams of CHO the food contains per standard serving and dividing this number by 100. For example, the GL of a medium apple, which contains 15 g CHO and has a GI value of 40, is determined as follows:

$$GL = (40 \times 15)/100$$

$$= 600/100$$

$$= 6$$

Foods with a GL greater than 20 are considered high-GL foods, whereas foods with a GL less than 20 are classified low-GL foods. In general, the higher the GL is, the greater the food elevates blood glucose. Eating diets composed of foods that maintain high GL levels contributes to the development of type 2 diabetes and coronary artery disease (CAD). Table 4.2 contains the GIs and GLs of some common foods. More complete tables are available from a variety of published sources, both in print and electronically.[5,6,9–11]

TABLE 4.2 The glycemic index and glycemic load of common foods

FOOD	GI	GL
Carrots	47	3
Green peas	48	3
Sweet potato	61	17
Baked potato	85	26
Orange	48	5
Apple	40	6
Banana	51	13
Skim milk	32	4
Cranberry juice	68	24
Cola	63	16
Long grain rice	41	16
White rice	53	20
Spaghetti	47	23
Wheat bread	52	10
Pancakes	102	22
Bagel	72	25

GI = glycemic index; GL = glycemic load.

Fat

Lipids include a broad group of energy-dense compounds that are made up of carbon, hydrogen, and oxygen and are insoluble in water. Often, the terms *fat* and *lipid* are used interchangeably, though these substances are different. Fats are **esters** formed when fatty acids react with **glycerol**, whereas lipids include fats and oils as well as fatty compounds such as **sterols** and phospholipids. The lipids of greatest importance in the body and the diet include triglycerides, fatty acids, phospholipids, and cholesterol. For the purposes of this chapter, the terms *fat* and *fats* are used to refer to dietary lipids.[12]

Weight gain is often associated with the ingestion of fats because fats contain far more energy per gram (approximately 9 kcal/g) than CHOs or PROs (approximately 4 kcal/g). Because of this, fats are often viewed in a very negative light, particularly when the role they play in the development of a variety of diseases is considered. However, fats serve many useful functions in the body. These functions include providing energy for tissues and organs, membrane makeup, nerve signal transmission, vitamin storage and transport, and cushioning and insulation for internal organs. In addition, in endurance athletes, fats are a vital fuel source for skeletal muscle.[3,4]

The primary fats found in large quantities in foods are triglycerides. Triglycerides are composed of three fatty acids and one glycerol molecule. Fatty acids are grouped by the amount of hydrogen they contain, otherwise known as *saturation*. Saturated fatty acid chains, referred to as *bad fats*, contain no double bonds; monounsaturated fatty acids contain one double bond; and polyunsaturated fats, or *good fats*, have multiple double bonds. Triglycerides typically contain a mix of these three fatty acid types, with the ratio of polyunsaturated to saturated fatty acids known as the *P/S ratio*. Animal fats usually have a low P/S ratio, whereas most vegetable oils (except tropical plant oils) have a high P/S ratio. Therefore, animal fats tend to have more saturated fats than do plant-derived fats.[8,12]

PEARL

Animal fats tend to have more saturated fats than do plant-derived fats because they have a lower P/S ratio.

The fatty acid makeup of the triglycerides is important to its metabolism in the body. For example, saturated fats increase cholesterol in the body, whereas unsaturated fats may have no effect or lower cholesterol. A sterol molecule, cholesterol, is an essential component of cell membranes. It is found in small amounts in food and is also naturally produced by the body. Cholesterol is transported in the bloodstream by lipid-protein complexes called *lipoproteins*. Lipoproteins transport fat in aqueous blood and come in three types: HDL, low density (LDL), and very low density (VLDL). A lipoprotein is designated as high, low, or very low based on the ratio of protein to fat within the compound. HDL maintains a higher percentage of protein, whereas LDL and VLDL have more fat. This means that LDL and VLDL are commonly referred to as *bad cholesterol* because they are the compounds that bind to arterial walls, contributing to conditions such as hypertension and CAD. They are usually found in foods that are high in saturated fats. HDLs, otherwise known as *good cholesterol*, are healthier compounds found in foods with higher concentrations of unsaturated fats. These compounds collect cholesterol from the arterial walls, transporting it to the liver for processing and excretion.[1,3,4,12]

PEARL

LDLs and VLDLs bind to arterial walls, whereas HDLs collect cholesterol from the arterial walls, transporting it to the liver for processing and excretion.

When advising patients on which fats to include in their diet, there are two types of fatty acids that require special attention. These are the essential fatty acids and trans-fatty acids. Essential fatty acids are fats not synthesized in the body.

Therefore, they must be ingested. These include linoleic (omega-6) and linolenic (omega-3), both 18-carbon fatty acids. Linoleic acid is found in oils of plant origin, whereas marine oils are a good source of linolenic acid. Otherwise known as *trans fats*, trans-fatty acids are oils that are solidified through a process known as **hydrogenation**, though some amounts are found naturally. Trans fats are in foods such as margarine, shortening, and some dairy products. In recent years, the reduction of trans fats has become a point of public scrutiny in places such as fast and packaged foods because, though they are unsaturated fats, they behave like saturated fats in the body as they promote a myriad of diseases, including heart disease, diabetes, and obesity.[1,2,4,13]

As with CHOs, advising patients on what to eat with regard to the fat concentration of a particular food can be challenging because it is difficult to relate to them all the information they need to know to make sound food choices. However, though there are exceptions, in general saturated fats are solid at room temperature, whereas unsaturated fats are liquid at the same temperature. Butter, lard, cream, and cheese are examples of foods high in saturated fat. Meanwhile, vegetable oils, such as olive, canola, corn, and sunflower, have primarily unsaturated fats. Exceptions to the room temperature rule include coconut and palm oils, which are high in saturated fats yet are liquid at room temperature. People should take in at least two-thirds of fat in the diet from unsaturated sources.[1,2,4,12]

Protein

Proteins are nitrogen-containing compounds composed of up to thousands of **amino acids**. Amino acids are joined by peptide bonds, and several amino acids joined together become a **polypeptide**. Polypeptide chains then bond together and form various proteins. Chemically, PROs are divided into two groups: simple and conjugated. Simple PROs contain only amino acids or their derivatives. More recognizable to the nutritionist are conjugated PROs, which contain some nonprotein substance, such as sugar molecules (glycoproteins), lipids (lipoproteins), or phosphate groups (phosphoproteins).[4,13]

For nutritional purposes, amino acids can be divided into two general groups: essential and nonessential. Determining whether an amino acid is essential or nonessential hinges on whether the body synthesizes sufficient amounts to meet its own needs (nonessential) or whether the diet must provide them (essential). Essential and nonessential amino acids are listed in Table 4.3. The most important of the essential amino acids are the branched chain amino acids (BCAAs). The BCAAs are made up of leucine, isoleucine, and valine. These amino acids are available for uptake directly by the skeletal muscle, without having to be metabolized by the liver. Indeed, many protein supplements on the market today, which are commonly used by people who exercise and play sports, either supplement whole protein with BCAAs or simply market a product that contains only BCAAs.[3,4,14]

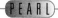

On average, the human body is composed of 18% PRO, with these compounds providing bodily tissues such as skeletal muscle, connective tissue, bone, and organs

TABLE 4.3 Essential and nonessential amino acids

ESSENTIAL	NONESSENTIAL
Histidine*	Alanine
Isoleucine	Arginine
Leucine	Asparagine
Lysine	Aspartic acid
Methionine	Cysteine
Phenylalanine	Glutamic acid
Threonine	Glutamine
Tryptophan	Glycine
Valine	Proline
	Serine
	Tryosine

*Some adults may be able to synthesize histidine.

with structure. As previously mentioned, PROs also provide the body with approximately 4 kcal/g of energy. In addition, nonstructural PROs act as hormones, catalysts (enzymes), buffer systems, cellular water balance regulators, lubricants, and immunoregulatory cells. Noting these numerous functions, the value of PROs in the body cannot be underestimated. However, in contrast to CHOs and fat, the body has no physiologic reserve of PRO stores. Therefore, if the body is not sufficiently supplied with PRO, it catabolizes tissue PROs, resulting in a loss of cellular function.[3,4,13]

A helpful stratification of dietary PROs is by whether the PRO is complete or incomplete. Primarily found in animal products, PROs that contain the proper quantity and balance of essential amino acids are known as complete PROs. Meat, fish, eggs, milk, and cheese are all good sources of complete PROs. In contrast, incomplete PROs lack one or more essential amino acids or are imbalanced with regard to the composition of their essential amino acids. Though a few animal products maintain incomplete PROs, these are primarily found in plant PRO sources such as grains, beans, and vegetables.[3,4,14]

When advising patients on protein intake, realize that recommendations are based on a person's age and weight. The Recommended Dietary Allowance (RDA) for an adult is 0.8 to 1.0 g PRO/kg body weight per day, whereas infants, children, and pregnant and lactating women may require additional daily PRO based on increased metabolic and/or developmental status. A person can easily create the proper balance of PROs at each meal by complementing incomplete sources of PROs with complete PRO sources. Because the Western diet is abundant in meat and dairy products, most people in the United States have little trouble in getting essential amino acids through diet. However, it may be a challenge for vegetarians to obtain proper amounts of all essential amino acids because this population must eat incomplete PROs in proper combinations and amounts to fulfill complete PRO requirements. These patients may also have a slightly greater total PRO requirement than omnivores.[1,3,4,14]

Micronutrients

Micronutrients come in the form of **vitamins** and **minerals**, which are nutritionally essential substances needed for the body to function properly. Although they do not provide the body with energy, micronutrients do play specific roles in energy transfer. Thus, these nutrients, which are needed in only relatively small amounts, are no less critical in contributing to a person's optimal health than are the macronutrients.

PEARL

Though important to maintaining health, vitamins and minerals do not
provide the body with energy.

Vitamins

Vitamins are organic compounds that function in the body as coenzymes for reactions, as antioxidants, and to synthesize hormones. A broad classification system includes two primary types of vitamins: fat soluble and water soluble. Table 4.4 lists these vitamins and also identifies the major sources and functions of each.

As their name indicates, the fat-soluble vitamins are stored in fat. Thus, they do not need to be ingested every day. Indeed, ingesting too much of any one fat-soluble vitamin over a period of time can cause a toxic reaction. Also, the body can naturally produce vitamins A, D, and K, albeit in small amounts. In contrast, water-soluble vitamins must be ingested because the body cannot manufacture them, nor can they be stored. Thus, excess amounts of these vitamins are excreted from the body through the kidneys. Though this prevents water-soluble vitamins from reaching toxic levels, it also means that they need to be ingested on a regular basis. Though not unheard of, incidences of vitamin deficiency are fairly rare in the United States, especially when most people in this country consume enough calories to ensure adequate vitamin intake. However, it is important to remind patients that more is not always better. Even unnecessarily high levels of the water-soluble vitamins can be detrimental to health. For example, excessive intakes of antioxidants, such as vitamin C, can act as pro-oxidants and cause cellular damage under situations of physiological stress. Ingesting 100% of the RDA value is normally sufficient unless otherwise determined by a health care professional. A more comprehensive look at vitamins can be accessed electronically and from most nutrition textbooks.[2,4,14-16]

Minerals

Minerals are distinguished from vitamins by their inorganic, rather than organic, nature. The body needs to ingest at least 20 different minerals to perform vital functions

TABLE 4.4 Vitamin functions and dietary sources

VITAMIN	COMMON NAME	SOLUBLE	MAJOR SOURCES	MAJOR FUNCTIONS
A		Fat	Dark green, yellow, and orange vegetables; fruits; liver; eggs; cheese	Maintains skin, hair, mucous membrane health; bone growth; night vision; tooth development.
D		Fat	Milk, eggs, liver; produced naturally in skin when exposed to sunlight	Tooth and bone development; needed for calcium and phosphorus absorption.
E		Fat	Green leafy vegetables, whole-grain cereals, breads, vegetable oils	Helps forms cells of the body.
K		Fat	Green leafy vegetables, potatoes, liver, cereals, peas, cauliflower	Helps with blood clotting and bone metabolism.
B_1	Thiamin	Water	Liver; oysters, pork, whole-grain cereals, pasta, bread	Helps with nervous system health.
B_2	Riboflavin	Water	Dairy products, liver, dark green vegetables, whole-grain cereals, bread, peas, beans	Maintains mucous membranes.
B_3	Niacin	Water	Poultry, meat, fish, eggs, whole-grain cereals, bread, pasta, nuts	Assists cells to produce energy.
B_6	Pyridoxine	Water	Green leafy vegetables, bananas, nuts, potatoes, whole-grain cereals, bread, poultry, liver	Helps PRO to be absorbed. Assists in PRO and fat metabolism. Aids in the creation of RBCs.
B_{12}	Cobalamin	Water	Eggs, milk, meat, liver, fish, oysters	Produces genetic material. Helps with nervous system health. Aids in the creation of RBCs.

VITAMIN	COMMON NAME	SOLUBLE	MAJOR SOURCES	MAJOR FUNCTIONS
C	Ascorbic acid	Water	Citrus fruits, dark green vegetables, potatoes, strawberries, melon, tomatoes	Forms collagen. Helps with bone, teeth, and capillary health.
Pantothenic acid		Water	Eggs, liver, mushrooms, broccoli	Assists with fat metabolism and storage.
Biotin		Water	Peanut butter, cheese, liver	Aids in glucose formation and fat storage.
Choline		Water	Peanut butter, liver, lettuce	Helps with nervous system health and amino acid regeneration.
Folacin	Folic acid	Water	Dark green leafy vegetables, liver, peas, dried beans	Produces genetic material. Helps create hemoglobin in RBCs.

PRO = protein; RBC = red blood cell.

such as forming bone and signaling cells. Some minerals also act as electrolytes, which play an important role in fluid balance. Minerals are classified as either major, of which the body needs a minimum of 100 mg/d, or trace, of which the body needs less than 100 mg/d (Table 4.5). As with vitamins, most minerals are required in small amounts, and, for the majority of people in the United States, the risk of suffering from a mineral deficiency is uncommon. A more comprehensive look at minerals can be accessed electronically and from most nutrition textbooks.[2,4,14,16,17]

Water

Water, which is present in almost all foods, is arguably the body's most important nutrient, because it is needed for nearly all bodily functions. Indeed, it is the largest component of the body, representing 45% to 70% of a person's body weight. Though the average fluid requirement for adults is estimated at 1.9 to 2.6 liters per day, by sweating, fluid losses increases with exercise. This means it is vital that fluid be consumed before and replaced during exercise, because a 3% to 5% loss in body weight resulting from water loss during an exercise session can strain the cardiovascular system and impair the body's ability to dissipate heat. Ultimately, this can lead to extreme weakness and possible unconsciousness. Though these concerns are usually reserved for people who exercise in hot and humid conditions, these problems can occur in anyone who exercises in the heat who is not well hydrated or **acclimatized** to the environment. In these situations, patients should

TABLE 4.5 The major and trace minerals

MAJOR MINERALS	TRACE MINERALS
Sodium	Iron
Potassium	Zinc
Chloride	Copper
Calcium	Manganese
Phosphorus	Selenium
Magnesium	Iodine
Sulfur	Chromium
	Fluoride

liberally consume cool liquids before, during, and after exercise and should carefully monitor body weight before and after the exercise session.[12,18]

People who exercise should be encouraged to drink water before, during, and after exercise.

Because of factors including genetics, level of fitness, and level of acclimatization, it is difficult to make one recommendation for how much a person should drink during exercise. In addition, patients with certain conditions, such as congestive heart failure, may have varying fluid requirements, making it important to tailor hydration recommendations to each individual based on circumstance and health status. However, as a general rule, a person who becomes thirsty before or during exercise is already well on the way to becoming dehydrated. This highlights the importance of patients' understanding the need to stay properly hydrated when participating in sports or exercise.[18]

Nutrition and Body Weight

Various definitions are used—often incorrectly—to describe a person's body weight status. For example, the terms *overweight* and *obesity*, discussed in Chapter 3, are often used interchangeably. This can lead to confusion when working with patients desiring to lose or gain weight. However, as shown in Chapter 3, the Centers for Disease Control and Prevention (CDC) has more clearly defined the terms overweight and obesity, basing these definitions on a person's body mass index (BMI). In addition, Chapter 3 also points out that people who carry excess body weight are at risk of developing a number of serious medical conditions. These patients also have an overall increased risk of mortality. It is critical, therefore, that primary health care providers understand the concepts of optimal body weight, the physiology of weight control, and how a person's nutritional status affects body weight.[1]

The Physiology of Weight Control

Determining why some people experience weight gain more easily than others, and why some have an easier time losing weight, cannot be attributed to a single cause. Rather, multiple factors ultimately contribute to what a person's weight is. For example, as discussed in Chapter 3, the amount a person exercises directly affects the amount of weight he or she may lose. However, the effect exercise has on a person's net weight loss is directly affected by the person's caloric intake. Likewise, other physiological factors, such as a person's resting metabolic rate (RMR), an individual's genetic makeup, and the aging process, influence a person's ability to lose or gain weight. Additionally, it should be noted that fat is significantly less dense than muscle, at times making a fit 130-pound person who exercises regularly appear thinner than a 105-pound person who has less lean body mass (LBM) and does not exercise.

Using Proper Nutrition to Obtain and Maintain a Healthy Body Weight

When advising patients on how to lose, maintain, or gain weight, keep in mind that everyone's body is different, meaning that no two people react to a nutrition plan the same way. Thus, any weight loss program constructed needs to be person specific and modified periodically. Furthermore, implementing a successful weight loss plan typically necessitates that an appropriate exercise program also be prescribed and that behavior modification techniques be implemented to help with patient compliance (discussed in Chapter 3). Remember that when attempting to implement such lifestyle changes, the patient may have to be referred to other health care professionals, such as a licensed dietitian, to achieve desired goals. Also, recognize that in most cases it takes a number of years for a person to become overweight or obese. Thus, it is illogical to assume that the same person can shed excess pounds quickly.

PEARL

Implementing a successful weight loss plan necessitates that an appropriate diet and exercise program be prescribed and that behavior modification techniques be implemented to help with patient compliance.

Determining Caloric Intake Needs

Possibly the most important piece of the nutritional puzzle is determining the right amount of calories and macronutrients a person should consume. After all, knowing what the macronutrients are does patients little good if they do not know how much they need to ingest to maintain a healthy body weight.

When determining what a person's macronutrient intake should be, initially consider the goals of the nutritional design. That is, is the patient's goal to maintain, lose, or gain weight? Or is it to gain LBM and lose fat mass? In addition, the patient's current and desired activity levels must be considered, because a highly active person is able, and likely needs, to consume more calories than someone who is sedentary. The same applies to pregnant and lactating women. Finally, physiologic factors such as size, age, and gender play a role in caloric needs, as does the macronutrient distribution of calories. For example, older athletes may need higher protein intake to prevent muscle loss and/or bone resorption, whereas highly active women, who are at risk for amenorrhea, may need to increase caloric intake and fat consumption.

Determining the macronutrient needs for a patient starts with determining the total amount of energy a person expends, otherwise known as the person's *total energy expenditure* (TEE). This figure represents the total amount of calories a person needs to ingest to maintain body weight and is based the individual's

• RMR,
• exercise energy expenditure (EEE),
• **thermogenesis**, and
• activities of daily living (ADLs).

A person's total energy expenditure represents the total amount of calories the person needs to ingest to maintain body weight and is based on the individual's resting metabolic rate, exercise energy expenditure, thermogenesis, and activities of daily living.

Accounting for the greatest percentage of calorie expenditure, a person's RMR is positively correlated with the size and amount of LBM a person has. Though the exact percentage of TEE from RMR depends on a person's fitness and activity levels, in general this figure accounts for 60% to 70% of TEE. However, as a person becomes more active, RMR begins to account for a slightly lower percentage of TEE. Indeed, RMR values below 50% of TEE have been reported in male endurance athletes. The simplest and most accessible method for determining RMR is to use the Harris and Benedict equations. These formulas take into account height (centimeters), weight (kilograms), and age (years) to predict daily RMR. These formulas, which are gender specific, are as follows (figures are rounded)[19,20]:

$$\text{Males: RMR (kcal/d)} = 66 + (13.7 \times \text{wt}) + (5 \times \text{ht}) - (6.8 \times \text{age})$$

$$\text{Females: RMR (kcal/d)} = 665 + (9.6 \times \text{wt}) + (1.8 \times \text{ht}) - (4.7 \times \text{age})$$

For example, the RMR for a 30-year-old woman who weighs 57 kg and is 165 cm tall is determined as follows:

$$\text{RMR (kcal/d)} = 655 + (9.6 \times 57) + (1.8 \times 165) - (4.7 \times 30)$$

$$= 655 + 547.2 + 297 - 141$$

$$= 1358 \text{ kcal/d}$$

Because the amount of a person's LBM is omitted from these equations, people with leaner bodies may need to ingest more calories than their less-lean counterparts. Practically speaking, then, this equation is accurate in all but extremely muscular and very obese people. In these cases, calorie needs are respectively underestimated and overestimated by using these equations. Although these equations do not take LBM into account, they have been reported to predict RMR within 200 kcal/d in persons of both genders.[21]

Determining a person's TEE and energy expended performing ADLs is typically considered under the umbrella of energy expended during physical activity (defined in Chapter 3). Caloric expenditure tables, which are easily accessible both electronically and in print, provide estimates of the energy requirements for many activities per unit of time (e.g., minute, hour) based on a person's body weight. For example, by using these tables, it can be determined that a 150-pound person who walks 3 miles an hour for 30 minutes burns 120 kcal, whereas a 200-pound person bicycling 10 mph burns 8.5 kcal/min. These tables are an excellent resource to use with patients because they provide them with tangible evidence regarding the amount of energy being expended during physical activity.[17,22]

The final component of TEE is thermogenesis. The most important form of thermogenesis is the thermic effect the digestion process has on energy expenditure, because this increases metabolic rate. Fats and simple sugars have the lowest metabolic cost, whereas PROs and complex CHOs take more energy to digest. In general, the thermic effect of digestion accounts for 5% to 10% of TEE.

Though more complex and precise methods of determining a person's TEE exist, a simple and easy-to-use method entails multiplying a person's RMR by a factor based on the person's activity level (Table 4.6). For example, the TEE for the same 30-year-old woman in the previous example who is classified as having a light activity level is determined as follows:

$$TEE = RMR \times \text{activity factor}$$

$$= 1358 \times 1.5$$

$$= 2037$$

Thus, this patient needs to consume 2037 kcal each day to maintain body weight. If, however, a decrease in body weight is desired, the patient must adjust daily caloric intake downward and/or become more physically active. Because 1 pound of fat is equivalent to 3500 calories, a 3500-calorie deficit over a given period of time results in a loss of 1 pound, whereas a 3500 calorie excess over the same period of time results in a 1-pound weight gain. For most people, safe weight loss/gain guidelines generally recommend weight change of 1 to 2 lb/wk. So, to achieve a weight loss of 1 lb/wk, people need to consume 500 fewer kcal/d than TEE, or they must burn 500 kcal/d through physical activity. Certainly, if it is warranted, patients should be encouraged to both decrease caloric intake and increase physical activity. However, if gaining LBM is the goal, fewer than 500 kcal/d need to be ingested because LBM has a lower caloric density than does adipose tissue. In general, adding 2500 additional calories in the diet results in the addition of 1 pound of LBM, assuming the diet includes the proper foodstuffs and the patient participates in an exercise routine consisting of resistive exercises as outlined in Chapter 3.[3,19,22]

For most people, safe weight change guidelines recommend changes of no more than 1 to 2 pounds per week.

TABLE 4.6 Activity factors for determining total energy expenditure

ACTIVITY LEVEL		ACTIVITY FACTOR	
		MALE	FEMALE
Sedentary	Minimal movement, largely sitting or lying down Activities: watching TV, reading	1.3	1.3
Light	Day consists of sleeping 8 hours with 16 hours of office work, sitting, and standing Activities: usually include 1 hour of moderate activity such as doing laundry, playing golf or table tennis walking on level ground at 3 mph	1.6	1.5
Moderate	Light manual labor throughout the workday Activities: walking 3.5 to 4 mph, carrying moderately heavy loads, cycling, tennis, dancing, weeding and hoeing	1.7	1.6
Very active	Physically active throughout the workday Activities: agricultural labor, steel work, military work, carrying heavy loads up stairs or inclines, rock and mountain climbing, intense aerobic and anaerobic sports	2.1	1.9
Extremely active	Intense physical activity throughout the workday Activities: lumberjack work, construction work, coal mining, full-time athletics	2.4	2.2

Determining Macronutrient Intake Needs

Once you have determined a patient's daily caloric intake level, educate the person on what foods to eat. Although each patient has individualized needs, a good starting point for prescribing macronutrient intake is to recommend a diet that is 60% CHOs (with the majority coming from complex CHOs), 15% protein, and 25% fat. These numbers should be slightly adjusted based on the needs of the person. For example, a renal patient may need to decrease the amount of protein in his or her diet, whereas a person with a muscle wasting disease may need to increase protein intake. Certainly, diets with various macronutrient mixtures have been shown to be effective for athletes in optimizing training and performance.[23–25]

A second factor to consider when determining a patient's macronutrient intake is daily recommendations for CHOs and PROs. As previously mentioned, the recommended amount of PRO intake for the general population is approximately 0.8 to 1 g/kg body weight per day. However, these levels should increase to as much as 2 to 2.5 g/kg body weight per day during pregnancy and periods of rapid growth, such as infancy and puberty. In addition, people involved in endurance exercises, such as long-distance running, need approximately 1.2 to 1.4 g PRO/kg body weight daily, whereas persons engaging in frequent resistance training likely need anywhere from 1.7 to 2.0 g PRO/kg body weight per day. Though the general recommendation for CHO intake is 6 to 8 g/kg body weight per day, endurance athletes need between 8 and 10 g/kg body weight per day to restore depleted muscle and liver glycogen levels caused by involvement in such taxing activities.[2,4,13,16,22,26]

Once you have determined the total amount of PROs and CHOs a patient needs to ingest, multiply each factor by 4 to find the total number of calories the person should ingest from each. For example, the total amount of PROs and CHOs for the 57-kg, 30-year-old woman who is advised to ingest 1 g PRO/kg body weight per day and 6 g CHO/kg body weight per day is determined as follows:

$$PROs = 4(1 \times 57)$$

$$= 4 \times 57$$

$$= 228 \text{ kcal}$$

$$CHO = 4(6 \times 57)$$

$$= 4 \times 342$$

$$= 1368 \text{ kcal}$$

Once this is completed, the total amount of calories needing to come from fat in the diet is determined by subtracting the totals of the PRO and CHO calories from the person's TEE. Using the 30-year-old woman with a TEE of 2037 as an example:

$$\text{Fat kcal} = \text{TEE} - (\text{PRO kcal} + \text{CHO kcal})$$

$$= 2037 - (228 + 1368)$$

$$= 2037 - 1596$$

$$= 441 \text{ kcal}$$

Finally, determine the total number of fat grams to be consumed per day by dividing the number of fat calories by 9 because fats provide approximately 9 kcal/g/d:

$$\text{g/fat/d} = \text{kcal fat}/9$$

$$= 441/9$$

$$= 49$$

What to Eat: Simplified

Once a patient is aware of how many total calories and how much of each macronutrient he or she needs to ingest, the person needs to know how to make proper dietary choices. This is likely the most difficult step in nutrition guidance for the primary health care provider and the patient. The U.S. Department of Agriculture (USDA) provides some simple rules to follow when doing this (Box 4.1). In addition, in 2005, the USDA reconfigured the old food-guide pyramid to include physical activity. They also made the pyramid more interactive for users. Unlike the original pyramid, this new "MyPyramid" offers a person the opportunity to develop a custom-made eating plan based on individual needs such as energy expenditure. This eating plan[27]

- personalizes the diet by offering a variety of food choices,
- infuses physical activity into the plan,
- considers the proportionality of serving sizes,
- modifies individual food intake,
- plans and tracks personal dietary information, and
- provides detailed food group information.

The MyPyramid guide to healthy eating also offers the following advice regarding daily food consumption[27]:

- Grains: Eat primarily whole-grain breads, cereals, rice, or pasta. Whole grains should compose half of a person's total grain consumption.
- Vegetables: Eat those which are dark green and orange in color. Dry beans and peas can also be consumed.
- Fruits: Eat a variety of fresh, frozen, or dried fruits. Minimize the consumption of fruit juices.
- Milk: Drink low-fat or fat-free milk.
- Meat and beans: Eat low-fat meat and poultry. These foods should be baked, broiled, or grilled. Other choices include fish, beans, peas, nuts, and seeds.

One major advantage to using this method of developing an eating plan is that people can directly access the MyPyramid Web site, allowing them to plan and track dietary information, access detailed food group information, count servings, plan menus, and rate a diet regimen. Having a patient become actively involved in developing an eating plan in this fashion increases the likelihood that the patient will adhere to the plan. In addition, primary health care providers should encourage and aid patients in reading food labels and creating food logs to document dietary habits. With the availability of online calorie calculators, patients can become more aware about the content, variety, and volume of food consumed in their diet.[27]

BOX 4.1
U.S. DEPARTMENT OF AGRICULTURE DIETARY RECOMMENDATIONS FOR GENERAL HEALTH

Eat a variety of foods.
Balance the food you eat with physical activity—maintain or improve your weight.
Choose a diet with plenty of grain products, vegetables, and fruits.
Choose a diet low in fat, saturated fat, and cholesterol.
Choose a diet moderate in sugars.
Choose a diet moderate in salt and sodium.
If you drink alcoholic beverages, do so in moderation.

Shaw A, Fulton L, Davis C, et al. Using the Food Guide Pyramid: a resource for nutrition educators. U.S. Department of Agriculture, Food, Nutrition, and Consumer Services Center for Nutrition Policy and Promotion, 1995. Retrieved from: http://www.cnpp.usda.gov/Publications/MyPyramid/OriginalFoodGuidePyramids/FGP/FGPResourceForEducators.pdf#xml=http://65.216.150.153/texis/search/pdfhi.txt?query=food+guide+pyramid&pr=MyPyramid&sufs=2&order=r&cq=&id=4592b7130. Accessed 7/29/08.

Additional Issues

There are a number of nutritional issues primary health care providers encounter on a regular basis. For example, some patient populations require specific dietary intake advice based on the nature of a disorder or disease, whereas athletes may have questions regarding the role nutrition plays in increasing athletic performance. Though important, providing information on a range of topics such as these is beyond the scope of this discussion. Indeed, referral to another health care professional, such as a registered dietician or sports nutritionist, is typically warranted for these patients. Thus, this section concentrates on eating disorders primary health care providers are likely to encounter consistently in the clinical setting.

Eating Disorders

Most people tend to associate the term *eating disorder* with an obsession with being thin. Indeed, many people who live in today's society, females in particular, are obsessed with thinness, seeing thin body shapes as being the ideal. With media images, such as the use of wafer-thin models to sell clothing, reinforcing these perceptions, some people resort to abnormal eating practices that may lead to both morbidity and mortality. Unfortunately, these eating disorders, primarily in the form of anorexia nervosa, usually referred to as *anorexia*, and **bulimia nervosa**, known simply as *bulimia*, are all too common among female athletes. This is particularly true for people who participate in weight-dependent sports, such as gymnastics and figure skating. In recent years, this fact led to the identification of a condition known as the *female athlete triad* and to the American Psychiatric Association's (APA) recognition of disorders associated with caloric restriction as medical conditions. Indeed, in addition to anorexia and bulimia, the APA also recognizes the existence of a condition otherwise referred to as *eating disorders not otherwise specified* (EDNOS). This disorder was added so that people who did not meet the criteria to be diagnosed as anorexic or bulimic, but clearly were on their way to either or both of these conditions, could be identified. Diagnosing someone as having an ENDOS is analogous to identifying a person with angina as the step before the occurrence of a major cardiovascular event, such a myocardial infarction.[28]

Anorexia Nervosa and Bulimia Nervosa

Though historically anorexia and bulimia has been believed to occur mostly in females between the ages of 12 and 19, it is now known that all females, regardless of age, are at risk for developing one or both of these disorders because altered eating patterns can emerge at any age. In addition, males are not precluded from developing an eating disorder because these conditions also occur in response to conditions such as **body dysmorphic disorder.**[14]

Though separate conditions, anorexia and bulimia have overlapping symptoms. For example, both anorexic and bulimic patients have a distorted sense of body image, refusing to maintain a normal body weight because they have a fear of becoming fat. Both conditions also provide patients with a measure of control over their life, which they often perceive as being absent. Though these similarities do exist between people with these conditions, differences also exist. For example, anorexics use methods such as fasting and constantly exercising to avoid gaining weight. In contrast, people with bulimia exhibit a cyclic behavior of binge eating followed by purging, a compensatory behavior that includes self-induced vomiting combined with the use of laxatives, diuretics, and enemas. Table 4.7 compares these conditions by listing clinical indicators associated with each.[14,28]

Though many factors contribute to the development of eating disorders, too often people who are physically active and, in particular, those involved in competitive athletics are given signals by those in authority, such as coaches and sports judges, that they need to be thin to compete. To further complicate matters, certain sports, such as gymnastics and figure skating, place as much emphasis on the aesthetic value of the participant as on the person's ability to perform. Indeed, many who have an eating disorder seek to please those in authority, often willing to engage in abnormal eating behaviors to do so. When caring for such patients, emphasize that using quick weight loss techniques and depriving the body of food are not only unhealthy, but also serve only to hinder athletic performance by

TABLE 4.7 Clinical indicators associated with anorexic and bulimic patients

CLINICAL INDICATOR	ANOREXIC	BULIMIC
Has a distorted sense of body image	√	√
Participates in excessive exercise	√	√
Has low self-esteem	√	√
Presents with a lower-than-average body weight	√	
Avoids meals	√	
Exhibits perfectionist behaviors	√	
Wears baggy or large clothing	√	
Maintains low levels of energy	√	
Has amenorrhea	√	
Eats large amounts of foods in short periods of time		√
Makes frequent trips to the bathroom after meals		√
Purges after eating		√
Uses laxatives, enemas, and diuretics		√
Presents with tooth decay (caused by excessive vomiting)		√

depriving working muscles of needed energy. These practices also dehydrate the body, cause electrolyte imbalances, disturb homeostasis, and place the athlete at risk for injury. Be aware that careful monitoring of patients by the primary health care provider can help detect those with an eating disorder. To help providers do this, the CDC publishes age-appropriate clinical growth charts for adolescents that can be accessed through the CDC Web site.[14,29,30]

PEARL

Females who participate in sports such as gymnastics and figure skating, which place as much emphasis on the aesthetic value of the participant as on the person's ability to perform, are at an increased risk of developing an eating disorder.

Female Athlete Triad

The female athlete triad is a syndrome derived from the interrelated problems caused by disordered eating, amenorrhea, and osteoporosis. As previously mentioned, people who have an eating disorder are more likely than their healthy counterparts to exercise for great periods of time, either in the form of extended exercise sessions or by participating in multiple exercise sessions in a given day. Partaking in this type of excessive exercise regimen, coupled with depriving the body of food and/or purging ingested foodstuffs, results in a negative caloric imbalance. That is, those who engage in such activities expend more calories than they bring in. This cycle eventually disturbs the normal hormonal balance within the body. As the stress of exercise and poor diet persists, estrogen levels taper off, resulting in a disruption of the menstrual cycle. Because of a lack of estrogen production, bone growth is affected, first resulting in **osteopenia** and eventually progressing to osteoporosis. A person of slight build, regardless of the individual's level of physical activity, also maintains a higher risk of developing osteoporosis. This may predispose the female athlete to a rapid decline in bone density later in life. In addition, people with this triad are at great risk of fractures, particularly to the bones of the lower extremities.[31,32]

PEARL

The female athlete triad is a syndrome derived from the interrelated problems caused by disordered eating, amenorrhea, and osteoporosis.

Frequently Asked Questions

Can I get rid of fat cells?

No, fat cells cannot be lost once formed. However, the size of a fat cell can be shrunk by burning the fat that is within the cell. For most people, the number of cells in the body remains constant, though the number of cells can be increased in people who are obese. This happens when all existing fat cells have reached maximal storage capacity, necessitating that the body produce more cells. Though the reason why this happens is not completely understood, the fact that it happens makes it much more difficult for some patients to lose weight as compared with others.[33-35]

I'm genetically predisposed to obesity. Is there anything I can do about it?

Patients often blame a weight problem solely on genetic makeup. Though it is generally accepted that genetics account for approximately 25% of the variance in fat mass and percent body fat, many other modifiable factors are at play. Thus, rarely can a person's weight control problem be fully blamed on the "heredity factor."[36]

How does aging affect body weight?

Most people, particularly those entering the fifth decade of life and beyond, lose LBM as they age. A lower LBM means that RMR is decreased, making it easier to gain weight. Though the aging process cannot be reversed, people in the fifth decade of life and beyond can slow weight gain by participating in a regular exercise program, as described in Chapter 3, and through healthy eating.

What is my ideal body weight?

Historically, determining someone's optimal body weight was based on comparing the person's age, height, and frame size with a standardized weight table. Originally published by the Metropolitan Life Insurance Company in 1959 and revised in 1983, these tables are still used today to identify whether someone is underweight, the correct weight, or overweight. In theory, a person who falls within the normal weight category is considered to be at his or her optimal body weight. Though this is one way to determine whether a person is at the correct weight, these types of tables do not take into account certain factors, such as how active a person is. For example, when these types of tables are used to determine the weight of competitive athletes, some athletes are classified as underweight, as in the case of distance runners, who are typically of thin stature, or overweight, as in the case of weight lifters. This is because these tables do not evaluate certain factors, such as body fat percentage, which are considered much more accurate in determining a person's overall health status. Indeed, those who lift weights on a regular basis typically have more muscle mass than fat mass, which increases their total body weight because muscle weighs more that fat. Based on this information, a patient's BMI, waist circumference, and body fat percentage (all discussed in Chapter 3) should be used to determine what a person's optimal body weight should be, because these measurements are much more reliable in determining how healthy a person is.[37]

How do I lose weight from my waist, hips, and thighs?

Spot reduction refers to the reduction of subcutaneous fat in a body region as a result of exercising that area. For example, if spot reduction were to occur, performing sit-ups would decrease the amount of subcutaneous fat around the abdomen. Unfortunately, exercising a specific body part by itself does not cause a reduction of fat stores in that region. Rather, the reduction of body fat in a specific body area occurs only as part of a comprehensive weight loss program in which adipose tissue is reduced throughout the body.[38]

Should I take diet pills?

In general, most over-the-counter diet pills contain mild stimulants, such as caffeine, which have been touted as mild appetite suppressants. Though they may help reduce weight initially, if changes in behavior and lifestyle are not included with their use, a person is most likely to regain the weight. Indeed, scientific evidence does not support the use of diet pills as part of an ongoing weight loss program for the general population, because known risks outweigh potential benefits in those with a BMI of 30 or less. However, those who have obesity-related conditions, such as type 2 diabetes and hypertension, may benefit from prescription diet pills because it is advantageous for these patients to lose weight fairly quickly to help control their disease.[39]

Does eating a large meal before bedtime cause me to gain weight?

Remember that weight gain is based on calorie intake versus energy expenditure and not on the time of day food is consumed. Thus, other than stimulating the digestive process before sleep, which has the potential of causing discomfort, eating a large meal before bedtime has no greater effect on weight gain than eating at any other time. Anecdotally, many people report that the time between dinner and going to bed is the most difficult time to control eating. Therefore, any excess calories consumed at this time probably have more to do with weight gain than eating a late night meal.

Is cellulite different from fat?

Cellulite is not different from fat, nor is it a different type of fat. Rather, cellulite is fat that has projected out of the adipose tissue and into the dermis. This dimples the skin, making it appear that a specialized type of fat exists. Contrary to popular belief, cellulite appears in both obese and nonobese people, and the efficacy of medicated creams marketed to reduce cellulite have not been scientifically supported. However, some research suggests that though medicated creams cannot decrease the amount of cellulite, these creams can "firm" or "tense" skin overlying subcutaneous fat, causing a decrease in the skin's dimpling appearance.[40,41]

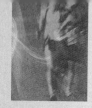

CASE STUDY
Nutrition for the Primary Health Care Provider*

SCENARIO
A 19-year-old female college student presents in your office for her first college pre-participation examination before beginning gymnastics practice as part of the college team.

PERTINENT HISTORY
Medications: None. Denies use of supplements and does not take a multivitamin.

Family History: Denies family history of sudden death before age 50 and any history of Marfan's syndrome, hypertrophic cardiomyopathy, or other heart disease.

PERSONAL HEALTH HISTORY
Tobacco Use: Has never smoked.

Alcohol Intake: Drinks 1 glass of red wine each Sunday at the weekly family meal.

Caffeinated Beverages: Has 4 caffeinated diet sodas per day.

Diet: Eats an apple for breakfast, a salad without dressing for lunch, and usually vegetables and a little chicken for dinner. Drinks diet sodas and plain water for fluids. Does not like milk or cheese products.

Exercise: 3 hours of aerobic exercise 6 days a week, with weight training 1½ hours three times per week. Increased over past year since she developed concerns about her weight.

Past Medical History: Unremarkable, has never had any surgery, had usual one or two colds per year but otherwise healthy. No history of asthma. No sports-related injuries.

Cardiopulmonary: Denies shortness of breath or wheezing with exercise. Within the past year, has had two episodes of light-headedness and palpitations after aerobic exercise in hot weather.

Reproductive History: Sexually active with one partner since age 17.

Birth Control: Uses condoms 100% of time. Up until a year ago she was taking Ortho Tri-Cyclen Lo, but stopped taking it because of an initial 6-pound weight gain. She says her boyfriend was upset by her discontinuing the use of oral birth control, and she proudly notes that she quickly lost 10 pounds by increasing her exercise and limiting her diet. This resulted in a loss of her period, a fact she "really likes," as does her boyfriend. She is trying to lose "at least another 10 pounds."

PERTINENT PHYSICAL EXAMINATION
Blood pressure: 92/60 mm Hg. Heart rate: 60 bpm. Respiratory rate: 14 breaths/min. Height: 68 inches. Weight: 119 pounds. Body mass index (BMI): 18.1.

Appearance: Muscular, thin build. Not emaciated.

Skin: Pink, dry. Hair dull, no thinning. No pitting edema, no lanugo, no knuckle calluses.

*Because of space limitations, these cases are not meant to be comprehensive but are used as exemplar cases for the point being illustrated.

Head, Eyes, Ears, Nose, and Throat (HEENT): Throat pink; no petechiae, mouth sores, eroded enamel, or enlarged parotids.

Cardiovascular: Heart rate 60 bpm; regular, no murmurs, no pitting edema in extremities. No orthostatic changes in blood pressure or pulse.

RED FLAGS FOR THE PRIMARY HEALTH CARE PROFESSIONAL TO CONSIDER

From history and physical examination, she is borderline for female athlete triad: eating disorder, amenorrhea, and osteoporosis. Examination and history point toward risk for anorexia nervosa: comments from boyfriend, weight loss, calorie restriction, excessive exercise, amenorrhea, and absence of signs of bulimia nervosa. However, although weight of 119 pounds and BMI of 18.1 (below 18.5 is underweight) put her in the category of underweight, she does not meet the criteria for anorexia nervosa. History of light-headedness after exercise may indicate cardiovascular complications.

RECOMMENDED PLAN†

- Delay approval for athletic participation pending further evaluation and consultation.
- Diagnostic tests include the following:
  - Electrocardiograph to rule out QT prolongation, which has been associated with sudden death.
  - Laboratory tests: Complete blood count to evaluate for anemia, leukopenia, and thrombocytopenia. Fasting blood sugar. Thyroxine and thyroid-stimulating hormone. Estrogen, luteinizing hormone, and follicle-stimulating hormone.
  - Electrolytes to assess for decreased potassium, sodium, and magnesium.
  - Bone density to evaluate for osteoporosis.
- Early diagnosis and intervention are important. At minimum, this athlete needs education and referral to the eating disorders team at the college. Monitoring by the athletic trainers and health care providers is essential. Appropriate referral for counseling is essential.

†Anorexia nervosa is a complicated, potentially life-threatening condition requiring an interdisciplinary team approach. All of these tests may not be initially indicated for this patient but may be indicated as the workup proceeds. As appropriate to nurse practitioner scope of practice in your state, you should consult with the responsible physician as needed.

REFERENCES

1. Summerfield L. *Nutrition, Exercise, and Behavior: An Integrated Approach to Weight Management.* Beverly, MA, Wadsworth Publishing, 2001.
2. Thompson JA, Manore M. *Nutrition for Life.* New York, NY: Pearson, Benjamin Cummins, 2006.
3. Powers S, Howley E. *Exercise Physiology, Theory and Applications*, 6th ed. New York, NY: McGraw-Hill Co., 2006.
4. Wardlaw G, Hampl J. *Perspectives in Nutrition*, 7th ed. New York, NY: McGraw-Hill Co., 2007.
5. Foster-Powell K., Holt SH, Brand-Miller JC. International table of glycemic index and glycemic load values. *Am J Clin Nutr* 2002;76:5.
6. Ludwig D. Dietary glycemic index and obesity. *J Nutr* 2000;130:280S.
7. Franceschi S, Dal ML, Augustin L. Dietary glycemic load and colorectal cancer risk. *Ann Oncol* 2001;12:173.
8. Toeller M, Buyken AE, Heitkamp G, et al. Nutrient intakes as predictors of body weight in European people with type 1 diabetes. *Int J Obes Relat Metab Disord* 2001;25:1.
9. Liu S, Willett W, Stampfer M, et al. A prospective study of dietary glycemic load, carbohydrate intake, and risk of coronary artery disease in U.S. women. *Am J Clin Nutr* 2000;71:1455.
10. Jenkins DJA, Wolever M, Taylor RH, et al. Glycemic index of foods: a physiological basis for carbohydrate exchange. *Am J Clin Nutr* 1981;34:362.
11. Home to the Glycemic Index. Retrieved from: http://www.glycemicindex.com/. Accessed 7/29/08.
12. Remiers K, Ruud J. Nutritional factors in health and performance. In: *Essentials of Strength and Conditioning*, 2nd ed. Champaign, IL: Human Kinetics, 2000.
13. Duyff RL, American Dietetic Association. *American Dietetic Association Complete Food and Nutrition Guide*, 2nd ed. Hoboken, NJ: John Wiley & Sons, 2002.
14. Hogan MA, DeLeon E, Gingrish MM, et al. *Nutrition and Diet Therapy*, 2nd ed. Upper Saddle River, NJ: Prentice Hall, 2007.
15. Finaud J, Lac G, Filaire E. Oxidative stress: relationship with exercise and training. *Sports Med* 2006;36(4):327.
16. United States Department of Agriculture. Dietary guidance. Retrieved from: http://fnic.nal.usda.gov/nal_display/index.php?info_center=4&tax_level=3&tax_subject=256&topic_id=1342&level3_id=5142&level4_id=0&level5_id=0&placement_default=0. Accessed 7/29/08.
17. NutriBase. Retrieved from: http://www.nutribase.com/exercala.htm. Accessed 7/29/08.
18. American College of Sports Medicine, Sawka MN, Burke LM, et al. American College of Sports Medicine Position Stand: exercise and fluid replacement. *Med Sci Sports Exerc* 2007;39:377.
19. Thompson JL, Manore MM, Skinner JS. Resting metabolic rate and thermic effect of a meal in low- and adequate-energy intake male endurance athletes. *Int J Sport Nutr* 1993;3:194.
20. Harris JA, Benedict FG. *A Biometric Study of Basal Metabolism in Man*, vol. 279. Philadelphia, PA: JB Lippincott Co., 1919.
21. Thompson JL, Manore MM. Predicted and measured resting metabolic rate of male and female endurance athletes. *J Am Diet Assoc* 1996;96:30.
22. Berning JR, Steen SN. *Nutrition for Sport and Exercise*, 2nd ed. Gaithersburg, MD: Aspen Publishers, 1998.
23. Muoio DM, Leddy JJ, Horvath PJ, et al. Effect of dietary fat on metabolic adjustments to maximal VO_2 and endurance in runners. *Med Sci Sports Exerc* 1994;26:81.
24. Pendergast DR, Horvath PJ, Leddy JJ, et al. The role of dietary fat on performance, metabolism, and health. *Am J Sports Med* 1996;24:S53.
25. Phinney SD, Bistrian BR, Evans WJ, et al. The human metabolic response to chronic ketosis without caloric restriction: preservation of submaximal exercise capability with reduced carbohydrate oxidation. *Metabolism* 1983;32:769.
26. American College of Sports Medicine, American Dietetic Association, Dietitians of Canada. Joint Position Statement. Nutrition and athletic performance. *Med Sci Sports Exerc* 2000;32:2130.

27. MyPyramid. A means of menu planning. Retrieved from: http://www.mypyramid.gov/. Accessed 7/29/08.
28. American Psychiatric Association. *Diagnostic and Statistical Manual of Mental Disorders,* 4th ed. Washington, DC: American Psychiatric Association, 1994.
29. Reimers K. Eating disorders and obesity. In: *Essentials of Strength and Conditioning,* 2nd ed. Champaign, IL: Human Kinetics, 2000.
30. Centers for Disease Control and Prevention. Clinical Growth Charts. Retrieved from: http://www.cdc.gov/growthcharts/. Accessed 7/29/08.
31. Nattiv A, Loucks AB, Manore MM, et al. Position stand of the American College of Sports Medicine: the female athlete triad. *Med Sci Sports Exerc* 2007;39:1867.
32. Sherman RT, Thompson RA. Practical use of the International Olympic Committee Medical Commission position stand on the female athlete triad: a case example. *Int J Eat Disord* 2006;39(3):193.
33. Garaulet M, Hernandez-Morante JJ, Lujan J, et al. Relationship between fat cell size and number and fatty acid composition in adipose tissue from different fat depots in overweight/obese humans. *Int J Obes* 2006;30:899.
34. Farnier C, Krief S, Blache M, et al. Adipocyte functions are modulated by cell size change: potential involvement of an integrin/ERK signaling pathway. *Int J Obes Relat Metab Disord* 2003;27:1178.
35. Le Soazig L, Krief S, Farnier C, et al. Cholesterol, a cell-size dependent signal that regulates glucose metabolism and gene expression in adipocytes. *J Biol Chem* 2001;276:16904.
36. Bouchard C. The response to long-term overfeeding in identical twins. *N Engl J Med* 1990;322:1477.
37. Healthy Life Project. 1983 Metropolitan Life Insurance Company Height and Weight Chart. Retrieved from: http://healthfullife.umdnj.edu/editor/METROLIFE_table.htm. Accessed 7/29/08.
38. Kostek MA, Pescatello LS, Seip RL, et al. Subcutaneous fat alterations resulting from an upper-body resistance training program. *Med Sci Sports Exerc* 2007:39:1177.
39. Keeping weight-loss drugs in perspective: if you're dangerously overweight, diet pills may help—but not without major lifestyle changes. *Harv Womens Health Watch* 2006;13(8):1.
40. Rao J, Gold MH, Goldman MP. A two-center, double blinded, randomized trial testing the tolerability and efficacy of a novel therapeutic agent for cellulite reduction. *J Cosmet Dermatol* 2005;4(2):93.
41. Piérard-Franchimont C, Pierary GE, Herny F, et al. A randomized, placebo-controlled trial of topical retinol in the treatment of cellulite. *Am J Clin Dermatol* 2000;1:369.

SUGGGESTED READINGS

De Lorenzo A, Gobbo VD, Premrov MG, et al. Normal-weight obese syndrome: early inflammation? *Am J Clin Nutr* 2007;85:40.
Miles JM. A role for the glycemic index in preventing or treating diabetes? *Am J Clin Nutr* 2008;87:1
Weinsier RL, Nagy TR, Hunter GR, et al. Do adaptive changes in metabolic rate favor weight regain in weight-reduced individuals? An examination of the set-point theory. *Am J Clin Nutr* 2000;72:1088.

WEB LINKS

http://dietary-supplements.info.nih.gov/index.aspx. Accessed 7/29/08.
   The National Institutes of Health Office of Dietary Supplements Web site containing a wide array of information about dietary supplements. Useful for both patients and practitioners.

http://www.cdc.gov/nccdphp/dnpa/nutrition/. Accessed 7/29/08.
   Centers for Disease Control and Prevention Web site maintaining all things about nutrition. Also has a Resources for Professionals link.

http://health.nih.gov/result.asp/474. Accessed 7/29/08.
   National Institutes for Health nutrition Web site maintaining a variety of nutrition topics. Links to professional organizations with an interest in nutrition, including alternative therapies, are included.

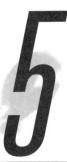

The Inflammation Process

● **Brian J. Toy, PhD, ATC**

Derived from the Latin *inflammare* ("to set on fire"), inflammation is one of the many outcomes produced by musculoskeletal trauma that must be managed for almost all soft tissue conditions. The inflammatory process involves a complex series of interrelated physiological, cellular, and molecular events and includes both local and systemic symptoms. Clinically, an inflammation is defined by the five cardinal signs listed in Box 5.1, whereas systemic manifestations include an increased white blood cell count, lethargy, and muscle catabolism. However, all of these are not always present. Furthermore, an *acute inflammation* is characterized by quick onset that lasts for a relatively short period of time, whereas inflammation that lingers for an extended period is referred to as *chronic inflammation*.[1,2]

The inflammatory process begins as soon as an injury occurs and, depending on circumstances, it takes days, weeks, months, or even years to come to full resolution. Thus, when a patient reports with a history consistent with that of musculoskeletal injury, it is safe to assume that the inflammatory process has been initiated. Maintaining a thorough understanding of the processes that produce the telltale signs of inflammation is essential when determining the proper course of treatment for musculoskeletal injury. Recommendations to use physical modalities, such as cold and heat, and the prescribing of pharmacological agents, such as over-the-counter and prescription strength analgesics (all discussed in Chapter 6), must be grounded in this knowledge. By making sound treatment decisions, patients can return to sports participation safely.

Inflammatory Process

Most people, and some practitioners, incorrectly associate the term *inflammation* with a negative outcome of musculoskeletal injury. Nothing could be further from the truth, because inflammation is a normal response to bodily trauma, making it vital to the healing process. It is not clear, however, whether it is best to try to limit the amount of inflammation after injury or whether it is best to allow the inflammatory process to proceed unimpeded. What is known is that inflammation produced beyond what is needed for proper healing can have negative consequences, such as leading to chronic inflammation and delayed recovery. Other factors that affect healing are listed in Box 5.2. Thus, one of the primary challenges practitioners face when treating musculoskeletal injury is determining how to allow the inflammatory process to occur without making the condition worse. This can be accomplished by using the injury management techniques outlined in Chapter 6 and by implementing body part–specific therapeutic exercises presented throughout Part II of this text.[3–6]

BOX 5.1
CARDINAL SIGNS OF AN ACUTE INFLAMMATION

Heat (calor)	Pain (dolor)
Redness (rubor)	Loss of function (functio laesa)
Swelling (tumor)	

BOX 5.2
FACTORS WHICH AFFECT TISSUE HEALING

Type of tissue damaged	Patient's nutritional status
Severity of the damage	Treatment the patient received after
Patient's overall health status	the injury
Genetics	Tissue vascularity
Hormonal changes	Patient's age
Tissue innervation	Patient's fitness level

PEARL

The inflammatory process must occur for proper healing to take place.

The inflammatory process is divided into three phases: reactive, repair/regeneration, and maturation. Though it is customary to offer a duration time for each phase, the duration of each is not distinct, because an overlap usually occurs from the end of one phase to the beginning of the next[7] (Fig. 5.1).

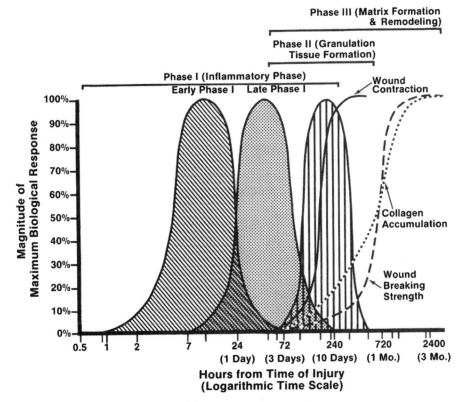

FIGURE 5.1 The reactive phase of the inflammatory process.

Reactive Phase

In the reactive, or *inflammatory response*, phase, body tissue reacts to an injury or irritant. On average, this phase lasts for about 72 hours or less; however, it can last longer. When injury occurs, soft tissues located in the area of injury are either destroyed or badly damaged. For example, a basketball player who sprains an ankle experiences immediate damage to the ligaments and connective tissues in the injured area. After this initial injury, the body undergoes a series of vascular and cellular changes. These changes are mediated by the release of chemicals produced from injured **mast cells** located in surrounding connective tissues. This phase is also marked by the clotting of injured blood vessels.[2,7,8]

On average, the initial inflammatory response to injury lasts for 72 hours.

Vascular, Cellular, and Chemical Responses

One of the initial responses to musculoskeletal injury is the tearing of blood vessels that supply the involved and closely surrounding tissues. This results in hemorrhaging, which usually subsides after a few minutes. This initial bleeding primarily stops in response to three factors[8–10]:

• the release of the chemical serotonin, which causes surrounding arterioles to undergo a period of transient vasoconstriction;
• the crushing of local capillaries caused by swelling in the region; and
• the clotting process (discussed later in this chapter).

Both arteriole vasoconstriction, which lasts no longer than 10 minutes, and the crushing of local capillaries cause damaged and healthy cells in the immediate and surrounding areas to be deprived of oxygen. Because all cells need oxygen to survive, any extended period of oxygen deprivation causes cell death. This type of cell death by **secondary hypoxia** is responsible for a continuing of the injury response process. Even with the most prompt care, there is nothing anyone can do to prevent the damage caused by the initial injury incident. However, the steps taken immediately after an injury can help determine the amount of further damage caused by secondary hypoxia.[11]

The vascular response of arteriole vasoconstriction occurs for the first 10 minutes after acute musculoskeletal injury.

After the initial period of blood vessel vasoconstriction, the chemical mediators **histamine** and **prostaglandin** are released. Prostaglandin is responsible for perpetuating the inflammatory cascade that follows the initial period of transient vasoconstriction. It is also responsible for stimulating nociceptive free nerve endings, which causes the patient pain. Prostaglandin and histamine both cause intact arterioles surrounding the injured area to dilate, resulting in increased blood flow to the region. Although vasodilation increases the amount of blood delivered, this process coincides with a prolonged period in which the blood's rate of flow is greatly diminished. This allows **plasma exudate** to accumulate in the intact vessels. During this time, histamine and prostaglandins, along with the chemical **bradykinin**, increase the permeability of the walls of these vessels. Eventually, the buildup of plasma exudate within these capillaries exerts enough pressure to cause the exudate to penetrate the vessel walls. As it moves from an area of higher concentration to an area of lower concentration, the plasma exudate accumulates in the injured area's interstitial spaces, producing the characteristic swelling associated with musculoskeletal injury. Because the amount of exudate created depends, in part, on the severity of injury, the most severe soft tissue injuries usually produce the greatest amount of swelling.[2,9,12,13]

PEARL

Swelling is primarily caused by the release of plasma exudate into interstitial spaces.

One of the body's responses to inflammation is the manufacturing and transportation of leukocytes to the region. These cells are normally located in the blood's central portion. However, because of the decrease in the blood's rate of flow, the increased concentration of leukocytes in the blood, and the release of the chemical mediator **leucotaxin**, these cells move from the center and align along the walls of the surrounding intact vessels in a process known as **margination**. Once aligned, mediators such as the chemical **necrosin** attract leukocytes to the injured area via a process known as **chemotaxis**. Once attracted to the injury site, leucotaxin allows the leukocytes to pass through the walls of the capillaries in a process known as **diapedesis**.[2,12–14]

Among several types of leukocytes, those most involved in musculoskeletal inflammation are neutrophils and monocytes. Neutrophils are small, exist in great numbers, arrive at the injury site first, and last for only a few hours. Part of their function is to produce collagenase, an enzyme that breaks down dead tissue in the area. In contrast, monocytes are large, exist in smaller numbers, and arrive at the injury site after the neutrophils. These leukocytes concentrate in great numbers in areas of greatest tissue damage. After they move into the affected area, monocytes mature into **macrophages**. These leukocytes live for months and can reproduce, enabling them to provide continuous, ongoing protection and to remove most of the waste products produced in the reactive phase. Once at the injured area, leukocytes, which are phagocytic, engulf foreign particles and cellular debris through **phagocytosis**, a process mediated by the chemical necrosin. After foreign particles have been phagocytized, **lysosomes** fuse with the now formed phagocytic vesicle. Once fused, lysosomes dump digestive enzymes into the vesicle, causing the phagocytized particles to be digested. The phagocytic waste products are ejected from the phagocytes and removed from the injured area via the lymph system. The effectiveness with which tissue debris is removed is a major factor in determining how successfully the body will repair and regenerate the injured tissue.[2–5,10,13] Figure 5.2 illustrates this process.

Though the release of neutrophils in an injured area is an important aspect in controlling the amount of inflammation produced by soft tissue trauma, neutrophils are also responsible for releasing high concentrations oxygen free radicals, molecules that maintain **cytotoxic** properties, in the injured region. This process is designed to act in

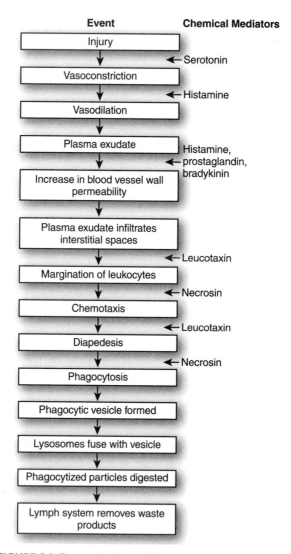

FIGURE 5.2 The reactive phase of the inflammatory process.

an antimicrobial capacity to ward off infection at the site of injury. Unfortunately, this can result in damage to otherwise healthy soft tissues surrounding the site of injury, referred to as the *secondary damage process*. Though they are also produced in response to musculoskeletal trauma, the role macrophages play in damaging healthy tissue in an injured region is less understood.[2-5]

The fact that neutrophils are responsible for both the removal of foreign particles and the destruction of healthy tissue raises the following question: Is it best to allow the inflammatory process to proceed unimpeded, or is it best to intervene with the goal of blocking neutrophil recruitment to decrease the effects of the secondary damage process? As was previously stated, one of the challenges in treating musculoskeletal injury is determining how to allow the inflammatory process to occur without making the condition worse. Chapter 6 attempts to answer this question.

Clotting Response

Blood vessels broken as a result of musculoskeletal injury cause blood to hemorrhage into the same interstitial spaces in which plasma exudate invades. Whereas exudate seeps into the tissue spaces for a period of hours or days, because of the body's clotting response time hemorrhage stops within minutes. Indeed, hemorrhagic exudate, which contains a large number of red blood cells, is usually present in only the most severe cases of inflammation. Thus, though bleeding does contribute to the swelling experienced after musculoskeletal injury, the amount it contributes to this process is usually negligible.[2,10,15]

PEARL

Blood vessels injured from musculoskeletal trauma typically clot within a few minutes after injury, making the amount of blood located in the swelling of most acute musculoskeletal injuries negligible.

Blood clotting is initiated by the transient vasoconstriction experienced after injury. This allows platelets, the first elements to materialize when a wound is created, to appear at the injury site. Though in normal circumstances platelets flow freely through blood vessels, in response to injury they adhere to each other and to the vascular wall at the site of injury. This aggregation and coagulation of platelets "plugs" the injured blood vessels. This temporary fix, which forms within 3 to 7 minutes after the appearance of platelets, helps to localize the injury response while the body initiates a more permanent clotting process.[2,4,10]

While the platelet plug develops, a second process begins to form a more permanent seal. Thromboplastin, a blood coagulant released from damaged cells, causes prothrombin, a plasma protein coagulation factor, to be changed into the enzyme thrombin. This enzyme causes the protein fibrinogen to unwind into individual fibrin protein filaments. These filaments form strands that interlace over the damaged vessels in a matrix arrangement, forming a fibrin clot. As it develops, the clot contracts, making it stronger. Ultimately, the formation of the fibrin clot begins about 12 hours after injury and is completed by 48 hours.[8-10] Figure 5.3 illustrates this process.

Repair and Regeneration Phase

As the reactive phase nears completion, the repair and regeneration phase begins. Clinically, this transition occurs when the cardinal signs of inflammation, swelling and pain in particular, begin to subside or level off. In general, this phase lasts for approximately 6 to 8 weeks.[7]

As its name implies, the objective of this phase is the repair and regeneration of damaged tissue. Regeneration occurs when damaged tissue is replaced with healthy tissue, whereas repair replaces injured tissue with scar tissue. Though desirable, soft tissues, unlike bone, are unable to mend entirely through regeneration. Thus, these tissues rely on both the regeneration process and the repair process to heal injury. This makes the formation of scar tissue essential to healing, a fact that is particularly true

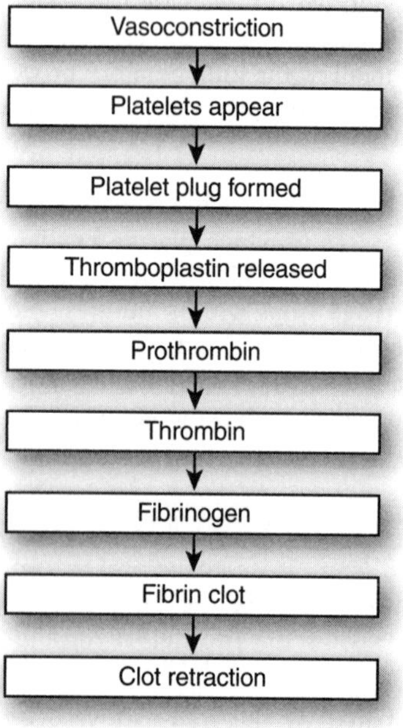

FIGURE 5.3 The clotting process.

for tissues that have a limited capacity for regeneration (Table 5.1). Furthermore, the ability of the body to repair and regenerate soft tissues decreases with age, though the extent to which this happens is unknown.[7,16]

PEARL

The development of scar tissue is necessary for complete musculoskeletal tissue healing.

TABLE 5.1 Regeneration properties of soft tissues

TISSUE	REGENERATION PROPERTIES	HEALING TIME	SCAR TISSUE FORMATION
Muscle/tendon	Limited	Fast	Increased
Ligament/joint capsule	Moderate	Moderate	Moderate
Connective tissue	Good	Slow	Decreased
Peripheral nerves	Good (if ends are opposed)	Slow	Decreased
Skin	Excellent	Very slow	Little

Revascularization

For tissue to regenerate or repair, the body must first reestablish normal blood flow to the area. Doing so brings oxygen and other much needed healing nutrients to the injured tissue. This begins once a mature fibrin clot has formed, because it is the lack of oxygen in the clot that initiates this process. This lack of oxygen causes small, granular bodies to develop within the clot, with each granule representing a new capillary outgrowth. These outgrowths come from healthy capillaries surrounding the area. Eventually, through the process of **granulation**, the clot forms into a well-vascularized mass of tissue. This granular tissue formation is the first step in scar development at the wound site and indicates that the healing process is occurring as it should.[17,18]

Scar Formation and Wound Contraction

Scar formation begins as the fibrin clot begins to break up. At this time, strands of immature connective tissue cells called *fibroblasts* are attracted to the area by the presence of macrophages. These cells infiltrate the area and are laid down parallel to the developing capillaries. Through a process known as **fibroplasia**, fibroblasts produce collagen, a strong, fibrous protein that is deposited within the developing scar. The result is the development of immature scar tissue. Though formed by the end of the first week after injury, immature scar tissue does not begin to mature until the third week. It is important to note that because immature scar tissue is very weak and unable to function as well as the original tissue or as well as mature scar tissue, it is critical to ensure that patients protect the affected body part from reinjury until mature scar tissue develops. As fibroblasts continue to produce and lay down collagen, by week three myofibroblasts, fibroblasts that contain the contractile element actin, appear in the immature scar. When these elements contract, the tissue shrinks and strengthens. By week six, the wound has almost entirely contracted, and a mature scar begins to fully emerge. However, realize that although the process of producing scar tissue begins only weeks after injury, it may take up to a year for scar tissue to fully mature.[2,9,18,19] Factors that affect tissue healing, as presented in Box 5.2, also contribute to the total amount of time it takes for a scar to fully mature.

PEARL

Because immature scar tissue is very weak and unable to function as well as the original tissue or as well as mature scar tissue, it is critical to ensure that patients protect the affected body part from reinjury until mature scar tissue develops.

Because it takes longer for tissues to regenerate than to repair, tissues that heal by forming scar tissue can return to function more quickly than tissues that rely solely on the regeneration process. This means that athletes with certain soft tissue injuries (e.g., strain) may be able to return to participation more quickly than athletes with other conditions (e.g., sprain). Realize, though, that although a person with a second degree muscle strain may be able to return to participation more quickly than a person with a second degree ankle sprain, the patient with the muscle strain maintains greater functional deficits and has a higher risk of reinjury because of the soft tissue's increased scar formation.[2,18,19]

The more a tissue heals by regeneration, the longer it will take the tissue to gain maximum strength.

Maturation Phase

The appearance of myofibroblasts within the scar marks the transition from the repair and regeneration phase to the maturation phase. This phase is marked by a decrease in wound size and the continuous breakdown and synthesis of the scar's collagen matrix. Each time the scar is remodeled in this fashion, it becomes stronger, with the amount of strength developed directly related to the tensile forces placed upon it. Thus, if appropriate force is applied, the scar matures and develops properly. For example, for a recovering knee injury, implementing a therapeutic exercise program that maintains the appropriate combination and amount of resistance training, range-of-motion (ROM) exercises, and functional activity properly strengthens the maturing scar. In contrast, if the patient is not prescribed or does not perform physical therapy after injury, it will take longer for the scar to reach its full strength. If the patient places undue stress on the scar by doing too much activity before the scar's tensile strength is ready for such stress, the scar will most likely be injured. In such a scenario, the entire inflammatory process restarts from the beginning.[20,21]

Although the total amount of time it takes for a scar to fully mature varies, maturation of the repair site can occur by month four. Commonly, it takes 6 to 12 months before complete maturation is realized. Be aware that even mature scar is never as strong or as functional as the tissue the scar is replacing.[7,22] This is primarily because of the characteristics of mature scar tissue, which are listed in Box 5.3.

It may take up to a year before the complete maturation of scar tissue is realized.

Common Problems of Soft Tissue Healing

Regardless of tissue injured or extent of injury, most patients recover fully from soft tissue trauma caused by sports participation. This is particularly true if the injury is evaluated in a timely fashion and if the patient follows proper initial and long-term

BOX 5.3
PROPERTIES OF MATURE SCAR TISSUE

Fibrous	Insensitive
Inelastic	Strong*
Avascular	

*Not as strong as original tissue.

management protocols. At times, this includes withholding the patient from participation or modifying the activity for a period of time before a return to full activity is
allowed. However, patients do not always follow proper treatment advice. Subsequently, problems such as scar tissue proliferation, **adhesion** development, and
chronic inflammation occur.[23]

Scar Tissue Proliferation and Adhesion Development

Problems arise during the healing process if too much scar tissue develops. Otherwise known as *scar tissue proliferation*, this usually occurs when an initial injury is not
allowed to heal properly. This typically happens when an athlete returns to participation too soon after an injury. As previously discussed, excessive stress or reinjury
causes the inflammatory process to restart before full healing has occurred. In these
cases, fibroblastic proliferation occurs. This increased production of fibroblasts leads
to an increased production of collagen, making scar formation widespread. On the
skin, excessive scar formation can be seen as a **keloid** scar. Internally, scar tissue can
cause two adjacent soft tissues to adhere. These adhesions can limit mobility and
function. **Adhesive capsulitis**, described in Chapter 11, is a condition in which
adhesion development severely limits the ROM within the shoulder.[17,19,23]

Chronic Inflammation

Chronic inflammation results when the body is unable to eliminate the cause of
injury and restore normal function to the traumatized tissue. It usually develops from
repeated acute microtraumas and overuse, and is most associated with an initial treatment plan that is too aggressive or a patient failing to follow a sound injury management plan. For example, if, during the treatment of an acute ankle sprain, the patient
returns to participation prematurely and reinjures the ankle, the inflammatory
process restarts. This results in the continuation of the production of inflammatory
mediators and phagocytic leukocytes, causing the symptoms of acute inflammation to
persist. This, in turn, delays healing and interferes with the ability of the affected tissue to repair and regenerate. Each occurrence of reinjury prolongs the total amount
of time needed for complete healing. A predominance of monocyte and macrophage
activity at the site of injury signals the beginning of chronic inflammation. Thus, it can
take months or years for even the mildest injury to fully heal if chronic inflammation
sets in. Clinically, chronic inflammation is characterized by constant pain, muscle
spasm, muscle atrophy, and muscle weakness. Pitting edema, signified by a depression, or "pit," left in the skin after compressing the area with a finger, is typically present. The injured tissues may also develop adhesions. Because in these instances
normal tissue is replaced with tough, fibrous tissue, fibrosis and scaring are almost
guaranteed outcomes of chronic inflammation.[2,7,24,25]

REFERENCES

1. Scott A, Khan, KM, Cook JL, et al. What is "inflammation"? Are we ready to move beyond Celsus? *Br J Sports Med* 2004;38:248.
2. Copstedd LE, Banasik JL. *Pathophysiology*, 3rd ed. St. Louis, MO: Elsevier, 2005.
3. Toumi H, Best TM. The inflammatory response: friend or enemy for muscle injury. *Br J Sports Med* 2003;37:284.
4. Scott A, Khan, KM, Roberts CR, et al. What do we mean by the term "inflammation"? A contemporary basic science update for sports medicine. *Br J Sports Med* 2004;38:372.
5. Tidball JG. Inflammatory process in muscle injury and repair. *Am J Physiol Regul Integr Comp Physiol* 2005;288:R345.
6. Baumert PW. Acute inflammation after injury: quick control speeds rehabilitation. *Postgrad Med* 1995;97(2):35.
7. Leadbetter WB. Cell-matrix response in tendon injury. *Clin Sports Med* 1992;11:533.
8. Kloth LC, Miller KH. The inflammatory response. In: Kloth LC, McCulloch JM, Feedor JA, eds. *Wound Healing: Alternatives in Management*, 3rd ed. Philadelphia, PA: FA Davis Co., 2002.
9. Wong ME, Hollinger JO, Pinero GJ. Integrated processes responsible for soft tissue healing. *Oral Surg Oral Med Oral Path Oral Radiol Endod* 1996;82:475.
10. Jorgensen L, Borchgrevink CF. The platelet plug in normal persons, I: the histological appearance of the plug 15-20 minutes and 24 hours after the bleeding and its role in the capillary haemostasis. *Acta Pathol Microbiol Scand* 1963;57:40.
11. Knight KL. Effects of hypothermia on inflammation and swelling. *Athl Train J Natl Athl Train Assoc* 1976;11:7.
12. Porth CM. Cellular adaptation/injury and wound healing/repair. In: Porth CM, ed. *Pathophysiology*, 4th ed. Philadelphia, PA: Lippincott Williams & Wilkins, 1994.
13. Knight KL. *Cryotherapy in Sport Injury Management*. Champaign, IL: Human Kinetics, 1995.
14. Binliff S, Walker BE. Radioautographic study of skeletal muscle regeneration. *Am J Anat* 1960;106:233.
15. McFarland RG. Normal and abnormal blood coagulation: a review. *J Clin Pathol* 1948;1:113.
16. Ji LL. Exercise at old age: does it increase or alleviate oxidative stress? *Ann NY Acad Sci* 2001;928:236.
17. Davidson JM. Growth factors, extracellular matrix, and wound healing. In: Kloth LC, McCulloch JM, eds. *Wound Healing: Alternatives in Management*, 3rd ed. Philadelphia, PA: FA Davis Co., 2002.
18. Hebda PA. Mast cells and myofibroblast in wound healing. *Dermatol Clin* 1993;11:685.
19. Chettibi S, Ferguson MWJ. Would repair: an overview. In: Gallin JL, Snyderman R, eds. *Inflammation: Basic Principles and Clinical Correlates*. Philadelphia, PA: Lippincott Williams & Wilkins, 1999.
20. Van der Meulen JH. Present state of knowledge on processes of healing in collagen structures. *Int J Sports Med* 1982;3:4.
21. Russel B, Dix DJ, Haller DL, et al. Repair of injured skeletal muscle: a molecular approach. *Med Sci Sports Exerc* 1992;24:189.
22. Frank C, Woo S-L, Amiel D, et al. Medial collateral ligament healing. *Am J Sports Med* 1983;11:379.
23. Pearsall AW, Speer KP. Frozen shoulder syndrome: diagnostic and treatment strategies in the primary care setting. *Med Sci Sports Exerc* 1998;30(4 suppl):S33.
24. Houghton PE. Effects of therapeutic modalities on wound healing: a conservative approach to the management of chronic wounds. *Phys Ther Rev* 1999;4(3):167.
25. Barbe MF, Barr AE, Gorzelany I, et al. Chronic repetitive reaching and grasping results in decreased motor performance and widespread tissue response in a rat model of MSD. *J Orthop Res* 2003;21:7.

SUGGESTED READINGS

Butterfield TA, Best TM, Merrick MA. The dual role of neutrophils and macrophages in inflammation: a critical balance between tissue damage and repair. *J Athl Train* 2006;41:457.

Merrick MA. Secondary injury after musculoskeletal trauma: a review and update. *J Athl Train* 2002;37:209.

Sandrey MA. Acute and chronic tendon injuries: factors affecting the healing response and treatment. *J Sport Rehabil* 2003;12:70.

WEB LINKS

http://rdh.b.home.att.net/inflamm/. Accessed 7/29/08.
   A PowerPoint presentation that provides an excellent overview of the inflammatory process.

http://en.wikipedia-org/wiki/Inflammation. Accessed 7/29/08.
   A website that provides a detailed look into the inflammatory process.

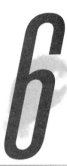

Therapeutics

● **Brian J. Toy, PhD, ATC, and Phyllis F. Healy, PhD, BC-FNP, CNL, RN**

W hen a patient requires treatment for musculoskeletal injury, it is proper to recommend appropriate physical modalities and pharmacological agents for the specific injury. Unfortunately, many clinicians base treatment decisions on what has been done traditionally rather than on what evidence-based practice supports. Furthermore, some practitioners apply a "one size fits all" treatment plan to all patients with musculoskeletal injury, prescribing the same physical modalities or oral medications when caring for people with a variety of conditions and ages. This chapter helps avoid these practice errors and bases treatment decisions on factors such as observed and reported signs and symptoms, inflammatory stage of the injury, and ability of the patient to comply with the treatment plan.

Many physical modalities are available to choose from when developing a management plan for musculoskeletal injury. These modalities are classified as follows:

• thermal (cold, heat),
• electrical (muscle stimulation, nerve stimulation), and
• mechanical (compression, massage, traction).

Because accessibility to deep heating (e.g., ultrasound), electrical, and most mechanical modalities usually requires referral to a certified athletic trainer, licensed physical therapist, or other health care professional with special training, the discussion here is limited to those things that can be included in a home care program. As with the physical modalities, there are a variety of choices when using pharmacotherapy to treat musculoskeletal injury. This chapter is limited to the most commonly used agents.

Goals of Physical Modality and Pharmacotherapy Interventions

The use of any physical modality or pharmacotherapy does not speed the healing process. Rather, the goal of these interventions is to aid the body to heal itself and to alleviate pain and discomfort. It does this by removing the factors that impede healing. This, in turn, produces an optimal healing environment. Simply put, if the severity of an injury dictates a 6- to 8-week recovery time, nothing can be done to speed this up. However, through physical modality and oral medication use, combined with such methods as protecting the body part from further injury and implementing appropriate rehabilitative exercises, the body can heal itself in the shortest time possible. Though it would be nice to be able to inform patients at the initial visit exactly how long an injury will take to get better, this is not possible because no two injuries or individuals heal at the same pace. Understanding this concept helps when working with physically active people who usually want to return to the next exercise session, practice, or contest as quickly as possible.

PEARL

The goal of using physical modalities and pharmacotherapies in the treatment of musculoskeletal injury is to alleviate pain and discomfort while producing an optimal environment to allow the body to heal itself.

Initial Treatment of Inflammation

The initial treatment provided during the reactive phase of inflammation directly affects the healing process. Treatment goals during this phase include

* protecting the injured area from further insult,
* decreasing pain,
* decreasing the amount of tissue affected from secondary hypoxic injury, and
* limiting the amount of swelling.

These goals can be achieved by treating acute musculoskeletal conditions with the following interventions, commonly identified by the PRICE acronym:

* *P*rotect
* *R*est
* *I*ce
* *C*ompress
* *E*levate

Use Patient Teaching Handout (PTH) 6.2 when providing this information to patients as part of a home care management program for acute musculoskeletal injury.

Protect

Until the extent of injury has been determined and a proper course of action has been decided on, protect a patient from further injury by immobilizing the traumatized area. Do this by applying a splint or soft cast to the region. In the case of lower extremity injury, fit the patient with crutches as described in PTH 6.1 if he or she cannot walk without a limp. Apply a sling immobilization brace for patients with an upper extremity condition if the unsupported extremity causes the person discomfort (Fig. 6.1). Though immobilization is an important component of initial musculoskeletal treatment, prolonged immobilization is contraindicated for most soft tissue injuries because it can lead to a loss of joint range of motion (ROM) and the development of adhesions (discussed in Chapter 5) in the region. Even in some of the most severe soft tissue injuries, such as a third degree knee sprain, protecting the body part usually occurs in conjunction with a regimen of active rest, described below.

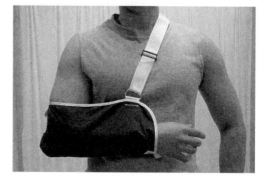

FIGURE 6.1 Sling immobilization of the upper extremity.
From Beam: *Orthopedic Taping, Wrapping, Bracing and Padding.* 2006. Philadelphia: F.A. Davis Company, Fig. 8–11C, pg 251, with permission.

Rest

Rest is an important component of managing musculoskeletal trauma. This is particularly true in the early phases of injury. However, in most cases, the patient is able to perform some type of rehabilitative exercises fairly early in the inflammatory process. The chapters in Part II of this book provide examples of ROM and strengthening exercises, known as *active rest*, that can be prescribed during the initial and subsequent phases of healing.

Ice

The use of ice as a **cryotherapy** technique is common in the treatment of acute musculoskeletal trauma. An in-depth look at the role cryotherapy plays in the treatment of musculoskeletal injury is provided later in this chapter.

Compress

The goal of compression is to decrease swelling by hindering fluid loss from injured vessels and reducing the amount of interstitial space available for fluid infiltration. A compression bandage works best on acute swelling if it is applied before swelling occurs (Fig. 6.2). However, once fluid from an acute injury infiltrates a region, applying pressure to the area cannot significantly reduce it. Nevertheless, the application of a compression bandage is indicated even after acute swelling is present because it helps limit any additional swelling that may occur. Compression wraps also stimulate pressure receptors in the area, which help decrease the perception of pain by competing with pain receptors for space on afferent pathways traveling to the brain.

Achieve compression by placing an elastic wrap on the involved extremity. Apply the wrap in a spiral fashion working distal to proximal (Fig. 6.2). Place more pressure distally and lessen as the wrap ascends the leg. This helps fluid to travel toward the heart and helps to avoid a pooling of fluid in the distal extremity. Overlap each wrap layer by one-half. This assures that no holes appear between each layer.

After application, place an index and middle finger underneath the distal and proximal portions of the wrap. If more than two fingers can fit, the wrap is too loose, making it ineffective in trying to control swelling. If two fingers cannot fit underneath

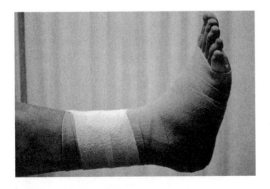

FIGURE 6.2 Spiral compression wrap of the foot and ankle.
From Beam: *Orthopedic Taping, Wrapping, Bracing and Padding.* 2006. Philadelphia: F.A. Davis Company, Fig. 4–10A, pg 110, with permission.

the wrap, it is too tight, which may hinder distal circulation and prevent movement of unwanted fluids away from the injured area. To assure that circulation has not been compromised, check for capillary refill and for a distal pulse.

Once applied, instruct the patient to remove a compression wrap before bedtime. A patient should never sleep with such a wrap applied to the body, because an increase in swelling under the wrap during sleep may go unrecognized. This increase in pressure may decrease circulation distal to the wrap, resulting in tissue damage or necrosis. Teach the patient or a caregiver how to properly apply the compression wrap so that it can be reapplied as needed.

PEARL

**A patient should never sleep with a compression wrap applied
to the body.**

Elevate

When compared with ice and compression, elevation is far superior in removing swelling from an injury site. This is because elevating an extremity higher than the level of the heart places the body part in a gravity-independent position (Fig. 6.3A). This prevents fluid from pooling distally and maximizes the ability of the lymph and venous systems to remove fluid from the region. When a limb is placed in a gravity-dependent position (Fig. 6.3B), it is harder for the venous and lymph systems to function efficiently. As shown in Figure 6.4, when a body part is elevated, gravity actually aids the lymph and venous systems to remove fluids from the distal extremities.

PEARL

**Elevating a body part after injury can significantly reduce swelling
by aiding the lymph and venous systems in removing fluids
from an injured area.**

Unlike ice and compression, elevation can be used on a continuous basis. Thus, for patients to take full advantage of gravity when treating musculoskeletal injury to an extremity, tell them to elevate the injured limb as much as possible. Though it is best for an injured extremity to be elevated to a point where it is perpendicular to the ground, as shown in Figure 6.4, doing so can be uncomfortable for most patients. Thus, instruct patients to elevate an injured extremity to a 45° angle, because most people can do this comfortably. Make sure patients understand the importance of supporting the entire extremity while the body part is elevated. For example, when elevating the lower extremity, the ankle, thigh, knee, and leg regions must be supported, as shown in Figure 6.3A. This prevents placing undue stress on these body parts. For injuries to the lower extremity, instruct the patient to elevate the distal end of the mattress while they sleep by placing a suitcase, or similar object, between the mattress and the box spring. Advise against placing the body part on a stack of pillows, because doing so typically causes the extremity to "roll off" the pillows during sleep.

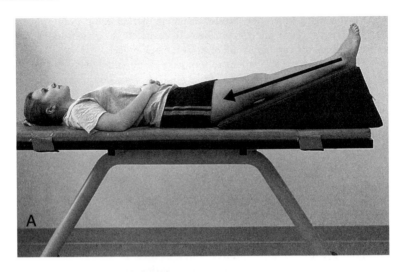

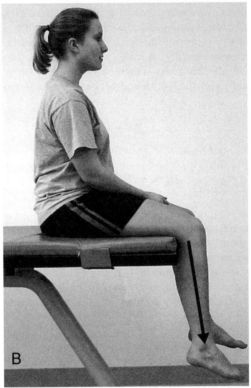

FIGURE 6.3 (A) Gravity-independent position. Gravity assists with lymph and venous return. (B) Gravity-dependent position. Gravity works against lymph and venous return. From Starkey: *Therapeutic Modalities*, 3rd ed. 2004. Philadelphia: F.A. Davis Company, Fig. 1-11, pg 20, with permission.

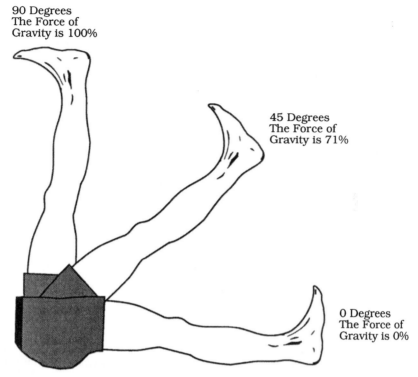

90 Degrees
The Force of
Gravity is 100%

45 Degrees
The Force of
Gravity is 71%

0 Degrees
The Force of
Gravity is 0%

FIGURE 6.4 Effect of gravity on lymph and venous drainage at various limb positions. From Starkey: *Therapeutic Modalities*, 3rd ed. 2004. Philadelphia: F.A. Davis Company, Fig. 1-13, pg 22, with permission.

Advise patients with a lower extremity injury to elevate the body part while they sleep by placing a suitcase or similar item between their bed mattress and box spring.

Cryotherapy

Cryotherapy is the most commonly used physical modality for the treatment of musculoskeletal injury. When applied to the body, cold produces a number of physiological effects that aid in healing, particularly in the injury's acute phase. It is also safe to use and easy to administer.[1,2]

Cryotherapy is the most commonly used modality in the treatment of musculoskeletal injuries.

Physiological Effects on Human Tissue

When cold is applied to the skin, underlying blood vessels constrict and cell permeability in the cooled tissues decreases. These two reactions explain how cold might help to control the amount of swelling experienced after acute musculoskeletal trauma. Though it may seem that these responses would significantly reduce swelling, as summarized previously in this chapter, swelling is mainly controlled via lymphatic and venous return, which is best achieved with elevation. Thus, if cryotherapy is used without elevation, minimal success is achieved in preventing swelling from occurring and in reducing existing swelling.[1]

Applying cryotherapy to an acute musculoskeletal injury without elevating the body part limits the success cold has in decreasing swelling.

If reduction of swelling is not the primary reason for applying cold to injured tissue, why is the application of cryotherapy so vital in the treatment of acute musculoskeletal trauma? The answer lies with the secondary hypoxic injury process.

Tissue Protection

The primary reason for using cryotherapy in the initial stages of musculoskeletal trauma is to protect the damaged and surrounding tissues from cell death caused by secondary hypoxic injury (described in Chapter 5). Cold does this by decreasing metabolic activity in the area, thereby reducing a cell's need for oxygen. This allows a cell to live longer after initial trauma. Less tissue damage results in less serious injury and a quicker recovery time.[1-5]

To illustrate this concept, consider the case of cold-water drowning. As with musculoskeletal tissue, brain tissue responds to cold with decreased metabolic activity. This enables brain cells to survive for an extended period of time without oxygen. The well-documented cases of victims who experience full neurological recovery after an extended period of time immersed in cold water can be attributed to this protective effect.

Preventing cell death caused by secondary hypoxic injury is the primary reason for using cryotherapy in the initial stages of musculoskeletal trauma.

Pain Reduction

As most practitioners already know, applying cold to an injured body part also decreases the amount of pain a patient experiences. Therefore, another primary use of cryotherapy is to decrease pain. Cold does this is in a couple of ways.[1,2]

Because pain is a perception processed by the brain, decreasing that perception can reduce the amount of pain an injured person feels. Cold does this by both slowing the depolarization rate of pain nerve fibers and decreasing the speed at which a pain stimulus travels along these fibers. Together, these actions limit the level of pain stimuli that reaches the brain, resulting in decreased pain perception. A total reduction of pain is realized when the nerve fibers are completely inhibited from depolarizing. If the brain does not receive a stimulus, it has nothing to process, resulting in analgesia.[1,6–8]

Other Effects

Other effects of cryotherapy include decreases in both muscle spasm and muscle strength. The process by which cold affects muscles is the same involved in pain relief. That is, cold decreases the depolarization rate of the nerves that stimulate muscle tissue. Because muscle spasm is, at times, a primary cause of pain, cold is an excellent modality to treat pain caused by muscle spasm. However, a decrease in muscle strength after cold application can be problematic if the patient engages in physical activity or a weight-bearing rehabilitation program immediately after cryotherapy treatment. Keep this in mind when developing an injury management plan that includes the use of cryotherapy.[9,10] A summary of the physiological effects of cold is presented in Table 6.1.

Treatment Misconceptions

Misconceptions regarding the use of cryotherapy as a treatment modality are plentiful. It is necessary for a primary health care provider to be able to distinguish fact from fiction to maximize the use of cold as a treatment modality. Some of the more common fallacies are discussed here.

Use a Barrier to Protect the Skin

To protect the skin from cold-induced injury such as frostbite, many health care providers believe, and teach, that a barrier, such as a dry or wet towel, must be placed between the cold source and the skin. This intervention is also recommended in primary care textbooks and journal review articles. The belief that a barrier is needed has so permeated the primary care setting that generations of health care providers, believing they are protecting patients, have significantly limited the effectiveness of cryotherapy treatments. The fact is, for human tissue to receive every physiological effect that cold has to offer, in most cases direct contact between the modality and the skin must

TABLE 6.1 Physiological effects of cold and heat	
COLD EFFECTS	HEAT EFFECTS
Vasoconstriction	Vasodilation
Decreased cell permeability	Increased capillary permeability
Decreased rate of cell metabolism	Increased cell metabolism
Decreased nerve depolarization rate	Increased nerve depolarization rate
Decreased nerve conduction velocity	Increased nerve conduction velocity
Decreased pain	Increased venous and lymph flow
Decreased muscle spasm	Increased tissue elasticity
Decreased muscle strength	Increased basal metabolic rate
	Increased nutrients
	Decreased pain
	Decreased muscle spasm

occur. Using a barrier between a cold modality and the skin only acts to insulate the target tissue from the cold. This ultimately affects the degree to which the tissue is cooled and, in many instances, renders the treatment useless.[2,11–13]

In most instances, placing a barrier between the cold modality and the skin renders the cryotherapy treatment useless.

Except in certain situations, the occurrence of cold-induced injury to the skin in response to properly administered cryotherapy is extremely remote. Conditions such as frostbite rarely occur when the skin is exposed to temperatures above 32°F. When the traditional cryotherapy treatment of an ice pack is used, its temperature is never less than freezing, virtually eliminating any potential risk for cold-related injury for most patients. However, when a patient's skin is more susceptible to cold-induced injury, such as in the case of the very young, the elderly, and people who are hypersensitive to cold, a barrier should be used when applying a cryotherapy treatment directly to the skin. A barrier should also be used when a modality's treatment temperature is less than 32°F.[2,13] A continuation of this discussion appears in the Modes of Application section of this chapter.

Except in certain situations, most forms of cryotherapy treatment can be safely applied to the skin without the fear of causing tissue damage.

Limit Treatment Duration

For years, many in the clinical setting have advocated limiting cryotherapy treatment time to 15- to 20-minute intervals. One of the primary reasons for this has been the belief that a treatment that lasts too long or gets the target tissue too cold causes reflexive vasodilation of the vessels being cooled. It has been theorized that this reflexive vasodilation, termed the *hunting response*, or *rebound phenomenon*, acts as a protective mechanism by increasing blood flow to overly cooled body tissues.[11,14,15]

The research on this matter shows that the hunting response probably does not exist as originally proposed, because it is questionable whether vessels vasodilate at all in response to prolonged cold exposure. If reflexive vasodilation does occur, the vessel's size probably remains smaller than it was before the cold application. This still makes vasoconstriction the net result of prolonged exposure to cold. Thus, advising a patient to remove a cryotherapy treatment too quickly does not prevent significant vasodilation, but does limit the cold's ability to provide all of its physiological benefits.[1,5,16]

Limit Treatment Days

As an injury transitions from the reactive phase to the repair and regeneration phase as discussed in Chapter 5, many health care providers recommend replacing cryotherapy with **thermotherapy** treatments (described later in this chapter). Indeed, instructing patients to apply heat 24 to 48 hours after musculoskeletal injury occurrence has become standard in many health care settings. Though using heat after the initial phase of inflammation has subsided is certainly indicated, often the use of cold is abandoned too quickly. This is particularly disturbing when a patient is responding well to cryotherapy. Thus, if a patient's condition improves with cold treatments during the first few days after injury, consider advising the patient to continue to manage the injury with cryotherapy. In some instances, patients heal without ever introducing heat treatments. This is true when treating patients with chronic, as well as acute, musculoskeletal conditions. Ultimately, determining the modality to which a patient responds better involves trial and error.

PEARL

Consider treating a musculoskeletal injury with cryotherapy beyond the first few days after injury.

Treatment Parameters

As previously mentioned, cryotherapy treatments applied in the clinical setting typically occur in 15- to 20-minute intervals. Although in some instances this may be appropriate, it is not necessarily correct for all patients or for all conditions. Thus, base the length of a patient's cryotherapy treatment on

- the goal of the treatment,
- how deep the target tissue is in relation to the skin, and
- the amount of adipose tissue located in the treatment area.

For example, if the goal of the treatment is to decrease pain, treatment can be terminated once the patient experiences numbness. This usually occurs fairly quickly because most people report numbness no later than 15 minutes into the treatment. If, however, the goal of the treatment is to decrease metabolic rate to reduce the chance of secondary hypoxic injury, or to maximize the depth to which the cold penetrates, treatment length must be much longer than the time it takes for analgesia to occur.[5,11,14,16,17]

The primary factor in determining the length of a cryotherapy treatment is the amount of adipose tissue located in the injured area. Because it acts as an insulator, the amount of adipose tissue present directly affects both the speed at which cold is conducted and the depths to which it penetrates. Simply put, the more subcutaneous fat a patient has, the longer the cryotherapy treatment should be. It stands to reason, then, that accurately gauging an appropriate duration of cryotherapy treatment is dependent on the amount of adipose tissue located in the treatment area. This can be determined by taking skinfold caliper measurements and comparing these results with the treatment guidelines presented in Table 6.2. In the absence of using this technique, prescribing cryotherapy for 30 minutes allows the physiological effects of cold to occur for most patients. Be aware that cooling continues to occur for a short period of time after the modality is removed, so the total treatment time is always slightly longer than the prescribed treatment duration. Although it is safe, and advised, to prescribe a longer treatment for those with excessive adipose tissue, when an increased treatment length is included as part of a home care management program, patient compliance decreases. Also, because children have low amounts of subcutaneous fat, in general the length of a cryotherapy treatment for a child can be shorter than that for an adult.[2,4,18,19]

TABLE 6.2 Recommended cryotherapy treatment duration times based on skinfold thickness of the treatment area

SKINFOLD THICKNESS, MM	TREATMENT TIME, MINUTES
<20	20
20–30	40
>30	60

Adapted from: Otte JW, Merrick MA, Ingersoll CD, et al. Subcutaneous adipose tissue thickness alters cooling time during cryotherapy. *Arch Phys Med Rehabil* 2002;83:1501.

Though the amount of adipose tissue present in a body region directly affects the ability of cold to cool a target tissue, a 30-minute cryotherapy treatment produces the desired physiological effects for most patients.

Although cold cannot be used continuously, it can be reapplied many times over the course of a day. In fact, it is essential that as many cryotherapy treatments as feasible be administered for an acute injury. However, 1 to 2 hours should separate treatment sessions. This allows the treated area to return to a normal state before the next scheduled treatment and provides the patient with a process he or she can reasonably implement as part of a home care management program.

Apply cryotherapy treatments at 1- to 2-hour intervals.

Patient Education

Before prescribing cryotherapy, teach the patient what normally happens when cold is applied to the body. It is particularly important that this is done for patients who have never experienced a cryotherapy treatment and for people who have had a negative cold treatment experience. Explain to the patient the sensations he or she should expect to feel when cold is applied to the body. Doing so helps ease the anxiety a cryotherapy treatment can create, makes the treatment more tolerable, and helps with patient compliance. The most commonly reported sensations occur in the following order[7,17]:

- cold;
- stinging or burning;
- aching, throbbing, or a "pins and needles" feeling; and
- numbness.

Be aware that not all patients feel all four sensations, whereas others may experience a number of other sensations, including freezing, penetrating, sharpness, and tingling. Tell the patient that they may never get to the numbness stage, because analgesia occasionally does not occur.[7,8]

When including cryotherapy as part of a home care management program, teach the patient how to inspect the skin periodically throughout the treatment. It is particularly important to do this if the patient has never had a cryotherapy treatment before. Explain that the patient should see **erythema** underlying the treatment modality. If any other response occurs, such as blistering, advise the patient to immediately discontinue treatment and have him or her report this reaction. If this occurs, the method of treatment administration should be changed. Altering parameters such as treatment length, frequency, and mode may allow the patient to continue cryotherapy treatments without adverse affects. If the skin continues to be irritated in response to cold application, permanently discontinue the cryotherapy treatments.

(PEARL)

Teach patients what they can expect to feel in response to placing cold on the body.

Modes of Application

There are many different ways to apply a cryotherapy treatment. Typical modes of application include **ice bag, ice massage,** and **cold immersion**. In addition, **cold gel packs** and some common household freezer items, such as a frozen bag of peas, can be used as a cryotherapy modality.

Ice Bag

The most common way to apply cryotherapy is with an ice bag, otherwise known as an *ice pack*. This treatment method is easy to apply, is readily available, and maintains a fairly high compliance rate among users. It also cools tissue quickly and provides deep penetration. Because it can be used in combination with compression and elevation, prescribe an ice bag treatment whenever ice, compression, and elevation are indicated for an acute injury.[2,20]

(PEARL)

Choose an ice bag for an acute musculoskeletal injury because this mode of cryotherapy treatment can easily be combined with compression and elevation.

Teach patients the proper method of applying an ice bag as follows. Fill a plastic bag with cubed, disk, flaked, or crushed ice. Crushed or flaked ice works best because these conform to the body better than the other products. Remove excess air from the bag and place the bag directly on the skin, securing it with an elastic wrap (Fig. 6.5). Doing this holds the bag in place and adds compression, increasing treatment effectiveness. Covering the ice pack with a wrap also reduces the amount of energy lost from the pack, increasing treatment effectiveness. Clinically, a wrapped ice bag has been shown to work better in combating swelling than compression alone. Remind patients always to place the ice bag on the body and never to place the body on the ice bag. Doing so increases the rate at which cooling occurs, which could lead to tissue damage. Also, be sure to tell patients never to sleep with an ice bag wrapped on the body, because this also can lead to tissue damage.[2,21]

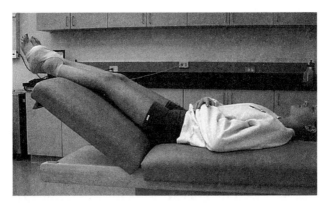

FIGURE 6.5 Ice bag application to the ankle.
From Starkey: *Therapeutic Modalities*, 3rd ed. 2004. Philadelphia:
F.A. Davis Company, Fig. 5-5, pg 113, with permission.

Ice Massage

Ice massage is another common way to apply cryotherapy. Although popular among health care providers, this treatment method is not the best choice for most acute conditions because it cannot be combined with compression, it is difficult to apply with elevation, and it treats a relatively small area. Nevertheless, it does work well with subacute and chronic conditions, is easy to prepare, and is easy to administer. It is also as effective as an ice bag in cooling tissue, as long as the treatment durations are the same.[22]

Teach patients to prepare an ice massage treatment as follows. Fill a 5- to 10-ounce paper cup with water and place it in a freezer (if a smaller cup size is used, the ice melts before the recommended treatment length of 30 minutes passes). After the water freezes, peel the top half of the cup away. Rub the ice on the body in longitudinal and circular strokes, with each stroke overlapping the previous stroke by one-half (Fig. 6.6). Cover an area no more than three times the size of the cup. Advise that a towel be available throughout the treatment.[1]

Cold Immersion

Cold immersion is the least used of the traditional cryotherapy techniques because it cannot be combined with elevation or compression. It is also limited to treating the distal parts of the extremities: foot, ankle, leg, elbow, forearm, wrist, and hand. One advantage of using cold immersion as a treatment modality is the patient's ability to perform ROM exercises during the treatment. If prescribed, cold immersion does provide prolonged, significant tissue temperature reduction.[23]

When prescribing cold immersion, instruct patients to place water in a bucket large enough to cover the treatment area. In most instances, patients have to add ice to arrive at the recommended treatment temperature of 55°F. Instruct them to sit comfortably and immerse the body part so that the injured area is fully submerged. Advise that a towel be available to dry the extremity after the treatment (Fig. 6.7).

Cold Gel Packs and Common Household Freezer Items

Commercially produced cold gel packs have become popular as a way to provide cryotherapy. In part, their popularity is due to their ability to be refrozen

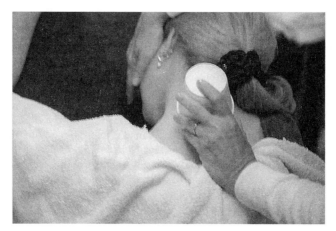

FIGURE 6.6 Ice massage application to the posterior neck. From Michlovitz and Nolan: *Modalities for Therapeutic Intervention*, 4th ed. 2005. Philadelphia: F.A. Davis Company, Fig. 3-6, pg 53, with permission.

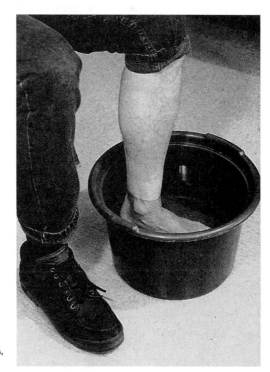

FIGURE 6.7 Cold immersion to the foot and ankle. From Michlovitz and Nolan: *Modalities for Therapeutic Intervention*, 4th ed. 2005. Philadelphia: F.A. Davis Company, Fig. 3-7A, pg 54, with permission.

and reused as needed. Educate patients regarding the limitations and dangers of using these packs.

Once frozen, cold gel packs become stiff, making it challenging for them to conform to irregular body surfaces such as the ankle. This causes an uneven transfer of energy, predisposing bony prominences to a greater cooling effect than other areas. During treatment, cold gel packs warm more quickly than an ice bag, ice massage, or cold immersion bath. In fact, most packs are unable to maintain the necessary treatment temperature long enough to produce all the desired cryotherapy effects. The use of these packs can also cause tissue damage due to the pack's initial treatment temperature being equivalent to the temperature of the freezer in which it was stored. For the typical home freezer, this is usually 10°F, and anything placed directly on the skin at this temperature will damage tissue (Fig. 6.8). If this form of cryotherapy is used, advise patients to place a thin, wet barrier between the gel pack and the skin[20,24] (Fig. 6.9).

To prevent tissue damage, advise patients to place a thin, wet barrier between a cold gel pack and the skin.

Many primary health care providers advise patients to use items found in the average household freezer, such as a bag of frozen peas, for use as a cryotherapy modality. Indeed, such frozen foods conform well to the body and work better than chemical gel packs. If patients use this treatment method, be sure to advise them to place a thin, wet barrier between the package and the skin because, as with chemical gel packs, frozen foods are used at a treatment temperature that has the potential to harm the skin.[24]

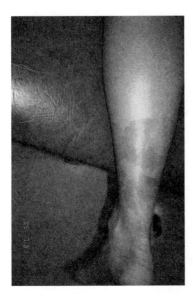

FIGURE 6.8 Tissue damage resulting from applying a commercial gel pack directly to the skin.

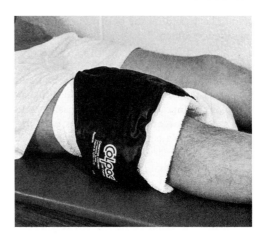

FIGURE 6.9 Commercial cold gel pack applied to the thigh. Note that a barrier is placed between the pack and the skin. From Michlovitz and Nolan: *Modalities for Therapeutic Intervention*, 4th ed. 2005. Philadelphia: F.A. Davis Company, Fig. 3-7B, pg 54, with permission.

Contraindications and Precautions

As with any modality, relevant precautions must be taken before prescribing cryotherapy for patients. For example, instruct patients to watch for signs, such as the development of blisters, that indicate that the treatment should be terminated. However, be aware that the discomfort most people experience with cold application differs vastly from a tissue-damaging situation. Use caution when applying cold to people older than 60 years because these patients experience a reduced vasoconstriction response when exposed to cold. Elderly patients also have a dulled sensitivity to decreases in air temperature. This may reduce an older person's ability to recognize adverse affects of a cryotherapy treatment.[25,26]

Contraindications include areas of decreased circulation and decreased sensation. In addition, do not use cryotherapy for patients with a known hypersensitivity to cold, such as **cold urticaria** or **cold erythema**. Recognize, however, that many people do not realize they suffer from such sensitivity until they receive their first cryotherapy treatment. Fortunately, the welts and hives associated with cold urticaria usually remain local and disappear after treatment is terminated. However, a systemic reaction resulting in respiratory distress and unconsciousness could occur, particularly if a cold treatment is allowed to continue after hives and welts have developed. Children are more likely to develop cold erythema because they are more sensitive to cold than are adults.[1,16,17]

In addition to cold hypersensitivities, vasospastic disorders, such as **Raynaud's phenomenon,** can result from the application of cold to the body. Furthermore, if cold is applied inappropriately over nerves that lie close to the body's surface, neuropathies can result, sometimes with devastating affects.

Raynaud's Phenomenon

Raynaud's phenomenon most commonly happens to the hands, feet, nose, and ears. The blood flow restriction associated with this condition results in a blue, gray, or purplish discoloration of the skin and is usually accompanied by burning, tingling, or numbness. This condition can be transient and is more common in women and people younger than 40 years. Patients who experience Raynaud's phenomenon cannot keep cold on the body long enough for the treatment to produce the desired therapeutic effects.[16,17]

Superficial Nerve Neuropathies

Superficial nerves are especially vulnerable to injury from cold because these structures lack the surrounding soft tissues that protect deeper nerves. These nerves are especially vulnerable when compression is used in conjunction with an ice bag or cold gel pack because this increases both the pressure on the nerve and the rate of nerve cooling, causing neuralgia (discussed in Chapter 1). Although cold can injure any superficial nerve, the nerves most at risk are the common peroneal (fibula head), ulna (medial elbow epicondyle), and lateral femoral cutaneous (lateral hip). Symptoms of nerve palsy include decreased strength of the muscles innervated by the involved nerve and paresthesia over the area served by the nerve's afferent component. Usually symptoms are transient, but they can be permanent.[1,27]

If the condition being treated requires the use of an ice bag with compression over the area of a superficial nerve, cover the region with a small cloth or layer of elastic wrap. Decrease the amount of pressure placed over the area when applying the compression wrap. Refer any incidence of neuropathy to a neurologist for further evaluation.

When applying an ice pack treatment in the area of a superficial nerve, cover the region with a small cloth or layer of elastic wrap to prevent a neuropathy from developing.

Superficial Thermotherapy

As with cryotherapy, the use of superficial thermotherapy for the treatment of musculoskeletal injury is quite extensive. Just as most primary health care providers equate treatment of acute injury with cold, they also associate the treatment of chronic conditions with heat. Whereas this thinking may not do justice to the scope cryotherapy plays in the management of musculoskeletal injury, it is much more accurate for the role heat plays in the treatment process.

Physiological Effects on Human Tissue

The physiological effects thermotherapy has on human tissue are, for the most part, the exact opposite of those effects produced by cryotherapy (Table 6.1). Because thermotherapy produces effects such as vasodilation and increased cell metabolism, the application of heat is contraindicated for the treatment of acute musculoskeletal injury. Shared effects include a reduction in pain and muscle spasm. Factors that affect a thermotherapy modality's ability to produce these physiological effects include the intensity of the treatment, the amount of adipose tissue in the treatment area, and the duration of the treatment.[9,14]

For the physiological benefits of heat therapy to occur, the intensity of the treatment must be between 104° and 112°F. If the treatment temperature is less than 104°F, the desired effects do not occur, because at lower temperatures the body is able to dissipate heat faster than the target tissue can absorb the energy. The net result is a useless treatment. In contrast, if the treatment temperature rises above 112°F, the body is unable to dissipate the heat quickly enough to protect the tissue from harm. This results in tissue damage that manifests itself as a superficial burn.[28,29]

The temperature range for superficial thermotherapy is between 104° and 112°F.

Like cryotherapy, the amount of adipose tissue in the treatment area directly influences the effectiveness of a superficial thermotherapy treatment, because heat produced by superficial modalities penetrates the body to a depth of only 1 inch. Contrary to cryotherapy, increasing treatment time for people with excessive subcutaneous fat does not make the treatment more effective. Nevertheless, a superficial heat treatment can still be recommended for people with 1 inch or more of subcutaneous fat over the injured tissue, because these patients can benefit from the analgesic effect of heat therapy. In addition, underlying injured tissue may be heated indirectly if it is in direct contact with overlying adipose tissue. However, without producing effects such as increased capillary permeability, cell metabolism, and lymph flow, superficial thermotherapy is ineffective in aiding the healing process.[28,29]

Treatment Parameters

Treat patients for 20 minutes with all modes of superficial thermotherapy treatment described below. By 20 minutes, the physiological effects of heat occur, and after 20 minutes, in the case of some moist heat modalities, the modality has most likely cooled to the point where it is no longer transmitting heat to the body. Although multiple treatments can be performed over the course of a day, prescribe only one treatment per day, because the use of thermotherapy should occur in conjunction with rehabilitative exercises. This prolongs the total amount of time needed to complete a proper home care management program.[29]

Apply superficial thermotherapy treatment 20 minutes per day.

Patient Education

Review with patients the normal sensations associated with thermotherapy treatment. Tell patients they should feel uniform warmth throughout the treatment area. Instruct them to remove the modality if it becomes too hot. Emphasize that "if it feels like it's burning, it's burning." Teach patients how to inspect the skin periodically throughout the treatment. Erythema of the skin is a normal response that spreads evenly around the treatment area. If any other response occurs, such as **mottling**, advise the patient to discontinue treatment immediately, because this a precursor to a burn. Approximately 10 minutes into the treatment, the warmth originally felt by the patient slowly disappears. This is a normal response as the body accommodates to, or gets used to, the treatment temperature. Explain that the treatment is still working and advise the patient not to add additional heat during this period. Increasing the intensity of the treatment during this period of accommodation subsequently increases the risk of a superficial burn.

Modes of Application

Though there are many ways to administer a superficial thermotherapy treatment, in general, the use of moist heat is recommended because it is more effective than dry heat at transmitting energy to the target tissue. This discussion is limited to those superficial thermotherapy modalities most used in the clinical setting and implemented as part of home treatment programs.[29]

Moist heat works better than dry heat in providing the physiological benefits of thermotherapy.

Moist Heat

The use of a moist heat pack is a highly versatile and easy-to-use method of applying superficial thermotherapy to the body (Fig. 6.10). When applying this treatment, advise patients to purchase a moist heat pack from a drug, sports, or surgical supply store. Have them place the pack in a pot of water at 170°F for 30 minutes. Instruct them to remove and wrap the pack in six to eight layers of towels. The towel-wrapped pack is then placed on the injured area. Patients should place the pack on the body and not place the body on the pack, because placing the body on the pack increases the risk of burning.

Another way to perform a moist heat treatment is with warm immersion. As with cold immersion, instruct the patient to fill a bucket large enough to cover the treatment area with warm water between 104° and 112°F. Instruct the patient to sit

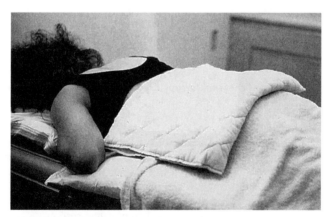

FIGURE 6.10 Moist hot pack application to the low back.
From Michlovitz and Nolan: *Modalities for Therapeutic Intervention,* 4th ed. 2005. Philadelphia: F.A. Davis Company, Fig. 4-6, pg 68, with permission.

in a comfortable position and immerse the body part so that the injured area is fully submerged. ROM exercises can be performed in the water during the treatment. Advise that the patient keep a towel available to dry the extremity after the treatment.

Dry Heat

Traditionally, prescribing the use of an electric heating pad has been popular among primary health care providers when developing a home care management program for patients with musculoskeletal injury. More recently, commercially made gel and bead packs, which can be heated in a microwave oven, have become options for both patients and providers. Average household items, such as rice wrapped in a cloth bag, can also be heated and used as a form of dry heat. Indeed, the use of rice in this capacity can be cheaper and potentially safer than using a commercial product.

When advising patients to use dry heat, do so cautiously because heating pads can easily cause a superficial burn if the unit's intensity is set too high or if the pad is left on too long, a scenario that typically happens when a patient falls asleep with the unit on. The same concern regarding superficial burns holds true for commercial and homemade heating packs—though unlike an electric heating pad, these modalities cool over time, making it unlikely to cause a superficial burn by leaving it on the body for too long.

Contraindications and Precautions

Contraindications to thermotherapy treatment are presented in Box 6.1. Use caution when treating diabetics, the elderly, and the very young, because these populations may be more sensitive to the application of heat to the body. In these instances, decrease treatment intensity and monitor the patient's reaction to the treatment. In addition, for all patients, decrease treatment intensity when treating areas of new skin growth, such as developing scars. The chance of burning the skin with thermotherapy is much greater than the chance of frostbiting the skin with cryotherapy. Thus, use more caution when prescribing thermotherapy. Never apply heat to an injury while it is in the reactive phase of the inflammation process.

Never apply heat to an acute injury, and use caution when treating diabetics, the elderly, and the very young.

 BOX 6.1
AREAS OF THE BODY AND CONDITIONS WHERE THE USE OF THERMOTHERAPY IS CONTRAINDICATED

Genitals	Acute injuries
Eyes	Tumors
Pregnant abdomen	Bleeding disorders
Areas of decreased sensation	Previously burned areas
Areas of decreased circulation	

Contrast Therapy

Managing musculoskeletal injury with **contrast therapy** entails switching between heat and cold modalities during a single treatment session. Although this method of treating musculoskeletal injury has been widely used for many years, its efficacy has come under scrutiny, which has led to a decrease in its use.[30,31]

Historically, the primary reason health care providers prescribed contrast treatments was to reduce swelling by vasodilating (hot) and vasoconstricting (cold) blood vessels, thus causing a "pumping"-type action within the area. However, as discussed in Chapter 5, this is not how the body removes swelling from an injured area, making contrast therapy ineffective for this purpose. Though contrast treatment has also reportedly been used to facilitate early movement in joints, to stimulate circulation, and as an aid in healing, its effectiveness for these purposes is also unsubstantiated.[30,31] So, the question arises, Why prescribe contrast as a treatment modality? Does it do any good? As with all physical interventions, the answer depends on the goal of the treatment.

Because heat and cold both have an analgesic effect on the body, contrast therapy can be an effective pain relief modality. It is theorized that contrast therapy relieves pain by stimulating more afferent nerve fibers as compared with treating the injury with just cold or just heat. However, contrast therapy should never be prescribed for pain control in the acute stage of injury, because this is a major contraindication for the application of heat. Contrast treatments also work well as patients transition from the acute stage of injury to the subacute and chronic injury stages. By monitoring the body's reaction during contrast sessions, the tissues' ability to safely progress from cryotherapy to thermotherapy treatments can be gauged.[30,31]

Never prescribe a contrast treatment for an injury still in the reactive phase of healing.

When using contrast therapy, initially prescribe a long period of cold treatment followed by a short period of heat treatment, such as a starting ratio of 4 minutes of cold to 1 minute of heat (4:1). When using contrast to transition a patient from cryotherapy to thermotherapy, with each passing treatment, slowly phase out the use of cryotherapy by decreasing the amount of time designated for the cold cycle and increasing the amount designated for the hot cycle. Though any heat and cold modality can be used, cold and warm baths are the easiest modalities to alternate. They also allow the patient to perform ROM exercises during the treatment.

Pharmacotherapy

Management of pain and inflammation that accompany musculoskeletal injury is complex, requiring far more than a variation on the old cliché, "Take two aspirin and call me in the morning." Patients have reasonable expectations that pain and discomfort can be relieved, and they are entitled to safe, evidenced-based care. When a patient experiences musculoskeletal pain, carefully reflect upon all therapeutic options available.

It is important that appropriate nonpharmacological treatments be immediately employed for patients who present with musculoskeletal injury. When needed, pharmacological agents can be used to complement these treatments.

In most instances, prescribing nonopioid analgesics is the primary health care provider's treatment of choice when drug therapy is indicated for mild to moderate pain. By and large, these include the NSAIDs and acetaminophen. At times, opioids are required to obtain effective analgesia, particularly in instances of severe pain.

NSAIDs

Available both over the counter (OTC) and by prescription, NSAIDs are among the most commonly used drugs in the United States. As a class, they have analgesic, anti-inflammatory, and antipyretic properties, though not all NSAIDs are used for all of these actions. The NSAID class of drugs has long been the mainstay in the management of pain and inflammation associated with musculoskeletal injury.[32,33]

Types of NSAIDs

NSAIDs are divided into two classifications: selective and nonselective. Of the nonselective NSAIDs currently on the market, acetylsalicylic acid, or aspirin, is arguably the best known. First introduced in the late 19th century, the effects aspirin has on the human body have been well studied. At one time, aspirin was commonly used and prescribed for musculoskeletal injury. Today, competition from newer, nonselective NSAIDs has decreased the use of aspirin among adults and children. This is largely because the newer NSAIDs have a slightly lower risk of causing gastrointestinal (GI) bleeding in adults and are not related to the development of **Reye's syndrome** in children. However, unlike other nonselective NSAIDs, aspirin is not highly protein bound, making it safer to use with other highly protein-bound drugs, such as phenytoin. In addition, aspirin is commonly the NSAID of choice for the elderly because it is safe to use with many medications used heavily by this population.[33-35]

Of the newer, nonselective NSAIDs, ibuprofen use has increased the most. Considered potentially the least damaging to the GI mucosa, ibuprofen is commonly recommended for treatment of acute musculoskeletal trauma. The use of naproxen has also increased over the past few decades. Available only in prescription strengths through the 1980s, the increase in use of both ibuprofen and naproxen is somewhat linked to their current availability as OTC medications.[33,35-38]

Ibuprofen and naproxen are popular nonselective **OTC NSAIDs** used to treat musculoskeletal injury.

Given the removal of selective NSAIDs from the market in the recent past, celecoxib (Celebrex) is the only selective NSAID currently available. It is prescribed for patients who require long-term NSAID use or are at risk for GI bleeding. However, use of this medication may increase the risk for cardiovascular (CV) events and potentially life-threatening GI bleeding. Consistent with 2005 U.S. Food and Drug Administration (FDA) actions, Celebrex remains on the market with boxed warnings about these potential risks and the need for close monitoring. Also in 2005, the FDA revised the labeling requirements for all prescription NSAIDs. This included the addition of boxed warnings highlighting the increased risk of CV events and the potentially life-threatening GI bleeding associated with the use of these drugs. The FDA also revised the labeling of OTC NSAIDs to include more specific information about the potential GI and CV risks. Recommendations for use of NSAIDs are in constant flux and continually updated.[39,40]

NSAIDs' Mode of Action

NSAIDs decrease pain by inhibiting the release of cyclooxygenase (COX), a necessary component of the prostaglandin inflammatory cascade. As explained in Chapter 5, musculoskeletal trauma initiates the release of prostaglandins and is partially responsible for stimulating nociceptive free nerve endings. Two forms of COX exist. COX-1 is responsible for prostaglandin "housekeeping" functions in the body, such as maintenance of the gastrointestinal mucosa. COX-2 is responsible for prostaglandin's inflammatory response. Nonselective NSAIDs affect both COX-1 and COX-2, whereas selective NSAIDs inhibit COX-2 only. Thus, nonselective NSAIDs exert analgesic and anti-inflammatory effects, but because they inhibit COX-1, they also have a number of adverse drug reactions (ADRs). As alluded to previously, their most notable ADRs are GI irritation and bleeding. When selective COX-2 inhibitors were introduced, they were touted as agents that could decrease pain and inflammation while eliminating GI concerns. This has not been the case, because COX-2 agents are associated with lessened GI bleeding, not the absence of GI bleeding.[33,35]

NSAID Adverse Drug Reactions

For many patients with chronic musculoskeletal and inflammatory conditions, such as osteoarthritis and rheumatoid arthritis, selective NSAIDs provide pain relief and decrease inflammation. Yet the removal of most selective NSAIDs from the market and the increased monitoring of Celebrex indicate that these drugs carry a serious risk profile. Box 6.2 lists the ADRs for both selective and nonselective NSAIDs. Although many of these reactions are rare, the absolute numbers can be large given the frequent use of these drugs. Furthermore, because older adults are more likely than younger people to seek relief from chronic musculoskeletal pain, NSAID use increases with age, just when comorbidities increase the likelihood of adverse reactions. A comprehensive list of known risk factors for NSAID ADRs is given in Box 6.3.[33,36,37,40,41]

BOX 6.2
ADVERSE DRUG REACTIONS FOR SELECTIVE AND NONSELECTIVE NSAIDS

Dyspepsia	Hypertension
Bleeding	Sodium retention with resultant fluid
Hepatitis	overload
Hypertension	Stevens-Johnson syndrome
Hepatic injury	Toxic epidermal necrolysis
Renal impairment	Cardiovascular events
Acute renal failure	Central nervous system abnormalities

BOX 6.3
KNOWN RISK FACTORS FOR **NSAID** ADVERSE DRUG REACTIONS

Age >60 years	Taking in combination with other
Hypertension	NSAIDs
History of GI bleeding	Warfarin or diuretics
Consuming 3 or more alcoholic	Heart disease
drinks per day	Kidney disease
Steroid use	

GI = gastrointestinal.

Because **NSAID** use increases with age, the potential for **NSAID**
adverse drug reactions in this population is increased.

Controversies Surrounding NSAID Use in Musculoskeletal Injury

In addition to the concerns surrounding ADRs, within the past 20 years, the efficacy of prescribing NSAIDs in the early stages of acute musculoskeletal trauma has come under scrutiny. As discussed in Chapter 5, inflammation is part of the healing process. When it is suppressed, healing is affected. Current research suggests that because NSAIDs interfere with the inflammatory process, early management of acute musculoskeletal injury with these medications may delay the rate at which soft tissues regenerate. Other concerns with early NSAID intervention include long-term decreases in the overall tensile strength of the involved tissue and increasing the potential of developing persistent pain. Ironically, the initial pain and swelling associated with acute musculoskeletal trauma responds positively to early NSAID intervention. Thus, using NSAIDs soon after injury occurrence may allow the patient to return to sport participation earlier than would be possible if NSAID treatment were not used. Unfortunately, following this course of action may interfere with providing the injured area with an optimal healing environment and may lead to long-term difficulties. Given the option, many patients involved in competitive athletics would rather be treated with NSAIDs early in the inflammatory process if it means they may return to participation sooner.[33,42–44]

Acetaminophen

Like NSAIDs, acetaminophen is a commonly used OTC medication. It is an analgesic and antipyretic but lacks anti-inflammatory properties because it is a weak central prostaglandin inhibitor. Historically, this limitation contributed to NSAIDs becoming the medication of choice immediately after musculoskeletal trauma. Although acetaminophen is regarded as safe for most patients because it is not likely to cause GI bleeding, it does come with its own limitations. Recent evidence suggests that, when the acetaminophen dose nears the maximum-allowed 4000-mg/d level, its GI toxicity potential approaches that of NSAIDs. Also, at doses above 4000 mg/d, acetaminophen is hepatotoxic and can cause liver failure. When used at maximal dose or when used chronically, it can also cause renal damage similar to that seen with NSAID use. Thus, patients who use acetaminophen must be closely monitored, particularly if the dose prescribed nears the maximum allowed; if the patient uses the drug for an extended period; or if the patient has a history of alcohol consumption, which increases the risk for liver failure. Also, minimize acetaminophen use in the treatment of bone and cartilage injury because some evidence indicates that suppressing central prostaglandins delays bone and cartilage healing, increasing the time for fractures to heal.[33,35,36,38,41,45]

Opioids

Used to relieve moderate to severe pain, opioids are natural and synthetic substances that act on the brain to decrease the perception of pain. They are most commonly used to manage chronic pain, and although their role in this process is important, it is controversial.

Opioids provide pain relief through their action on endogenous opioid peptide receptors present in the central and peripheral nervous system. Three opioid receptors exist: mu, delta, and kappa. Most therapeutic actions take place through agonist actions at the mu receptors. The FDA "schedule three" opioids (codeine, hydrocodone, propoxyphene, and oxycodone) are most commonly used for pain relief and are frequently used in combination with acetaminophen or ibuprofen. Of these opioids, hydrocodone and oxycodone provide the most effective pain relief, whereas codeine and propoxyphene are the least effective. In fact, acetaminophen administered by itself provides similar analgesic benefits when compared with codeine and propoxyphene. Acetaminophen is also a safer medication than those within the opioid class of drugs.[34,35]

In contrast to NSAIDs and acetaminophen, one benefit of using opioids is that they lack a ceiling effect. This means that the dose can be increased as needed to produce necessary analgesia. Any decision to titrate the dose upward must be balanced against the ADRs associated with opioids (Box 6.4). In addition, opioids that are used in combination drugs require even more careful monitoring for toxicity because safe doses of acetaminophen and NSAIDs, taken in conjunction with a combination drug, must be factored in before prescribing such opioids. Combining prescription levels of these medications with OTC dosages would most likely exceed safe dosage recommendations.[34,35]

Tolerance may develop both to the analgesic effects of opioids and to most of the ADRs, but tolerance does not develop to the constipating effects of opioids. Thus, increased fiber and water intake must be recommended for patients taking opioids. For patients who experience severe constipation for extended periods, prescribe stool softeners and stimulant laxatives, but do so cautiously because these can lead to **lazy bowel syndrome**. For those requiring long-term use of opioids, tolerance and physical dependence are concerns that must be considered. In contrast, addiction to opioids

BOX 6.4
ADVERSE DRUG REACTIONS FOR OPIOIDS

Respiratory depression	Vomiting
Central nervous system depression	Itching
Nausea	Constipation

prescribed for pain relief is extremely rare, making addiction less of a concern in these instances. However, the possibility of drug diversion is occasionally a legitimate concern, but proceed with caution before making assumptions about patients.[46,47]

Determining Drug and Dosage

Given the variety of analgesics and anti-inflammatory medications currently on the market, and taking into account the controversies and adverse affects surrounding certain drugs, determining which agent to prescribe for someone with an acute or chronic musculoskeletal injury can be challenging. However, based on current knowledge, prescribing NSAIDs in the initial stages of musculoskeletal injury should be avoided so the initial stages of the inflammatory process can proceed unabated. Thus, use acetaminophen for pain control until the reactive phase of the inflammatory process has subsided. If the patient responds well to acetaminophen, consider staying with this medication instead of automatically substituting an NSAID or other agent even after healing enters the repair and regeneration stage.[36,38,41]

PEARL

Prescribe acetaminophen, not anti-inflammatory medications, during the reactive phase of acute musculoskeletal injury.

Initially treat adult patients with musculoskeletal injury with 1000 mg acetaminophen every 6 hours. If pain relief is inadequate and the patient can tolerate an NSAID, prescribe an NSAID, such as ibuprofen (600 to 800 mg every 8 hours), after the reactive phase of healing has ended. Table 6.3 provides a synopsis of dosage recommendations for acetaminophen, ibuprofen, and naproxen. These recommendations include using these medications at the lowest possible dose for the shortest period of time.[32,35]

For patients who do not respond to the above treatment, prescribe an agent that combines hydrocodone and acetaminophen to decrease pain. This combination can also be used for patients who are unable to tolerate NSAIDs. Further evaluation and treatment with other drugs, including stronger opioids, and referral to a pain specialist may be

TABLE 6.3 Recommended NSAID and acetaminophen dosage	
DRUG	**DOSAGE**
Acetaminophen (i.e., Tylenol)	Adult: 1000 mg q6h Maximum: 4000 mg/24 h Children: use children or junior form
Ibuprofen (i.e., Advil, Motrin)	Adult: 600–800 mg q8h Maximum: 2400 mg/24 h Children: use children or junior form
Naproxen (i.e., Aleve, Naprosyn)	Adult: 250–500 mg q12h Maximum: 1376 mg/24 h Children: use children or junior form

needed if these analgesics do not provide adequate relief. Prescribe celecoxib in instances where long-term maintenance is needed for pain and inflammation.[35]

During the entire process of deciding the best agent to prescribe for someone with an acute or chronic musculoskeletal injury, keep in mind that NSAID-related GI bleeding is estimated to cause about 17,500 deaths per year in those receiving long-term therapy. When long-term NSAID use is warranted, particularly in high-risk populations, protecting the GI tract is essential. Achieve this protection by suggesting that patients take an OTC proton pump inhibitor, such as omeprazole (Prilosec). If this proves ineffective, use prescription medications, such as misoprostol (Cytotec). Be aware that H2-receptor antagonists have not proved beneficial in this regard. These combinations are considered at least as effective as the COX-2 inhibitors alone, and they do not carry the increased risk of unwanted cardiac events. Choosing the correct NSAID and GI protectant can be complicated by cost, tolerability, comorbidities, and differing patient responses necessitating an individualized approach to care.[35-37,47]

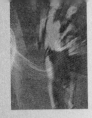

CASE STUDY
Therapeutics After Musculoskeletal Injury

SCENARIO

A 21-year-old male college senior presents to the student health clinic reporting ankle pain of about 18 hours' duration. He says he injured his ankle last night playing a game of pickup basketball with his friends. He states that he landed wrong after a layup shot and felt his left ankle twist under him. He heard a popping sound and immediately experienced pain and disability. He hobbled off the court, "walked off" the pain, and returned to play about 10 minutes later. He played for an additional 15 minutes, at which time play concluded. Afterward, he returned to his dorm room and placed ice on his ankle for about 20 minutes. He then went to a local bar with his friends. He reports having had 5 beers before returning to his dorm. He states that he "slept just fine." When he awoke this morning, his left ankle was very swollen, painful, and discolored. He went to his 10 o'clock class because he had to go, but he is now in to see you because of this injury.

PERTINENT HISTORY

Medications: No routine medications. Took two extra-strength acetaminophen (500 mg each) last night for pain and two ibuprofen (200 mg each) when he got out of bed to go to class this morning.

Family History: Paternal grandfather aged 66 with type 2 diabetes and cardiovascular disease. Otherwise no significant family illnesses reported.

PERSONAL HEALTH HISTORY

Tobacco Use: Denies smoking cigarettes or using oral tobacco.

Recreational Drugs: Denies use.

Alcohol Intake: Drinks about 9 to 10 beers per week. States that drinking 5 beers on one occasion, as on the previous night, is usual for him.

Caffeinated Beverages: 1 to 2 regular colas per day.

Exercise: Plays pickup basketball with friends twice a week and is on the college track-and-field team. Practice will start in 2 weeks.

Past Medical History: Generally healthy. Mononucleosis at age 16 and chicken pox at age 5.

PERTINENT PHYSICAL EXAMINATION

On physical examination, his left ankle is moderately swollen around the lateral malleolus. The site is also discolored and is so tender to palpation that he does not want you to touch the area. Because of the amount of pain he is experiencing, you are not able to perform the usual special/stress tests (described in Chapter 8) used to test the integrity of the underlying structures. He can engage in partial weight-bearing, but he walks with a pronounced limp.

(case study continues on page 156)

CASE STUDY
Therapeutics After Musculoskeletal Injury (continued)

RED FLAGS FOR THE PRIMARY HEALTH CARE PROFESSIONAL TO CONSIDER

- Basketball is commonly associated with ankle sprains. The physical examination is consistent is with a grade 2 ankle sprain.
- A popping sound may be associated with a fracture and would indicate a need for an ankle x-ray series.
- With this ankle injury, he should not participate in track-and-field practice.
- Excessive alcohol consumption while taking acetaminophen is contraindicated.

RECOMMENDED PLAN

- Immobilize the ankle.
- Obtain an ankle x-ray series to rule out fracture.
- Fit with crutches and teach a three-point walking gait as described in PTH 6.1.
- Provide the patient with the following information in writing by using PTH 6.2.

  Treat with PRICE for at least 72 hours. Crushed or flaked ice works best. Cycle ice treatments as follows: 30 minutes on, 1 to 2 hours off. Apply a compression wrap and instruct the patient to keep it on at all times during waking hours. Tell him to elevate the extremity above the level of the heart as much as possible. Advise the patient to elevate his mattress during sleep. Recommend 1000 mg acetaminophen q6h for up to 48 hours for pain. Be sure he knows how to properly apply PRICE and that he understands what the normal and unwanted outcomes of applying compression and ice to the body are. Make sure that he understands that it is not safe to drink more than 3 alcoholic beverages per day while taking acetaminophen. Also, explain to him not to take more than 8 acetaminophen capsules in a 24-hour period.

- Advise a follow-up visit in 3 days for reevaluation. If he should experience problems over the weekend, tell him to report to the local hospital emergency room for evaluation and treatment.
- Alert the college's certified athletic trainer regarding the situation. After your follow-up visit, refer to the athletic trainer for further treatment and rehabilitation.

REFERENCES

1. Knight KL. *Cryotherapy in Sport Injury Management.* Champaign, IL: Human Kinetics, 1995.
2. Merrick MA, Knight KL, Ingersoll CD, et al. The effects of ice and compression wraps on intramuscular temperature at various depths. *J Athl Train* 1993;28:236.
3. Knight KL. Effects of hypothermia on inflammation and swelling. *Athl Train J Nat Athl Train Assoc* 1976;11:7.
4. Merrick MA, Rankin JM, Andres FA, et al. A preliminary examination of cryotherapy and secondary injury in skeletal muscle. *Med Sci Sports Exerc* 1999;31:1516.
5. Knight KL, Aquino J, Johannes SM, et al. A re-examination of Lewis' cold induced vasodilation—in the finger and the ankle. *Athl Train J Nat Athl Train Assoc* 1980;15:238.
6. Yuka S. Effect of local application of cold or heat for relief of pricking pain. *Nurs Health Sci* 2002;4:97.
7. Misasi S, Morin G, Kemler D, et al. The effect of a toe cap and bias on perceived pain during cold water immersion. *J Athl Train* 1995;30:49.
8. Ingersoll CD, Mangus BC. Sensations of cold reexamined: a study using the McGill pain questionnaire. *Athl Train J Nat Athl Train Assoc* 1991;26:240.
9. Dontigny R, Sheldon K. Simultaneous use of heat and cold in treatment of muscle spasm. *Arch Phys Med Rehabil* 1962;43:235.
10. Johnson J, Leider FE. Influence of cold bath on maximum handgrip strength. *Percept Mot Skills* 1977;44:323.
11. Baumert PW. Acute inflammation after injury: quick control speeds rehabilitation. *Postgrad Med* 1995;97(2):35.
12. Smith SF, Duell DJ, Martin BC. *Clinical Nursing Skills: Basic to Advanced Skills,* 6th ed. Saddle River, NJ: Pearson, 2004.
13. LaVelle BE, Snyder M. Differential conduction of cold through barriers. *J Adv Nurs* 1985;10:555.
14. Fick DS, Johnson JS. Resolving inflammation in active patients. *Phys Sportsmed* 1993;21(12):55.
15. Lewis T. Observations upon the reactions of the vessels of the human skin to cold. *Heart* 1930;15:177.
16. Baker R, Bell G. The effect of therapeutic modalities on blood flow in the human calf. *J Orthop Sports Phys Ther* 1991;13:23.
17. Grant A. Massage with ice (cryokinetics) in the treatment of painful conditions of the musculoskeletal system. *Arch Phys Med Rehabil* 1964;45:233.
18. Myrer JM, Myrer KA, Measom GJ, et al. Muscle temperature is affected by overlying adipose tissue when cryotherapy is administered. *J Athl Train* 2001;36:32.
19. Otte JW, Merrick MA, Ingersoll CD, et al. Subcutaneous adipose tissue thickness alters cooling time during cryotherapy. *Arch Phys Med Rehabil* 2002;83:1501.
20. Merrick, MA, Jutte LS, Smith ME. Cold modalities with different thermodynamic properties produce different surface and intramuscular temperatures. *J Athl Train* 2003;38:28.
21. Levy AS, Marmar E. The role of cold and compression dressings in the postoperative treatment of total knee arthroplasty. *Clin Orthop* 1993;297:174.
22. Zemke JE, Anderson JC, Guion WK, et al. Intramuscular temperature responses in the human leg to two forms of cryotherapy: ice massage and ice bag. *J Orthop Sports Phys Ther* 1998;27:301.
23. Myrer JM, Measom G, Fellingham GW. Temperature changes in the human leg during and after two methods of cryotherapy. *J Athl Train* 1998;33:25.
24. Chesterton LS, Foster NE, Ross L, et al. Skin temperature response to cryotherapy. *Arch Phys Med Rehabil* 2002;83:543.
25. Smolande J. Effect of cold exposure on older humans. *Int J Sports Med* 2002;23:86.
26. Taylor NA, Allsopp NK, Parkes DG. Preferred room temperature of young vs aged males: the influence of thermal sensation, thermal comfort, and affect. *J Gerontol A Biol Sci Med Sci* 1995;50:M216-M221.
27. Covington DB, Bassett FH. When cryotherapy injures: the danger of peripheral nerve damage. *Phys Sportsmed* 1993;21(3):78.

28. Kaul MP, Herring SA. Superficial heat and cold: how to maximize the benefits. *Phys Sportsmed* 1994;22(12):65.
29. Halvorson GA. Therapeutic heat and cold for athletic injuries. *Phys Sportsmed* 1990;18(5):87.
30. Higgins D, Kaminski TW. Contrast therapy does not cause fluctuations in human gastrocnemius intramuscular temperature. *J Athl Train* 1998;33:336.
31. Myrer JM, Draper DO, Durrant E. Contrast therapy and intramuscular temperature in the human leg. *J Athl Train* 1994;29:318.
32. Thornton JS. Pain relief for acute soft-tissue injuries. *Phys Sportsmed* 1997;25(10):108.
33. Stovitz SD, Johnson RJ. NSAIDs and musculoskeletal treatment: what is the clinical evidence? *Phys Sportsmed* 2003;31(1):35.
34. Nicholson B. Responsible prescribing of opioids for the management of chronic pain. *Drugs* 2003;63(1):17.
35. Sachs CJ. Oral analgesics for acute nonspecific pain. *Am Fam Physician* 2005;71(5):914.
36. Pincus T. Managing the patient with musculoskeletal pain. In: *A Practical Approach to the Patient With Chronic Musculoskeletal Pain*, a supplement to *Clinical Advisor* 2005;8(520):15.
37. Simon LS. NSAIDs: Therapeutic use and variability of response in adults. *Up to Date* 2005;13(2). Retrieved from: www.uptodate.com. Accessed 7/29/08.
38. Biederman RE. Pharmacology in rehabilitation: Nonsteroidal anti-inflammatory agents. *J Orthop Sports Phys Ther* 2005;35(6):356.
39. FDA Public Health Advisory. Safety of Vioxx . September 30, 2004. Retrieved from: http://www.fda.gov/cder/drug/infopage/vioxx/PHA_vioxx.htm. Accessed 7/29/08.
40. FDA Public Health Advisory. FDA announces important changes and additional warnings for COX-2 selective and non-selective non-steroidal anti-inflammatory drugs (NSAIDs). April 7, 2005. Retrieved from: http://www.fda.gov/cder/drug/advisory/COX2.htm. Accessed 7/29/08.
41. Simon LS. NSAIDs: overview of adverse effects. *Up to Date* 2005;13(2). Retrieved from: www.uptodate.com. Accessed 7/29/08.
42. Obremskyt WT, Seaber AV, Ribbeck BM, et al. Biomechanical and histologic assessment of a controlled strain injury treated with piroxicam. *Am J Sports Med* 1994;22:558.
43. Jarvinen M, Leto M, Sorvari T, et al. Effect of some anti-inflammatory agents on the healing of ruptured muscle. *J Sports Traumatol Rel Res* 1992;27:2.
44. Reynolds JF, Noakes TD, Schwellnus MP, et al. Non-steroidal anti-inflammatory drugs fail to enhance healing of acute hamstring injuries treated with physiotherapy. *S Afr Med J* 1995;85:517.
45. Ruane JJ. On the front line: providing optimal management of pain. In: *A Practical Approach to Pain Management: A Therapeutic Update*, a supplement to *Clinical Advisor* 2005;8(10):3.
46. Antoin H, Beasley RD. Opioids for chronic noncancer pain: tailoring therapy to fit the patient and the pain. *Postgrad Med* 2004;116(3):37.
47. Williams GW. Determining the appropriate use of Cox-2 inhibitors in pain management. In: *A Practical Approach to Pain Management: A Therapeutic Update*, a supplement to *Clinical Advisor* 2005;8(10):9.

SUGGESTED READINGS

Deal DN, Tipton J, Rosencrance E, et al. Ice reduces edema. *J Bone Joint Surg Am* 2002;84:1573.

Merrick MA. Secondary injury after musculoskeletal trauma: a review and update. *J Athl Train* 2002;37:209.

Sweet BV, Townsend KA, Tsai CY. Risk assessment of NSAID-induced gastrointestinal toxicity in ambulatory care patients. *Am J Health Syst Pharm* 2004;61:1917.

WEB LINKS

http://www.ampainsoc.org. Accessed 7/29/08.
   American Pain Association Web site providing extensive pain information, including clinical guidelines for pain management, pain issues in children, clinical trial research, and measurement of pain.

http://www.pain.com. Accessed 7/29/08.
   Provides pain information and resources for both patients and professionals. Has an excellent section on musculoskeletal pain. Also provides access to continuing education activities for health care professionals.

http://www.painmed.org. Accessed 7/29/08.
   American Academy of Pain Medicine Web site providing consumer information, links to pain-related Web sites, publications, and many other professional pain-related resources.

2

ORTHOPEDIC CONDITIONS

7

Introduction to Orthopedic Evaluation

● **Brian J. Toy, PhD, ATC**

he goals of the orthopedic evaluation are to arrive at a differential diagnosis and to decide on a proper management plan. These goals can be achieved by developing a systematic process for assessing musculoskeletal injury. Such a process is outlined here. Subsequent chapters within this section implement this assessment process for specific regions of the body and review the most common traumatic and nontraumatic musculoskeletal conditions resulting from sports participation. Thus, be sure to combine information presented in this chapter with the information in the chapter appropriate to the patient's specific injury when assessing a patient with an orthopedic condition.

The parts of the orthopedic evaluation include the following:

• History of the injury, including pain assessment
• Physical examination
  ◦ Observation
  ◦ Palpation
  ◦ Range-of-motion (ROM) and strength testing
  ◦ Special and stress testing
• Musculoskeletal imaging

Although in most situations all parts of the evaluation can be implemented, certain circumstances dictate that some portions be excluded. For example, in instances in which a patient has a suspected ankle sprain, it is usually safe to perform a complete evaluation. However, in cases in which an ankle fracture is suspected, the ROM and strength testing portions of the evaluation should be delayed until x-rays have been obtained. Certainly, the history, pain assessment, and observation portions of the orthopedic evaluation can be performed for most musculoskeletal conditions.

History

When assessing a musculoskeletal injury, collect subjective data from the patient before performing a physical examination. Doing so allows for the patient's chief symptom to be better understood and lets you formulate a plan of action before initiating the physical examination. Thus, the history portion of the evaluation supports the goal of arriving at a differential diagnosis and deciding on the best course of action.

History of the Injury

Start the orthopedic evaluation by obtaining a complete history of the injury. Inquire about the mechanism of injury and about the presence, quality, and duration of any symptoms. Make sure to listen closely to what the patient has to say, ask for clarification as necessary, and adequately document the patient's answers. Use the questions listed in Box 7.1 as a guide when performing this portion of the evaluation.

Because macrotrauma injuries usually result from single episodic events, patients will usually be very clear about how the injury occurred. For example, those with a severe muscle strain or a sudden tearing of a tendon often relate hearing an audible "pop" at the time of injury. In contrast, patients with microtrauma conditions typically find it difficult to pinpoint the exact cause of injury. Thus, the history portion of the evaluation for these

BOX 7.1
QUESTIONS TO ASK WHEN EVALUATING ORTHOPEDIC CONDITIONS

When did the injury occur?

How did the injury occur?

Was it a contact or noncontact injury?

Did the symptoms come on quickly or gradually?

What position was the body part in when the injury occurred?

If a lower extremity injury, was the foot planted on the ground/floor at the time of injury?

Did you hear any sounds, such as pop, snap, or crack, when the injury occurred?

Have you ever injured this body part before? If so, what was the injury and what was its outcome?

What did you do for treatment immediately after the injury?

What could you do physically immediately after the injury?

Did you return to activity after the injury?

Has it gotten better or worse since the injury occurred?

What aggravates the injury?

What activities can you do/not do?

- For the lower extremity: walking? running? jumping? ascending stairs? descending stairs?
- For the upper extremity: raising the hand above the head? throwing a ball?

patients may be more involved. For example, what the patient does outside of sports, such as excessive typing or use of a computer mouse, common in patients in the high school and collegiate settings, may be a contributing factor in a patient with **carpal tunnel syndrome** (described in Chapter 12). Also bear in mind that symptoms produced by overuse can manifest in a body region distant from the area where the pathology originates. For example, chronic back pain reported by a patient may be caused by a structural abnormality of the feet. In such cases, the patient may not be aware of the pathology. This might lead to a situation where the history does not reveal key data. In these instances, an extensive physical examination is needed to arrive at the proper diagnosis. For example, the patient with chronic back pain may require an assessment of the entire lower extremity. A holistic evaluation helps avoid a situation in which the symptoms (e.g., low back pain) are treated but the cause (e.g., structural abnormality of the feet) is not.

Pain Assessment

After the history portion of the examination is completed, evaluate the patient's pain using the well-known "PQRST" mnemonic[1]:

- P: provocation, precipitating and palliative factors. Ask the patient to identify those things that make the injury feel better (e.g., rest? ice? elevation? stretching?) or worse (e.g., walking? sitting?). Determine what, if any, nonpharmacological and pharmacological measures the patient has already employed to treat the pain.
- Q: quality/quantity of the pain. Ask what type pain the patient is experiencing (e.g., stabbing? aching? burning? stinging?). Establish how often the patient experiences the pain.

- R: region/radiation. Ask where the pain is located and, if applicable, to where it radiates.
- S: severity of the pain. Use the numerical rating scale (NRS), presented in Figure 7.1, to evaluate pain severity. Have the patient circle or state their perceived level of pain, with 0 being no pain and 10 being the worst pain imaginable. The NRS can also be used to evaluate the effect of nonpharmacological and pharmacological agents on decreasing the patient's pain.
- T: time. Ask how long the patient has been experiencing the pain and how long a typical episode lasts.

Physical Examination

Maintaining a comprehensive understanding of the anatomy for the region being assessed is necessary to correctly perform a musculoskeletal examination. As presented in Chapter 1, important anatomical structures include bones, muscles, tendons, ligaments, cartilage, fascia, bursae, nerves, and retinacula. A detailed review of relevant anatomy for each body region is presented at the beginning of each chapter in this section. In general, the specific portions of a musculoskeletal physical examination include

- observation,
- palpation,
- ROM and strength testing, and
- stress and special testing.

Observation

The observation portion of the examination starts with the inspection of the injured body part and surrounding region. Visually compare and contrast with contralateral areas, being sure to observe the entire region, not just the injured area. For example, inspect the entire upper extremity of a patient who reports wrist pain, because its cause may be originating from somewhere other than the wrist. Look for obvious signs of injury, such as deformity, swelling, ecchymosis, and erythema.

Observe the entire body in the anatomical position from anterior, posterior, and lateral views, noting bony malalignments of the extremities and of the axial skeleton. In most cases, more information can be gathered from a posterior view than from any other. Notice whether an injured body part is being supported, such as when a patient holds one upper extremity with the other in a sling position as shown in Figure 6.1 on page 129. Have the patient walk away from you and then toward you. Look for gait abnormalities or a favoring of the injured body part, such as limping or an irregular gait pattern. In general, these abnormalities are more noticeable when the patient

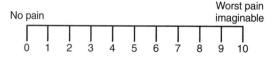

FIGURE 7.1 Pain numerical rating scale.

walks away from you. Complete the observation portion of the examination by viewing the injured body part from a seated position. Certain conditions may present differently in a non-weight-bearing position; document your findings before beginning palpation.

Palpation

Continue the physical examination by performing a systematic palpation of the region. To be able to make a comparison and to place the patient at ease, when you are able palpate the corresponding structures on the uninjured contralateral side first. When palpating, visualize the structures under your fingers to help determine what has been injured.

Palpate structures on the uninvolved side before evaluating
the involved area.

Palpate the involved region by starting several inches away from the site of injury and gently work toward the injured area. Doing so gains patient confidence and helps to assure that other injuries in the region are not overlooked. To avoid inflicting undo discomfort, which can cause patient apprehension, start with mild pressure, increasing the amount as the examination progresses. Note the presence of swelling, ecchymosis, calor, crepitus and/or muscle spasm, or defect in the region, because these signs are commonly associated with musculoskeletal injury. For example, a bulge of a muscle associated with muscle gapping immediately proximal or distal to the bulge is almost always present in patients with a second or third degree muscle strain (discussed in Chapter 1). Observe facial expressions and listen for patient feedback regarding pain and discomfort. Designate the site that produces the most pain as the area of point tenderness. This usually corresponds with the injury location.

Although no standard exists with regard to the order in which tissues are palpated, it is best to palpate bones first because bony point tenderness, bone clicking, and crepitus are signs of fracture. If a fracture is suspected early in the evaluation process, it is usually best to postpone the rest of the examination until x-rays of the region are obtained. An example of how to organize the palpation process is presented in Box 7.2.

Start the palpation portion of the physical examination by palpating
bones first.

BOX 7.2
ORDER IN WHICH STRUCTURES ARE PALPATED

Bones	Ligaments
Muscles	Other (bursae, nerves, retinacula)
Tendons	

Range-of-Motion and Strength Testing

In most instances, determining whether a joint's ROM and strength have been affected by injury can help you to formulate a differential diagnosis and management plan. Test ROM first because these findings reveal the range in which strength tests can be safely performed. When testing the extremities for ROM and strength, evaluate the uninvolved one first because doing so provides a baseline for comparison.

Test the **ROM** of a joint before strength testing the muscle groups that surround the joint.

Occasionally, it is not possible to test either ROM or strength. For example, neither ROM nor strength can be evaluated in a joint that has a significant amount of swelling, because the patient is usually in too much discomfort and/or is too apprehensive to allow for these assessments. Although this limits your ability to perform a complete examination, the simple fact that these functions cannot be evaluated is helpful information and can aid in determining how to manage the injury. When possible, evaluate ROM and strength as follows.

Range-of-Motion Testing

Evaluate the amount of primary motion present in a joint both actively and passively. Always test active ROM first because this revels the range in which a patient can safely move a joint. To test active ROM, have the patient move the uninjured contralateral joint through its range without assistance (Fig. 7.2). Then have the patient do the same for the injured joint. If a difference between the involved and uninvolved sides is observed, use a **goniometer** to measure the ROM in both joints (Fig. 7.3). Doing so allows you to objectively document the deficiency. Use these findings for comparison at follow-up visits and to track the effectiveness of treatment programs.

Test a joint's active **ROM** before testing the joint passively.

In certain instances, ROMs between involved and uninvolved joints should not be compared. For example, it may not be wise to compare the ROM of a recently injured

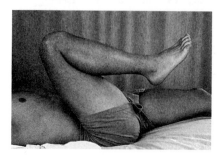

FIGURE 7.2 Active range-of-motion test for knee and hip flexion.
From Dillon: *Nursing Health Assessment: A Critical Thinking, Case Studies Approach.* 2003. Philadelphia: F.A. Davis Company, pg 630, with permission.

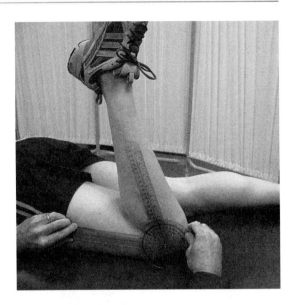

FIGURE 7.3 Using a goniometer to check knee flexion.

right elbow in a patient who presents with compromised ROM in the left elbow. In these cases, compare goniometer findings with normative ROM data. Also, use normative data to determine ROM deficits for nonpaired body regions, such as the cervical and lumbar regions. Normative ROM data for the major joints of the body are presented in each body region chapter in this section.

After testing active ROM, perform the same tests passively by asking the patient to relax the muscles in the region and then moving the joint through its range (Fig. 7.4). A passive ROM test may reveal deficiencies at the joint's extreme ranges not detectable by an active ROM test. When performing a passive ROM test, be careful when approaching the joint's extreme ranges, because going too far can cause pain and injury to the involved body part.

Strength Testing

After the amount of active and passive motion present is determined, test the strength of the muscle groups surrounding the joint. Although some providers test strength using resistance machines like those found in fitness and therapy centers, in the clinical setting the most practical method is through a **manual muscle test** (MMT). In an MMT, the patient moves a joint through its ROM against the examiner's resistance. Joint strength is determined by subjectively comparing the amount of force needed to resist the involved joint's motion with the amount of force needed to resist the same motion on the contralateral side.

To perform an MMT, apply resistance distal to the joint being tested and in a direction opposite the muscle group's line of pull. For example, when testing the strength of a patient's quadriceps (thigh) muscles, the primary knee extensors, push back on the tibia as the patient attempts to extend the knee from a seated position. Start the test by providing submaximal resistance during the beginning stages of motion. Then, increase resistance as the joint moves throughout its range until the

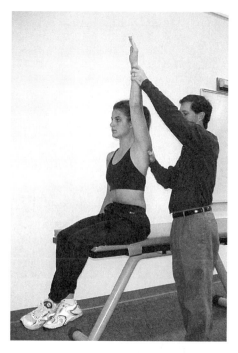

FIGURE 7.4 Passive range-of-motion test for shoulder flexion.
From Starkey and Ryan: *Evaluation of Orthopedic and Athletic Injuries,* 2nd ed. 2002. Philadelphia: F.A. Davis Company, Fig. 13-27A, pg 450, with permission.

maximal amount of resistance the joint can handle is determined. If the muscle group has been injured, decreases in strength are likely to be noted. In cases of a second or third degree muscle strain, an MMT typically accentuates muscle bulging and gapping associated with this injury. This is because as the test is performed, the proximal portion of the muscle contracts toward its bony origin, causing this portion of the muscle to bulge, leaving the distal, torn portion stationary. This produces a gap between the muscle's proximal and distal portions.[2,3]

Stress and Special Testing

Stress testing and special testing, two useful assessment tools, help determine the presence of injury and, in certain cases, the degree of injury. General considerations for their use are discussed here, whereas the specific tests for each body region are identified in the remaining chapters in this section. Initially, include all stress and special tests for a given body part in your evaluation. As you become more proficient in the orthopedic evaluation process, you will learn to choose the precise tests needed to help arrive at a differential diagnosis.

Incidentally, these tests require psychomotor skills that take time and practice to master. Become proficient in the administration of these tests before using them in the clinical setting.

Stress Testing

A stress test is an orthopedic evaluative technique used to determine the integrity of a joint's capsule and its associated ligaments. It is performed by applying force to the injured joint in a direction that mimics the way the original injury occurred. For example, as discussed in Chapter 1, a valgus force injures structures on the medial side. Thus, when using a valgus stress test to evaluate an injured joint's medial side, apply force laterally, because doing so mimics how the injury occurred. The amount of force needed when performing a stress test depends on the test being performed and the body part being tested. For example, to properly perform a valgus stress on the knee, as described in Chapter 9 and shown in Figure 9.10 on page 240, more force must be produced than what is required to properly perform a valgus stress test on the elbow, as described in Chapter 12 and shown in Figure 12.18 on page 379.

Stress tests are used to evaluate the integrity of ligaments and joint capsules and are administered by reproducing the mechanism of injury.

When testing the stability of a ligament, you need to determine the amount of joint laxity present. In other words, you need to decide whether any opening, or separation, of the bones that make up the joint is present. Do this by watching the reaction of the joint line and by palpating the joint line while performing the stress test. When stress is applied to a fully intact joint, no laxity and, thus, no joint opening occur. As the severity of the injury increases, the amount of joint laxity increases, which can be both seen and felt. Table 7.1 quantifies the amount of laxity present in first, second, and third degree ligament sprains (discussed in Chapter 1).

Swelling masks visible and palpable signs of joint laxity. Therefore, it is best to perform stress tests as soon as possible after the injury, before swelling develops. If a patient presents with significant swelling, wait a few days for it to subside before conducting a complete examination.

Perform stress tests as soon as possible after the injury, before swelling develops.

When performing stress tests, instruct the patient to relax all muscles surrounding the joint being tested, because muscle tension has the potential to affect the findings. For example, a contracted muscle or muscle group may prevent

TABLE 7.1 Grading the severity of ligament injury	
DEGREE OF INJURY	JOINT MOVEMENT, MM
First	<5
Second	5–10
Third	>10

you from seeing or properly feeling excessive joint laxity. This could lead to the determination that a ligament is healthy when, in fact, it is injured. This type of **false-negative** finding is a common mistake made by providers not experienced in orthopedic evaluation. Bear in mind that the inability of a patient to relax may be a sign that the patient is in pain and/or is apprehensive about being examined. In these cases, omit stress testing from the evaluation and rely on other findings to establish a differential diagnosis. Remember that stress testing comprises only one part of the evaluation, and a negative finding does not necessarily mean there is no injury. Always test the uninvolved extremity first and compare the findings with the contralateral side.

When administering a stress test, make sure all muscles surrounding
the joint are relaxed.

If it is determined that joint laxity exists, establish the type of **end-feel** present. Do this by gauging the type of resistance felt from the joint at the end of the test. A test that suddenly stops and does not allow the joint to be further separated has a firm end-feel. This occurs when the ligament's remaining, undamaged fibers stretch to their maximum length, verifying that at least part of the ligament is still intact. If this firm end-feel does not occur as further stress is applied, the joint keeps opening. This produces a soft, or mushy, end-feel, indicating that the ligament is no longer intact. This is indicative of a third degree sprain.

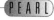

Determine the type of end-feel present in a joint with excessive laxity.

Special Testing

Special tests are used to determine whether nonligamentous structures, such as cartilage, nerves, muscles, or bones, are injured. They include a wide variety of tests unique to each body region, such as **McMurray's test** for meniscal tears of the knee (discussed in Chapter 9) and **Phalen's test** for carpal tunnel syndrome of the wrist (discussed in Chapter 12). Positive signs and symptoms associated with special tests include tingling, pain, clicking, popping, snapping, muscle weakness, and muscle tightness. The patient may also report these signs as symptoms during the history portion of the examination. As with stress tests, a negative finding is just one part of a complete evaluation, and does not necessarily rule out injury.

Special tests, used to determine whether nonligamentous structures
are injured, produce signs and symptoms such as tingling, pain,
clicking, popping, snapping, muscle weakness,
and muscle tightness.

Musculoskeletal Imaging

Diagnostic imaging plays a critical role in the assessment of musculoskeletal injury. Techniques available include **plain-film radiography, bone scan, computed tomography** (CT), and **magnetic resonance imaging** (MRI). However, determining which imaging test to order and when to order it can be a challenge for any health care provider. The intent of this section is not to make you an expert in these procedures. Rather, the goal is to provide enough information so that you know when and how to incorporate these techniques into the assessment process.

Plain-Film Radiography

The plain-film radiograph, otherwise known as a *standard radiograph, plain-film,* or *x-ray,* is the most common imaging technique used to evaluate orthopedic injury. In the primary care setting, it is usually the first test ordered after physical examination for patients with sports-related musculoskeletal trauma.

Plain-film radiography is the most common imaging technique used to evaluate musculoskeletal injury.

Radiographs are helpful for evaluating bone abnormalities such as dislocations and fractures, as well as avulsion injuries associated with tendons and ligaments. Although the bony attachments of these tissues are readily visible on x-ray, the bulk of these structures, and other soft tissues such as muscles and cartilage, do not show up well. Although obtaining an x-ray is indicated in many situations, remember that radiographic imaging should be pursued in conjunction with, and not in place of, a thorough musculoskeletal evaluation.[4-6]

Refer the patient for radiographs when the results of the evaluation suggest the possible presence of a bone abnormality. Indications for radiography include bony point tenderness, crepitus, or noted deformity as well as a recent history of traumatic injury. A routine radiographic examination entails the taking of at least two images, because a single image provides only a one-dimensional view of the structure. Adding a second image at a 90° angle to the first provides a three-dimensional view of the body part. Standard views include anteroposterior (or posteroanterior, depending on the body part) and lateral, with oblique and other views added to visualize joints (Fig. 7.5). Additional views include **stress radiographs,** which are taken while stress is applied to the joint. These views are helpful in confirming a clinical finding of a joint that is unstable as a result of ligament laxity.[4,7]

Although highly effective in revealing most bone abnormalities, plain-film radiography may not reveal all bone injuries. This is particularly true in cases of stress fractures. Whereas acute fractures appear quite readily on plain-film radiograph, in many instances it takes weeks, and sometimes months, for stress fractures to appear. When the clinical evaluation leads to a stress fracture being included as part of the differential diagnosis and when x-ray findings are negative, obtain a bone scan of the area.[4,7]

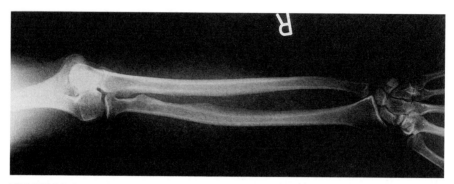

FIGURE 7.5 Anteroposterior radiograph view of the right forearm.
From McKinnis: *Fundamentals of Musculoskeletal Imaging*, 2nd ed. 2005. Philadelphia: F.A. Davis
Company, Fig. 3-25, pg 459, with permission.

Bone Scan

A bone scan is a nuclear imaging technique in which radioactive isotopes are injected
into the body. The isotopes are eventually absorbed by areas of bone that have been
compromised. The body is then scanned with a special x-ray film to identify areas
that show an increase in isotope uptake. Known as *hot spots*, these areas can be seen
as darkened spots on the scan and indicate regions of abnormal metabolic activity[4,7]
(Fig. 7.6).

   Although increased isotope uptake could be caused by any of a variety of abnormalities, in the case of sports-related injury it usually indicates a stress fracture.
Whereas a plain-film radiograph is typically unable to detect stress fractures for
several weeks or months after onset, a bone scan can identify the condition within a
few days. In addition, unlike other imaging techniques, a bone scan can precisely
locate the area of fracture. Nevertheless, because a bone scan cannot provide a definitive diagnosis, other reasons for an increase in isotope uptake, including metabolic
bone disease, metastatic tumor, infection, and avascular necrosis, should be considered. Combine the physical examination findings with bone scan results to form a
differential diagnosis.[4,7]

**A bone scan is the definitive diagnostic technique to detect
a stress fracture.**

Computed Tomography

Computed tomography scanning is a radiographic technique in which the radiography tube emits x-ray beams in a 360° circle around the patient's body, producing
image "slices" that are interpreted with computers. The images are three-dimensional,
and their resolution is much clearer than that of images produced by plain-film
radiography. Thus, CT allows for clearer identification of bone abnormality and, to
a lesser extent, musculoskeletal soft tissue injury. For these reasons, CT is usually
ordered when the results of plain-film radiography are inconclusive but physical

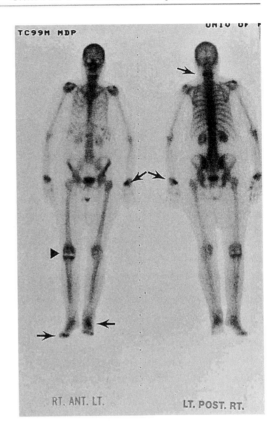

FIGURE 7.6 Whole-skeleton bone scan. Arrows indicate areas of increased isotope uptake.
From McKinnis: *Fundamentals of Musculoskeletal Imaging*, 2nd ed. 2005. Philadelphia: F.A. Davis Company, Fig. 1-37A, pg 34, with permission.

examination findings indicate the presence of pathology. It is also useful in demonstrating calcification formation.[4,7]

Magnetic Resonance Imaging

As its name indicates, MRI produces images from the interaction of a magnetic field with a radiofrequency signal. Whereas plain-film radiography and CT scanning expose the patient to ionizing radiation, MRI produces its images without radiation exposure. In addition, MRI creates images that are extremely detailed and are particularly effective in revealing differences between normal and injured soft tissues. MRI can also show interarticular lesions such as tears to the menisci of the knee. This makes MRI the preferred noninvasive technique for evaluating soft tissue injury, and it is used when soft tissue trauma is not detectable by either plain-film radiograph or CT scan.[4]

MRI is the preferred noninvasive imaging technique to evaluate soft tissue injury.

Although MRI can be used to determine whether a soft tissue is injured, it cannot reveal the degree of injury. Because MRI is limited in exposing fine bone detail and calcifications, the initial use of MRI is usually limited to soft tissue trauma. Furthermore, it should only be used after a complete musculoskeletal assessment has been performed and after plain-film radiographs have been obtained.[4-9]

REFERENCES

1. Brunton S. Approach to assessment and diagnosis of chronic pain. *J Fam Pract* 2004;53:S3.
2. Best TM, Garret WE. Hamstring strains: expediting return to play. *Phys Sportsmed* 1996;24(8):37.
3. Garrett WE. Muscle strain injuries. *Am J Sports Med* 1996;24:S2.
4. McKinnis LN. *Fundamentals of Musculoskeletal Imaging,* 2nd ed. Philadelphia, PA: FA Davis Co., 2005.
5. Onieal ME. Knee injuries: collateral ligament sprains. *J Am Acad Nurse Pract* 1993;5(6):271.
6. Onieal ME. Injuries to the anterior and posterior cruciate ligaments of the knee. *J Am Acad Nurse Pract* 1994;6(1):37.
7. Major NM. Sports medicine imaging. In: Garrett WE, Kirkendall DT, Squire DL, eds. *Principles and Practice of Primary Care Sports Medicine.* Philadelphia, PA: Lippincott Williams & Wilkins, 2001.
8. Calkins C, Sartoris DJ. Imaging acute knee injuries: direct diagnostic approaches. *Phys Sportsmed* 1992;20;(6):91.
9. Altchek DW. Diagnosing acute knee injuries: the office exam. *Phys Sportsmed* 1993;21(7):85.

SUGGESTED READINGS

Garrick J. Preparticipation orthopedic screening evaluation. *Clin J Sports Med* 2004;14(3):123.
Matheson GO. First, ask no harmful questions. *Phys Sportsmed* 2002;30(5):7.

WEB LINKS

http://www.radiologyinfo.org/content/mr_musculoskeletal.htm. Accessed 7/29/08.
   Provides a detailed description of MRI experience. A helpful resource for answering patient questions and concerns related to the MRI process.

http://www.orthoimaging.com/defaultFlash.htm. Accessed 7/29/08.
   National Orthopedic Imaging Associates Web site providing educational material and imaging resources. "Case of the Month" under the Educational Programs link is especially helpful for case studies and corresponding radiographic views.

http://www.auntminnie.com/index.asp?sec=sup&sub=ort. Accessed 7/29/08.
   Radiology news, education, and services. Books, links, education, careers, conference information, and much more.

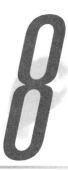

Conditions Involving the Foot, Ankle, and Leg

● **Brian J. Toy, PhD, ATC**

For the lower extremity to function efficiently, the foot, ankle, and leg must be healthy and work properly. This requires a complex coordination of activity among the many joints and muscle groups located in these areas. Unfortunately, when compared with other body regions, the incidence of sports-related foot, ankle, and leg injury is fairly high. Thus, when any of these regions become injured, the likelihood of pathology occurring in other structures, such as the knee and low back, increases. This makes the proper evaluation and subsequent management of foot, ankle, and leg conditions essential in preventing the development of associated pathologies.

Anatomy of the Foot, Ankle, and Leg

Important anatomical structures in these regions include bones, ligaments, muscles, tendons, fascia, and bursae. Knowing the arches of the foot is also important to those charged with evaluating musculoskeletal conditions of the foot, ankle, and leg.

Bones and Joints (Figs. 8.1 and 8.2)

The foot is divided into three distinct bony segments: tarsal, metatarsal, and phalangeal. The tarsal region consists of seven irregularly shaped bones. These include the large calcaneus, or heel bone; talus; navicular; cuboid; and medial (first), middle (second), and lateral (third) cuneiforms. Note that the talus is wider anteriorly than it is posteriorly. This feature plays a critical role in the mechanisms of injury (MOIs) in ankle sprains.

The metatarsal region contains five long bones. A prime metatarsal bony landmark is the tuberosity, or *styloid process*, of the fifth metatarsal. This can easily be palpated on the lateral side of the foot because the tuberosity protrudes more laterally than any other prominence. The phalangeal, or toe, region has 14 long bones. Except for the great, or first, toe, each remaining toe has three separate phalanges. Depending on their location, these bones are designated as a proximal, middle, or distal phalanx. The great toe has only a proximal and a distal phalanx.

With 26 bones, the foot maintains an abundance of articulations. As a group, the tarsal articulations are referred to as the intertarsal (IT) joints. These joints play an important role in maintaining proper foot function. Of particular note is the articulation between the talus and the calcaneus. Referred to as the **subtalar** (ST) **joint**, its importance is discussed in the motion and injury sections of this chapter. Some of the tarsal bones also articulate with the proximal portions, or bases, of the metatarsal bones to form the tarsometatarsal (TMT) joints. Distally, metatarsophalangeal (MTP) joints are formed by the metatarsal heads and proximal phalanges. For the second through fifth toes, the articulations between the phalanges are referred to as the proximal interphalangeal (PIP) and distal interphalangeal (DIP) joints. The joint between the proximal and distal phalanx of the great toe is known simply as the interphalangeal (IP) joint of the first toe.

The leg is the part of the body located between the knee and the ankle joint. In the clinical setting, this region is typically, and incorrectly, referred to as the *low leg*. In common usage, this area is also referred to as the *shin*. The bony anatomy of the

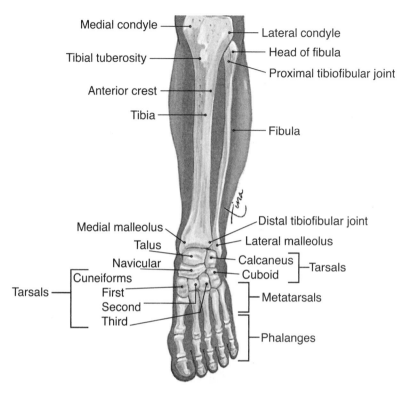

FIGURE 8.1 Bones and joints of the foot, ankle, and leg.
Adapted from Scanlon: *Essentials of Anatomy and Physiology*, 5th ed. 2007. Philadelphia: F.A. Davis Company, Fig. 6-14(A), pg 127, with permission.

leg includes two long bones: the larger, medially located, weight-bearing tibia and the smaller, laterally positioned, non-weight-bearing fibula. Important bony landmarks include the medial, or *tibial*, and the lateral, or *fibular*, malleoli. These protuberances represent the terminal ends of their respective bones and are located on either side of the talus. Note that the lateral malleolus is positioned more distal than the medial. Anteriorly, the shaft of the tibia can be palpated because it runs the length of the leg. In contrast, the shaft of the fibula cannot be easily palpated because it is covered by muscle and other soft tissue. The tibia's proximal portion maintains medial and lateral condyles, which help compose the knee's tibiofemoral joint, discussed in Chapter 9. The fibula's proximal portion, located laterally just distal to the knee, consists of the head of the fibula. The tibia and fibula articulate with each other at their proximal and distal ends, forming proximal tibiofibular (PTF) and distal tibiofibular (DTF) joints.

The ankle, or *talocrural*, joint, is the region located between the leg and foot. It is comprised of the talus, tibia, and fibula. More accurately, the malleoli surround the talus to form the ankle mortise. Be aware that some providers, and many published materials, incorrectly include the other six tarsal bones as ankle structures. This leads to a misunderstanding of how the ankle and IT joints function.

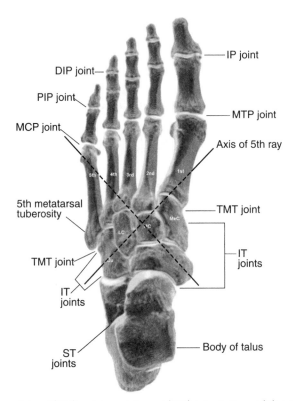

DIP joint—

PIP joint

MCP joint

5th metatarsal
tuberosity

TMT joint

IT
joints

ST
joints

IP joint

MTP joint

Axis of 5th ray

TMT joint

IT
joints

Body of talus

FIGURE 8.2 Tarsometatarsal (TMT), metatarsophalangeal (MTP), interphalangeal (IP), proximal interphalangeal (PIP), distal interphalangeal (DIP), intertarsal (IT), and subtalar (ST) joints of the foot. Cuboid (Cu), lateral cuneiform (LC), middle cuneiform (MC), and medial cuneiform (MeC) bones of the foot. Adapted from Levangie and Norkin: *Joint Structure and Function: A Comprehensive Analysis*, 4th ed. 2005. Philadelphia: F.A. Davis Company, Fig. 12-25, pg 458, with permission.

PEARL

The ankle joint is comprised of the talus, tibia, and fibula.

Motions

The IP joints of the toes all allow for the motions of flexion and extension, making them true hinge joints. Both the TMT and MTP joints are condyloid joints because they can flex, extend, abduct, and adduct. The IT articulations are gliding joints, and, with the exception of the ST joint, individually each of these joints maintains very little motion. However, when the amount of movement allowed by each IT joint is combined, the foot motions of **inversion** and **eversion** are produced. Most inversion and eversion comes from the ST joint, making its function critical in maintaining proper mechanics of the foot's tarsus region. Average ranges of motion (ROMs) for inversion and eversion are listed in Box 8.1.

BOX 8.1
ACTIVE ROMs OF THE ANKLE AND INTERTARSAL JOINTS

15°–20° Dorsiflexion (flexion)	20°–30° Inversion
45°–55° Plantar flexion (extension)	5°–15° Eversion

ROM = range of motion.

The ST joint is primarily responsible for motions of inversion and eversion.

The ankle is a hinge joint because it allows for the primary motions of flexion and extension. As you are probably already aware, the unique terms of **dorsiflexion** (flexion) and **plantar flexion** (extension) are used to describe these motions. Average plantar and dorsiflexion ROMs are also listed in Box 8.1. However, the ankle is not a true hinge joint, because slight amounts of ankle rotation and talar tilt also exist. That is, the talus can internally and externally rotate, and tilt within the mortise. This changes the ankle's classification from a true to a modified hinge joint.

The ankle, a modified hinge joint, allows for the primary motions of dorsiflexion and plantar flexion.

The PTF and DTF joints are slightly moveable articulations that allow the fibula to glide on the stationary tibia during ankle and foot movements. In addition, the DTF joint has the ability to widen when the ankle dorsiflexes, allowing the talus to fit snuggly between the malleoli in this position.

Ligaments

Because of the extensive number of joints located in the foot, ankle, and leg, it stands to reason that many ligaments are located in these regions. Those most involved in sports-related trauma are presented here.

Foot Ligaments

Not surprisingly, as a group, the ligaments supporting the IT joints are termed *IT ligaments*, and the ligaments supporting the TMT joints are termed *TMT ligaments*. Other pertinent foot ligaments include medial collateral ligaments (MCLs) and lateral collateral ligaments (LCLs) associated with each PIP, DIP, IP, and MTP joint. Remember that, as discussed in Chapter 1, all hinge and condyloid joints maintain collateral ligaments with each MCL, preventing valgus forces from injuring the associated joint, and each LCL, protecting the joint from varus force injury.

Ankle Ligaments

As a hinge joint, the ankle also maintains collateral ligaments. However, as with using the unique terms of *dorsiflexion* and *plantar flexion* to describe the motions of ankle flexion and extension, terms other than *MCL* and *LCL* are used to describe the ligaments supporting the ankle joint. For instance, the MCL of the ankle is termed the **deltoid ligament** (Fig. 8.3). This structure originates from the tibial malleolus and inserts on the talus, calcaneus, and navicular bones. It is responsible for preventing excessive eversion of the ST joint and medial tilting of the talus.

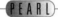

The deltoid ligament prevents excessive eversion of the ST joint and medial tilting of the talus.

Whereas one ligamentous structure provides medial ankle stability, three separate ligaments, all of which originate from the lateral malleolus, provide lateral ankle stability. These include the anterior talofibular ligament (ATFL), posterior talofibular ligament (PTFL), and calcaneofibular ligament (CFL) (Fig. 8.4). The ATFL, which runs anteriorly between the malleolus and the talus, prevents anterior translation of the talus, particularly when the ankle is plantar flexed. In contrast, the PTFL runs posteriorly from the malleolus to the talus as it prevents posterior translation of the talus. The CFL, which attaches the malleolus to the calcaneus, prevents lateral talar tilt and acts as a secondary restraint to anterior talar translation.

Both the ATFL and the CFL prevent anterior translation of the talus.

Leg Ligaments

The anterior inferior tibiofibular ligament (AITFL) supports the anterior aspect of the DTF joint, whereas the posterior inferior tibiofibular ligament (PITFL) supports the posterior aspect of this joint. The AITFL and PITFL combine with the interosseous membrane, a structure that connects the shafts of the tibia and fibula and attaches to these ligaments, to form the leg's **syndesmotic complex** (Fig. 8.5). Because this complex plays a vital role in the stability of the ankle mortise, a syndesmotic injury results in ankle instability. Furthermore, because the interosseous membrane serves as

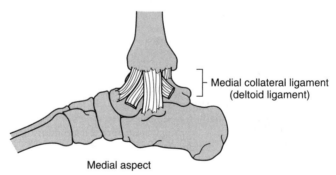

Medial collateral ligament
(deltoid ligament)

Medial aspect

FIGURE 8.3 Deltoid ligament of the ankle.
From McKinnis: *Fundamentals of Musculoskeletal Imaging,* 2nd ed. 2005.
Philadelphia: F.A. Davis Company, Fig. 11-3C, pg 370, with permission.

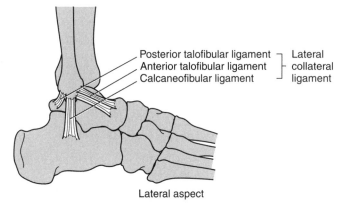

Lateral aspect

FIGURE 8.4 Lateral ankle ligaments.
From McKinnis: *Fundamentals of Musculoskeletal Imaging*, 2nd ed. 2005.
Philadelphia: F.A. Davis Company, Fig. 11-3A, pg 370, with permission.

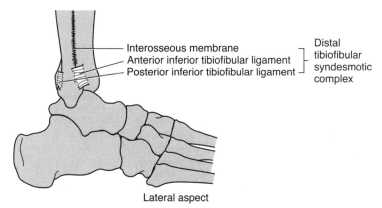

Lateral aspect

FIGURE 8.5 The distal tibiofibular syndesmotic complex is composed of the anterior inferior tibiofibular ligament, posterior inferior tibiofibular ligament, and interosseous membrane.
Adapted from McKinnis: *Fundamentals of Musculoskeletal Imaging*, 2nd ed. 2005.
Philadelphia: F.A. Davis Company, Fig. 11-3B, pg 370, with permission.

an attachment point for many leg muscles, this structure is commonly involved in acute and overuse leg conditions.

The syndesmotic complex is comprised of the AITFL, the PITFL, and the interosseous membrane.

Muscles and Tendons

Muscle groups in these regions are divided into to two categories: intrinsic and extrinsic. The location of a muscle's proximal attachment determines whether it is designated as an intrinsic or extrinsic structure. For instance, an intrinsic muscle's proximal attachment is located entirely within the structure of the foot, whereas this attachment site for an extrinsic muscle comes from the leg and/or thigh. All muscles in this region maintain their distal attachment within the foot. Most intrinsic muscles are located on the foot's plantar aspect, which, when palpated, gives the foot's bottom its fleshy, soft feeling. These intrinsic muscles act only to move the toes and, as a group, help support the multiple arches of the foot (discussed later in this chapter).

In general, the extrinsic muscles are located in one of three fascial compartments of the leg: anterior, posterior, or lateral (Fig. 8.6). All extrinsic muscles move the ankle, because their distal tendons all pass this joint as they proceed to their attachment site. Also, depending on where they insert, each extrinsic muscle helps to produce at least one foot motion (e.g., inversion, PIP and DIP flexion).

Anterior compartment muscles, which attach to the tibia, fibula, and interosseous membrane, are primarily responsible for producing the action of ankle dorsiflexion. The muscles of the lateral compartment, otherwise known as the *peroneals*, attach to the fibula and act to plantar flex the ankle and evert the foot. They also provide lateral ankle joint stability. Except for the gastrocnemius and plantaris muscles, which originate from the femur, posterior compartment muscles attach to the tibia, fibula, and/or

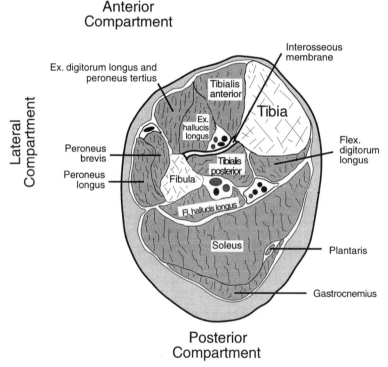

FIGURE 8.6 The extrinsic muscle compartments of the leg.
Adapted from Starkey and Ryan: *Evaluation of Orthopedic and Athletic Injuries,* 2nd ed. 2002. Philadelphia: F.A. Davis Company, Fig. 5-9, pg 141, with permission.

interosseous membrane. The gastrocnemius, soleus, and plantaris combine to form the **triceps surae**, the distal tendons of which unite to form the large **calcaneal**, or *Achilles*, **tendon**.

PEARL

The gastrocnemius, soleus, and plantaris muscles combine to form the triceps surae, the distal tendons of which unite to form the large calcaneal tendon.

Related Structures

Pertinent related structures in these regions include the arches of the foot, the **plantar fascia**, and the **calcaneal** and **retrocalcaneal bursae**.

Arches

The arches of the foot are formed by the tarsal and metatarsal bones and are supported by IT ligaments, TMT ligaments, intrinsic and extrinsic muscles, and the plantar fascia (discussed later in this chapter). The most prominent and best understood, the medial longitudinal arch (MLA) is the one most people associate with a singular "arch" of the foot (Fig. 8.7). It runs from the calcaneus to the heads of the medial three metatarsals. A properly functioning MLA is imperative to the well-being of the entire lower extremity and low back.

PEARL

The MLA is the structure most people associate with a singular "arch" of the foot.

Other arches include the lateral longitudinal arch (LLA) and the three transverse arches. The LLA runs the length of the foot's lateral aspect but produces a much less pronounced arc than does the MLA. The transverse arches include the tarsal arch, posterior metatarsal arch, and anterior metatarsal arch (AMA). The

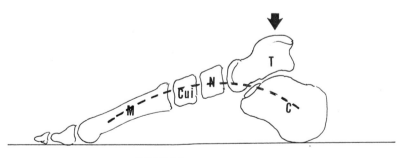

MEDIAL

FIGURE 8.7 The medial longitudinal arch of the foot is formed by the calcaneus (C), talus (T), navicular (N), cuneiforms (Cui), and three medial metatarsals (M).
From Cailliet: *Foot and Ankle Pain*, 3rd ed. 1997. Philadelphia: F.A. Davis Company, Fig. 1-17, pg 15, with permission.

AMA is formed by the heads of the metatarsals and is easily identified by the "dimple" it produces on the plantar aspect of the foot in the area of the second through fourth metatarsals.

Plantar Fascia

The tough, fibrous plantar fascia runs from the calcaneus to the heads of the metatarsals (Fig. 8.8). The fascia's calcaneal portion is a continuation of the calcaneal tendon, making calcaneal tendon conditions, such as decreased flexibility, contribute to plantar fascia injury. Functions of the plantar fascia include supporting the MLA, providing shock absorption for the lower extremity, and assisting in generating the power needed to push off in running and jumping activities.

Bursae

Bursae in these regions include the calcaneal and retrocalcaneal. The calcaneal bursa is located between the skin and the calcaneal tendon, whereas the retrocalcaneal bursa is located between this tendon and the calcaneus. These bursae protect the calcaneal tendon from injury.

Examination of the Foot, Ankle, and Leg

The musculoskeletal assessment of the foot, ankle, and leg regions can be challenging. Systematically approaching this process by combining this information with what is presented in Chapter 7 ensures that all essential aspects of the evaluation are covered.

History

One of the challenges in evaluating these regions is the thoroughness with which the history portion of the examination needs to be completed. Start by asking the patient

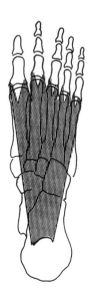

FIGURE 8.8 The plantar fascia.
From Cailliet: *Foot and Ankle Pain*, 3rd ed. 1997. Philadelphia: F.A. Davis Company, Fig. 1-42, pg 35, with permission.

pertinent questions from those listed in Box 7.1 on page 165. For suspected overuse conditions, concentrate questions on factors that increase the incidence of micro-trauma injury. As discussed in Chapter 1, these include sudden changes to training routine, playing surface, and footwear. Such alterations are particularly harmful to tissues of the foot and leg because they may not be able to adjust quickly enough to prevent the occurrence of injury.

For suspected macrotrauma injury to the foot or ankle, ask whether the injury was caused by a twisting-type force, because this is a very common way to acutely injure these regions. In these cases, the patient commonly states that his or her ankle "turned inward." Have the patient demonstrate, on the uninvolved limb, the position the involved extremity was in at the time of injury. During this reenactment, the patient usually places the ankle in plantar flexion and the foot in inversion, a common way to injure the foot and ankle. During this time, the patient reports lateral pain and discomfort. These signs are indicative of soft tissue damage such as a sprain.[1,2]

Ask whether the patient experienced blunt-force trauma to the foot, ankle, or leg, because this type of compression injury mechanism, such as what happens when the leg is kicked by an opposing player, is a common cause of macrotrauma injury. In these cases, a soft tissue contusion most certainly occurs, but you also may decide it necessary to rule out the possibility of a fracture. Conclude the history portion of the examination by asking whether any portion of the lower extremity or low back is in discomfort, because injuries to the foot, ankle, and leg regions—particularly those which cause the patient to walk with a limp—have the potential to affect other areas.

Physical Examination

As discussed in Chapter 7, begin the physical examination by observing the injured area. Follow this by palpating and testing ROM and strength of the joints. Complete the examination by applying specific stress/special tests for the foot, ankle, and leg.

Observation

Begin the observation portion of the examination by looking at the foot, ankle, and leg with the patient standing. Start with a posterior view, followed by lateral and anterior views. Determine whether any structural abnormalities of the foot exist. Do this by establishing the alignment of the calcaneal tendon in relation to the heel. Abnormal alignments include pronation, where the patient's calcaneus everts, and supination, where the calcaneus inverts (Fig. 8.9). Appreciate the importance of recognizing a pronated foot, because this condition contributes greatly to overuse pathology of the entire lower extremity and low back. To help you verify the presence of this condition, observe the wear pattern of the patient's shoes. An excessive wearing of the inside portion of the heel is indicative of pronation, whereas an excessive wearing of the heel's outer portion indicates supination.[3]

PEARL

Foot pronation contributes greatly to overuse pathology of the entire lower extremity and low back.

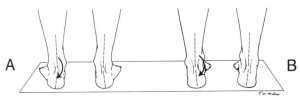

FIGURE 8.9 (A) Foot pronation. (B) Foot supination.
Adapted from Levangie and Norkin: *Joint Structure and Function: A Comprehensive Analysis*, 4th ed. 2005. Philadelphia: F.A. Davis Company, Fig. 12-3, pg 439, with permission.

After checking for pronation and supination, evaluate the MLA for pes planus, or *flat fleet*. This condition often occurs in conjunction with pronation and can also be a contributing factor in overuse injury. Pes planus can be congenital and is more prevalent in the African American population. It also can be acquired, which occurs when the MLA's supporting structures are not strong enough to support the patient's weight. This occurs in cases such as obesity and pregnancy.[3]

Conclude the observation portion of the evaluation by viewing the foot, ankle, and leg with the patient seated, knees flexed to 90° with the foot, ankle and leg hanging off the end of a table. Realize that certain structural abnormalities may present differently in this position. For example, pes planus may disappear in a non-weight-bearing position, also known as *flexible pes planus*, or it may be present in both weight-bearing and non-weight-bearing positions, otherwise known as *rigid pes planus*. With the patient in this seated position, evaluate structures such as the AMA that are hard to view with the patient standing. Look for signs of swelling, discoloration, and obvious bony deformity, which are more likely to be present in acute conditions than in chronic conditions.[2,3]

Palpation

With the patient in the same seated position, begin the palpation phase of the examination by palpating the bones of the leg, working your way distally to the bones of the foot. First, palpate the shafts of both the tibia and the fibula, ending at the medial and lateral malleoli. Working proximal to distal, palpate the dorsal aspect of the tarsal bones, the IT and TMT joints, and the shafts of the metatarsals. Direct palpation of the plantar aspect of these structures is difficult because of the abundance of soft tissue in this region. Palpate each toe by starting at its MTP joint and work distally through each phalanx and IP joint. Remember that bony point tenderness and crepitus are signs of fracture. Also, realize by palpating the foot bones in this fashion, the foot ligaments are being palpated at the same time.[1]

Return to the leg to start your palpation of the extrinsic muscles. From proximal to distal, palpate the anterior, lateral, and posterior compartments. Follow this by palpating the calcaneal tendon and the areas containing the calcaneal and retrocalcaneal bursae. Palpate the plantar aspect of the foot, beginning at the calcaneus and working toward the toes. Doing so assesses the health of both the intrinsic muscles of the foot and the plantar fascia.[1]

As discussed later in this chapter, the lateral ankle ligaments are injured more than the medial. Thus, if the patient reports lateral ankle pain and if the MOI leads you to suspect such an injury, first palpate the deltoid ligament, followed by the lateral ligaments. Move laterally and palpate the AITFL, PTFL, CFL, and ATFL. Reverse this order of ligament palpation if you suspect a deltoid ligament injury.[1]

Range-of-Motion and Strength Testing

To test active and passive ROM, instruct the patient to sit on a table, knees straight, with both ankles situated just off the table's end. Position your body lateral to, and facing, the ankle. With your proximal hand, grasp the leg just above the ankle joint. This stabilizes the lower extremity and ensures that the patient does not substitute hip rotation for the motions of inversion and eversion, a mistake commonly made by examiners. Ask the patient to actively dorsiflex, plantar flex, invert, and evert. To test active MTP and IP motion, instruct the patient to clench and spread his or her toes. Using your distal hand, dorsiflex, plantar flex, invert, and evert the ankle and foot, because this tests passive motion. Passive MTP and IP joint testing is not normally performed unless you note active differences. Be sure to test these motions on the uninvolved limb first and compare the findings between limbs.

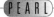
PEARL

When assessing active inversion and eversion of the foot, stabilize the lower extremity to ensure that the patient does not substitute hip rotation for these motions.

From the same patient and examiner positions, stabilize the patient's leg just above the ankle with your proximal hand, and place your distal hand on the dorsal aspect of the patient's foot. To test the strength of the ankle dorsiflexors, apply resistance with your distal hand as you instruct the patient to dorsiflex. Change the position of this hand to test the plantar flexors, invertors, and evertors. Because of the size and number of muscles located in the posterior compartment, it is very difficult to detect plantar flexion strength differences with a manual muscle test unless a severe deficit exists. If you suspect less than normal plantar flexion strength, instruct the patient to perform 20 one-leg toe raises. Decreased strength exists if the patient cannot complete the task or if fatigue experienced by the muscle group is greater than on the contralateral side.

Stress and Special Testing

Whereas stress tests used for these regions evaluate the integrity of the ankle and leg ligaments, most special tests are used to identify areas of fracture. For example, the foot percussion, or *vibration*, test, evaluates the integrity of the phalanges and metatarsals. When used to assess for a calcaneal, talar, tibial, or fibular fracture, this test is also known as the **bump**, or *heel tap*, **test**. To perform these tests, instruct the patient to sit on a table, knees straight, with the ankle situated just off the table's end. To test the phalanges and metatarsals, tap the end of each toe with one of your fingers. To perform a bump test, tap the plantar aspect of the patient's heel with the heel of your hand. When applying each test, start with little force, gradually increasing the magnitude of each tap until the bone vibrates. Vibration can also be achieved by applying a tuning fork to the end of the bone being tested. If the patient experiences localized pain anywhere along the bone, the test is positive for a possible fracture.[4,5]

The **squeeze test** is used to assess the integrity of the fibula. To perform this test, instruct the patient to sit on the edge of a table with the knees flexed to 90°. With your body positioned in front of the patient's leg, apply a compressive force to the tibia and fibula by squeezing them together (Fig. 8.10). Start proximally and work distally, being careful not to squeeze directly over any suspected fracture site. This test is positive if the patient experiences pain, or clicking occurs, anywhere along the shaft of the fibula. This test is also used to test for a **syndesmosis sprain**, discussed later in this chapter.[1]

PEARL

Use the percussion and squeeze tests to evaluate the bony integrity of the foot, ankle, and leg.

Musculoskeletal Imaging

Many musculoskeletal conditions of the foot, ankle, and leg are soft tissue in nature. Nevertheless, in certain situations, bony abnormalities, such as fractures, must be considered as part of the differential diagnosis. In these situations, ordering an imaging technique, such as an x-ray, should be part of the injury management plan. However, deciding when to do this can be confusing, because few guidelines exist for determining whether a patient with an injury in this region needs an x-ray. Thus, when the clinical evaluation reveals signs such as bony point tenderness, or if the patient cannot bear weight without limping, use the Ottawa Ankle and Foot Rules, presented in Figure 8.11, to help decide whether radiographs are needed. If x-rays are indicated, order anteroposterior, lateral, and mortise views. Be sure all relevant portions of the foot, ankle, and leg are included in the x-ray series, because doing so will help to avoid missing a fracture. For example, so as not to miss a **Jones fracture** (discussed later in this chapter), pain along the lateral ankle and foot caused by macrotrauma requires a thorough radiograph evaluation of the fifth metatarsal. Consider obtaining stress radiographs for suspected ligament injury to the ankle and leg. These are x-rays taken while stress tests are applied to the ankle joint. This concept is discussed in further detail in the ankle and leg sprain sections of this chapter.[2,6–8]

PEARL

Rely on the Ottawa Ankle and Foot Rules to help determine whether x-ray evaluation is needed for foot, ankle, and leg injuries.

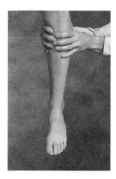

FIGURE 8.10 The squeeze test is used to identify fibula fracture and syndesmosis sprain.
From Gulick: *Ortho Notes: Clinical Examination Pocket Guide.* 2005. Philadelphia: F.A. Davis Company, pg 201, with permission.

Ottawa Ankle Rules

Radiographic series of the *ankle* is only required if one of the following are present:
- Bone tenderness at posterior edge of the distal 6 cm of the medial malleolus
- Bone tenderness at posterior edge of the distal 6 cm of the lateral malleolus
- Totally unable to bear weight *both* immediately after injury & (for 4 steps) in the emergency department

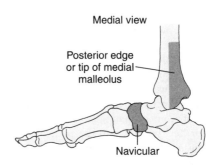

Medial view

Posterior edge or tip of medial malleolus

Navicular

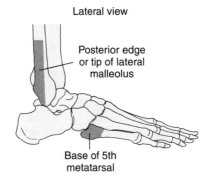

Lateral view

Posterior edge or tip of lateral malleolus

Base of 5th metatarsal

Ottawa Foot Rules

Radiographic series of the *foot* is only required if one of the following are present:
- Bone tenderness of the navicular
- Bone tenderness at the base of fifth metatarsal
- Totally unable to bear weight *both* immediately after injury & (for 4 steps) in the emergency department

FIGURE 8.11 Ottawa Ankle and Foot Rules.
From Gulick: *Ortho Notes, Clinical Examination Pocket Guide.* 2005. Philadelphia: F.A. Davis Company, pg 201, with permission.

Remember that radiographs are limited in their ability to diagnose suspected stress fractures, injuries that occur quite frequently in the foot and leg. Thus, in instances in which plain-film radiograph findings are negative but clinical findings suggest the presence of a stress fracture (described later in this chapter), consider ordering a bone scan. Also, consider obtaining a bone scan for macrotrauma injuries that do not respond to customary treatments and for microtrauma injuries that linger for longer than 2 to 3 weeks. Though certainly available, magnetic resonance imaging (MRI) is not usually used for the initial diagnosis of soft tissue injury in these regions. It is, however, used for patients with chronic ankle pain and instability and in cases in which an ankle sprain remains symptomatic for an extended period of time. In these instances, the patient should be referred to an orthopedist.[8,9]

Conditions of the Foot

Musculoskeletal foot injuries resulting from exercise and sports are caused by both traumatic and nontraumatic events. Typically, microtrauma conditions are associated with some type of structural abnormality, such as foot pronation and pes planus. Indeed, structural abnormalities of the feet can lead to a variety of lower extremity and low back conditions. Foot injuries that occur as a result of macrotrauma include strains, sprains, and fractures.

Pronation and Pes Planus

Once foot pronation or pes planus has been identified in a patient, advise the patient to replace worn-out athletic and everyday shoes with footwear that maintains good MLA support. Tell the patient to wear athletic shoes specifically designed to prevent the foot from pronating. If needed, add shoe inserts designed to support the MLA and/or heel wedges into the patient's shoes (Fig. 8.12). Off-the-shelf insoles can be purchased at any local pharmacy and at many sporting goods stores. Refer to an orthopedist or podiatrist those patients who have severe cases of pes planus and/or foot pronation and patients who do not respond to modifications performed in the primary care setting, because these patients require an extensive foot analysis and follow-up care.[10,11]

Traumatic Fractures, Sprains, and Dislocations

As you might imagine, macrotrauma incidents have the potential to fracture any of the foot's 26 bones or to sprain or dislocate any of the many foot joints. Of the foot's three regions, the metatarsals and phalangeals are particularly susceptible to traumatic fracture, whereas sprains and dislocations usually occur at the MTP and IP joints. People who experience a sprain, fracture, or dislocation that reduces spontaneously or is reduced by a lay person (e.g., parent, coach) commonly report to the primary care setting for evaluation and treatment. In contrast, patients with nonreduced dislocations almost always seek treatment through emergency medical means. This section focuses on the management of conditions typically seen in the primary care setting.

The MOIs for traumatic foot fractures, sprains, and dislocations are similar: any compression or twisting force placed on the foot has the potential to cause any of these conditions. For example, dropping something heavy on the dorsal aspect of the metatarsals or phalanges, such as a dumbbell weight, or a player forcefully stepping on the dorsum of another player's foot during competition, can cause a fracture. Striking

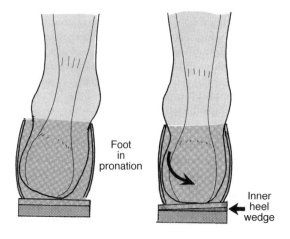

Foot in pronation

Inner heel wedge

FIGURE 8.12 A medial heel wedge to treat for foot pronation. Adapted from Cailliet: *Foot and Ankle Pain*, 3rd ed. 1997. Philadelphia: F.A. Davis Company, Fig. 4-8, pg 107, with permission.

an immovable object with the foot, such as what happens when someone stubs his or her toe, can also sprain, dislocate, or fracture a toe. Twisting the foot at the same time that a great deal of force is applied to the region, such as what happens when a person returns to the ground after jumping for a rebound in basketball, also places the metatarsals, the fifth in particular, at risk for traumatic fracture.

Any compression or twisting force placed on the foot has the potential to cause a foot fracture, dislocation, or sprain.

History and Physical Examination

Because traumatic fractures, dislocations, and sprains are macrotrauma conditions, the patient can usually recall the exact MOI and the acute pain he or she experienced at the moment of injury. In the case of fractures, the patient may also recount experiencing a period of transient paresthesia in the region soon after injury occurrence, especially if the area was subject to a compressive force.

Regardless of injury type, the patient usually states that the injured area is extremely painful and becomes worse when palpated. If severe enough, this causes the patient to walk with a noticeable limp. In cases of MTP or IP injury, pain also increases with toe movement. When observed, the injured site is easily identified by swelling and ecchymosis, particularly if the incident occurred more than 24 hours before evaluation. In cases of phalangeal or metatarsal fracture, the percussion test may be positive.

When a patient presents with pain around the base of the fifth metatarsal, consider that the patient has sustained either an avulsion fracture or a Jones fracture. Usually traumatized by either a compression or a twisting force, this area is particularly vulnerable to injury because it lacks the bony stability that the other metatarsal bases enjoy. A fifth metatarsal tuberosity avulsion fracture occurs when the tendon of the peroneus brevis, a muscle located in the leg's lateral compartment, avulses from its attachment site on the tuberosity, whereas a Jones fracture occurs at the proximal diaphysis of the bone, 1.5 cm distal to the tuberosity (Fig. 8.13). A Jones fracture is a troubling condition because it heals slowly, causes prolonged disability, and predisposes the area to reinjury. Even when treated properly, a Jones fracture maintains a high incidence of nonunion. It is for these reasons that you must pay particular attention to the base of the fifth metatarsal when evaluating all traumatic injuries to the foot and ankle.[12–15]

Pay particular attention to the base of the fifth metatarsal when evaluating all traumatic injuries to the foot and ankle.

Management

Immobilize all suspected foot fractures and joints that have been badly sprained or suffered a dislocation. Prescribe non-weight-bearing crutch use as outlined in Patient Teaching Handout (PTH) 6.1 for all with a suspected or confirmed metatarsal fracture. Recommend the same for patients with toe injuries who cannot walk without

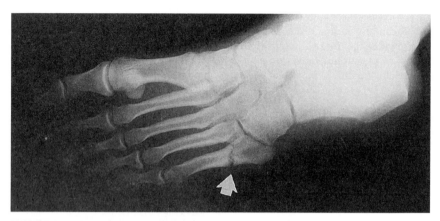

FIGURE 8.13 Radiograph of a Jones fracture.
From McKinnis: *Fundamentals of Musculoskeletal Imaging*, 2nd ed. 2005. Philadelphia: F.A. Davis Company, Fig. 11–63, pg 397, with permission.

a limp. Explain to these patients that even if the injury does not hurt too badly, walking with a limp can lead to the development of other conditions, such as knee or low back pain. Use the Ottawa Foot Rules, as presented in Figure 8.11, to help guide you when determining the need for radiographs. Always obtain x-rays when you suspect injury to the base of the fifth metatarsal. Refer patients with traumatic metatarsal fractures to an orthopedist. The standard course of treatment for a nondisplaced fracture is a short leg walking cast for 6 to 8 weeks. Surgical intervention may be indicated for displaced fractures, Jones fractures, and metatarsal fractures that do not respond to conservative treatment.[6,12,14–16]

PEARL

Always obtain x-rays when you suspect injury to the base of the fifth metatarsal.

Treat toe fractures, toe sprains, and reduced dislocations by splinting the affected body part. In many instances, taping the affected toe to its neighboring toes, known as *buddy taping*, is all the immobilization needed. The patient should progress from non-weight-bearing crutch use to a four-point, touch-down crutch gait as pain subsides. Discontinue crutch use as soon as the patient can walk without a limp. Recommend that he or she wear steel-toe shoes to protect the toe(s) during healing. Slowly return these patients to functional activity as pain and discomfort allow.

Metatarsophalangeal Joint Sprain of the First (Great) Toe

Remember that any MTP or IP joint of the toes can be sprained. Of note, however, is a sprain of the MTP joint of the great toe, because this joint is particularly vulnerable to traumatic forces. Otherwise known as **turf toe**, the increased incidence of this injury in sports directly relates to the use of synthetic playing surfaces since their introduction in the 1960s and their increased use since the 1970s. Although in recent years technology has made these surfaces safer, turf toe injuries continue to occur in those who play on these surfaces. However, this condition also occurs in people who participate on natural playing surfaces, such as grass.[17,18]

Turf toe occurs when the first MTP joint is forcefully hyperextended beyond its normal range, ultimately tearing the joint's ligaments and capsule on the plantar surface. This usually happens when the toe comes in contact with a nonyielding surface and most commonly occurs in people who participate in football. Because the great toe contributes significantly to standing balance and the forward propulsion associated with walking and running, injury to this joint is very disabling.[17,18]

PEARL

Turf toe is a very disabling condition that occurs when the first MTP joint is forcefully hyperextended beyond its normal range.

History and Physical Examination

A turf toe patient usually reports one macrotrauma incident that, as the person states, forced his or her big toe "backward." In some cases, the patient relates a history of smaller, multiple events of forced hyperextension. The person is unable to jump or run and may have difficulty walking without a limp. The toe is ecchymotic, swollen, and stiff. The plantar aspect of the MTP joint is point tender, and the patient's ability to actively hyperextend the great toe is decreased. Passive movement in this direction causes the patient the most pain.[17,18]

Management

Obtain radiographs of the foot to rule out fracture or associated joint pathology. Prescribe non-weight-bearing crutch use, as described in PTH 6.1, for patients who cannot walk without a limp. Instruct the person to wear metal-toe, hard-sole shoes because these protect the toe from direct trauma and prevent it from hyperextending. As symptoms subside, the patient can gradually progress to a four-point, pain-free touchdown crutch gait, followed by discontinuation of crutch use. Return the patient to pain-free activity as tolerated. To limit the toe's ability to hyperextend during exercise, advise the patient to add rigid sole inserts to his or her sports shoes. Avoid returning the person to full activity too soon, because prolonged disability may ensue. This can be a very frustrating injury because it might take months or even years for the toe to fully heal, particularly if the patient remains physically active during recovery.[17,18]

Metatarsal Stress Fractures

As with traumatic fractures, any foot bone can be injured as a result of microtrauma. However, it is the metatarsals that are most susceptible to development of a stress fracture, because these structures are responsible for the transmission of forces between the tarsal and phalangeal regions during walking and running. Indeed, people who participate in activities that place great stresses on the feet, such as distance running, basketball, soccer, and high-impact dance aerobics, are at an increased risk of sustaining a metatarsal stress fracture.[12,17,19]

Stress fractures of the foot most commonly occur in the shafts of the second and third metatarsals, otherwise known as **march fractures** because of their high prevalence in military personnel. These bones maintain higher stress fracture rates because they are less mobile than the other metatarsals. Because of its lack of bony stability as described earlier in this chapter, the base of the fifth metatarsal also maintains an increased stress fracture risk. In general, older people, Caucasians, and women who experience episodes of amenorrhea lasting longer than 6 months maintain a higher risk for development of metatarsal stress fractures.[17,19–23]

Stress fractures of the foot, which typically involve the shafts of the second and third metatarsals, commonly occur in older people, Caucasians, and women who experience episodes of amenorrhea lasting longer than 6 months.

History and Physical Examination

A patient with a metatarsal stress fracture usually reports that he or she recently increased the intensity and/or duration of an exercise program. This change usually does not cause a discrete injury, but, over time, the person experiences dull, non-specific foot pain associated with diffuse swelling. Initially, pain occurs only with activity and usually does not limit the person's exercise habits. As the fracture progresses, pain becomes more localized and is present while the person is walking and at rest. By this point, though the entire forefoot may be painful and swelling may disguise the exact area of injury, some patients may be able to precisely identify an area of point tenderness. In cases in which the patient's area of point tenderness is located around the base of the fifth metatarsal, be sure to consider a Jones fracture in the differential diagnosis. Use the history portion of the examination to differentiate between these injuries, because patients with a stress fracture report a long history of symptoms, whereas those with a Jones fracture report a specific macrotrauma event that caused the injury. Other signs of a metatarsal stress fracture include erythema or ecchymosis on the dorsum of the foot and a callus, corresponding with the shaft of the affected metatarsal, on the foot's plantar aspect. A callus forms in cases in which the fracture has been present for a long time.[12,17,19,20]

Management

If the clinical evaluation indicates a stress fracture, treat the patient conservatively by disqualifying him or her from participation until presence of a fracture can be confirmed or denied. Although x-rays do not always reveal the fracture's existence, initially obtain plain-film radiographs, because bone callous formation around the painful area may be present, particularly if the condition is more than a few weeks old. Remember, however, that up to 50% of all metatarsal stress fractures are never observed on plain films. If the x-ray findings are negative, order a bone scan, because this can show the fracture site as early as 2 to 3 days from the onset of symptoms.[12,17,19,20]

A bone scan can show a metatarsal fracture site as early as 2 to 3 days from the onset of symptoms.

Once confirmed, continue to treat all non–fifth metatarsal stress fractures conservatively by ordering complete rest from the offensive activity until the fracture is fully healed. As mentioned in Chapter 1, allowing a person to participate with a stress fracture increases the chance that the fracture will develop into a simple or compound fracture. Recommend that the patient use a stiff-soled shoe to protect the foot from moving excessively while walking. Prescribe only partial weight-bearing or non-weight-bearing crutch use, as shown in PTH 6.1, if discomfort causes the patient to walk with a limp. Order periodic plain-film radiographs to document healing. If this treatment is not successful, or if the fracture is diagnosed late, immobilize the foot by applying a short leg walking cast or boot for a period of 4 to 6 weeks. If further intervention is needed, prescribe non-weight-bearing crutch use, and refer the patient to an orthopedist. Except when occurring in the fifth metatarsal, most metatarsal stress fractures heal uneventfully after 6 to 8 weeks of conservative treatment.[12,17,19,20]

Immediately refer all patients with a suspected fifth metatarsal stress fracture to an orthopedist, because these injuries are prone to nonunion and refracture. In these cases, treatment includes short leg cast immobilization and no weight-bearing for a minimum of 6 to 8 weeks but may last as long as 6 months. If the fracture does not heal or if the orthopedist does not think the fracture will heal with conservative therapy, the patient is treated with intramedullary screw fixation with or without bone grafting.[12,14,17,19–21]

Metatarsalgia

Metatarsalgia can be caused by a number of things, including[12,17]

- Morton's toe, a condition that occurs when the second toe is longer than the first;
- an interdigital neuroma, or an entrapment of interdigital nerves located between the metatarsal heads with the nerve situated between the third and fourth metatarsal, otherwise known as a *Morton's neuroma,* most at risk of entrapment;
- an inflexible calcaneal tendon, which, in many cases, is brought on by the wearing of high-heeled shoes with a narrow toe box, placing the interdigital nerves under constant stretch;
- MTP joint inflammation from arthritis or synovitis; or
- **Freiberg's infraction** (discussed in detail later in this chapter).

Regardless of cause, the resulting metatarsalgia symptoms are similar among patients. The management plan is also similar.

History and Physical Examination

Patients with metatarsalgia have diffuse swelling, pain, and stiffness at one or more MTP joint. In the case of an interdigital neuroma, patients report an insidious onset of foot cramping, numbness, burning, and tingling. In severe cases, these symptoms radiate to the dorsal and plantar aspects of the foot. In most cases, patients with metatarsalgia report a decrease in symptoms once the offending footwear is removed and, in certain instances, when the forefoot is massaged. It is common to note when observing the foot of such a patient that the AMA has "fallen." That is, the dimple formed by the second through fourth metatarsal heads on the foot's plantar aspect is no longer present. Also, because of the increased pressure placed on the plantar aspect of the metatarsal heads, many times patients with this condition have development of a plantar callus in the affected area. Palpating each interdigital nerve with the eraser end of a pencil on the plantar aspect of the foot around the area of the metatarsal heads increases symptoms in those with an interdigital neuroma. Squeezing the metatarsal heads together may also increase symptoms.[12,17]

Management

The first step in managing a patient with metatarsalgia is to have the patient change footwear from a high-heeled shoe with a narrow toe box to a low-heeled shoe with a wide toe box. Remember to tell the person that all footwear, including nonathletic shoes, must have a toe box wide enough to relieve pressure on the involved area. Instruct the patient to apply a soft metatarsal adhesive pad to help spread the metatarsals and to support the AMA. These pads can be purchased at any local pharmacy. Prescribe calcaneal tendon and calf stretches as shown in PTH 8.1. Suggest that the patient modify activity until symptoms subside. If this conservative course of action does not resolve symptoms after a few months, refer the person to an orthopedist for possible corticosteroid injection and/or a custom foot orthotic fitting.[12,17]

Plantar Fasciitis

A very common overuse condition, **plantar fasciitis** is one of the most painful foot disorders occurring in adults and older adolescents who are physically active. It arises when the plantar fascia is exposed to repetitive microtrauma; happens most often in those who participate in sports that require a lot of running and jumping; and often develops as a result of sudden changes in training frequency, mode, and/or intensity. The fascia is usually injured near its attachment site on the calcaneus. Risk factors for development of this condition include foot pronation and pes planus. In addition, because the strands of the plantar fascia are actually a continuation of the calcaneal tendon, decreased flexibility and/or strength of this tendon and the triceps surae may also lead to plantar fasciitis.[3,24–27]

PEARL

Plantar fasciitis develops as a result of sudden changes in training frequency, mode, and/or intensity.

History and Physical Examination

Patients with plantar fasciitis report that the condition started as a dull ache in the plantar aspect of the foot just distal to the calcaneus and along the length of the MLA. They state that this initial symptom was aggravated by weight-bearing, particularly upon taking the first few steps after getting out of bed in the morning, but gradually subsided with increased activity. Unfortunately, by the time patients seek professional care, this dull ache has usually evolved into a sharp, knife-like pain upon arising after sleep. They also report increased pain with ascending stairs and when rising on the toes. Although they report that the amount of pain subsides as the day progresses, it is usually present throughout their waking hours, making this condition extremely disabling.[3,24,27]

When observed, the injured area of the person with this condition does not appear swollen, because, unlike other inflammatory conditions, plantar fasciitis does not normally produce visual swelling. However, regardless of the amount of pain the patient is experiencing or how long the injury has been present, the patient has extreme tenderness on the plantar aspect of the foot 1 inch distal to the calcaneus. Pain also increases when the patient jumps on his or her toes. Although diagnostic tools such as bone scans and MRIs are available to help determine its presence, rely on the results of the history portion of the examination and these clinical findings to make a diagnosis of plantar fasciitis. Reserve the use of imaging techniques for cases in which the differential diagnosis includes a more serious condition, such as **Sever's disease** (discussed later in this chapter).[3,24,27]

PEARL

A sharp, knife-like pain occurring 1 inch distal to the calcaneus on the plantar aspect of the foot, which is most intense upon arising in the morning, is indicative of plantar fasciitis.

Management

Treat plantar fasciitis symptomatically by reducing both the time the patient spends doing the offending activity and the intensity level with which the person participates. Indeed, the patient may have to stop participating altogether for a period of time. Emphasize that continuing to exercise through extreme pain may result in a complete rupture of the fascia or the development of a **calcaneal exostosis**, otherwise known as a *heel spur*. If indicated, correct for pronation and/or pes planus as previously described. To further support the plantar fascia, place a heel cup, which can be purchased at any local pharmacy, inside the patient's shoes. Immediately start the person on strengthening and stretching exercises for the foot, triceps surae, and calcaneal tendon, as shown in PTH 8.1. Although the use of any cold modality is indicated, ice massage is effective in treating plantar fasciitis, because this form of cryotherapy treats the entire length of the fascia and provides the area with a massaging effect. Consider using ice massage for an extended period of time, rather than changing to heat treatments, because plantar fasciitis responds very well to this modality.[3,24]

PEARL

Treatment for plantar fasciitis includes reducing the amount of time the patient spends doing the offending activity, as well as reducing the frequency and intensity of the activity; supporting the MLA; strengthening and stretching the area; and applying ice massage to the plantar aspect of the foot.

Once symptoms start to subside, gradually return the patient to activity. Unfortunately, it usually takes weeks, and sometimes months, for the symptoms of plantar fasciitis to fully disappear. Once the injury is fully healed, advise the patient to monitor for symptom reoccurrence, because this often happens when the patient returns to unrestricted activity.

Conditions of the Ankle

Though many ankle injuries result from sports participation, by far the most prevalent is the ankle sprain. Unfortunately, this injury is frequently treated very casually by physicians, coaches, parents, and patients. This means that in some instances, sound medical intervention is often replaced by a need to return athletes to play before the injury has adequately healed. The common refrain "it's just an ankle sprain" has so permeated the athletic culture that it is difficult to convince the injured patient that, treated improperly, an ankle sprain can cause chronic problems.[2,28]

Though both medial and lateral ankle sprains occur in sports, injury to the lateral ligaments occurs much more frequently than injury to the medial ligaments. This difference is attributed to these factors[9,28]:

- Shape of the talus: Because the talus is wide anteriorly and thin posteriorly, the wide portion of the talus fits snuggly between the malleoli in dorsiflexion, making the joint very stable in this position. Conversely, in the plantar flexed position, the talus's thin, posterior portion articulates in the mortise, making the ankle less stable.
- Position of the malleoli: The lateral malleolus lies more distal than the medial. Whereas this allows the talus to move freely during inversion, during eversion it comes into contact with the fibula. This limits the ability of the foot to evert as much as it can invert.
- Strength of the ankle ligaments: The four-part medial deltoid ligament is much stronger than the lateral three ankle ligaments.

From this information, it is easy to understand why the lateral ankle ligaments are injured more often than the deltoid ligament. When the ankle and foot are placed in their respective positions of plantar flexion and inversion, the talus is able to move freely, allowing the lateral ankle ligaments to become taut. As explained in Chapter 1, if a ligament is stretched beyond its capacity to elongate and is not strong enough to resist an external force, it will tear. Conversely, because the talus comes in contact with the distal fibula in eversion, the deltoid ligament does not become stretched, or stressed, to its maximum. This protects the deltoid ligament from becoming injured.

PEARL

A combination plantar flexion/inversion mechanism is the most common way to injure the lateral ligaments of the ankle.

Lateral Ankle Sprain

As just discussed, the lateral ankle ligaments are usually injured as a result of a plantar flexion/inversion mechanism. Indeed, 85% of all ankle sprains occur in these ligaments and result from this MOI. In general, sprains of this nature are commonly referred to as *inversion* ankle sprains. The lateral ligament injured most in this type of sprain is by far the ATFL. In fact, almost all lateral ankle sprains involve this ligament to some extent, because it is usually the first ligament to be traumatized in an inversion injury. In a first degree ankle sprain, the injury is isolated to this ligament. However, if the force placed on the ankle is great enough, the CFL may also be injured, resulting in a second degree, or two-ligament, sprain (Fig. 8.14). Though not often injured because of its location and its tensile strength, the PTFL may also be involved in severe plantar flexion/inversion injuries. Thus, injuries involving the ATFL, CFL, and PTFL are classified as third degree sprains.[1-3,9,28] Grading inversion ankle ligament sprains by the structures injured is summarized in Table 8.1.

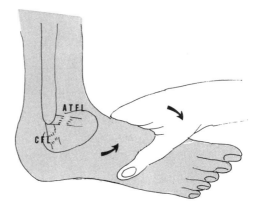

FIGURE 8.14 Two-ligament ankle sprain from a plantar flexed/inverted mechanism. ATFL = anterior talofibular ligament; CFL = calcaneofibular ligament. Adapted from Cailliet: *Foot and Ankle Pain*, 3rd ed. 1997. Philadelphia: F.A. Davis Company, Fig. 8-8, pg 209, with permission.

PEARL

The ATFL is the most common ligament injured in an inversion ankle sprain.

Because the ankle is very stable in dorsiflexion, inversion sprains are less likely to occur in the dorsiflexed ankle. If a dorsiflexion/inversion injury does occur, injury forces are more concentrated on the CFL. As discussed later in this chapter, an injury mechanism that includes a dorsiflexed ankle also places the syndesmotic complex at risk. In fact, a syndesmosis injury is more likely to occur from a dorsiflexed mechanism than from injury to the lateral ankle ligaments.[2] Table 8.2 summarizes the positions that place the ligaments of the ankle at risk for injury.

History and Physical Examination

Regardless of injury severity, the patient with an inversion ankle sprain commonly reports that his or her ankle "twisted inward" at the time of injury. The patient may also

---

TABLE 8.1 Lateral ankle ligament injury severity in differing degrees of ankle sprains

ANKLE SPRAIN SEVERITY	SEVERITY OF LIGAMENT INJURED		
	ATFL	CFL	PTFL
First degree	Mild	None	None
Second degree	Moderate	Mild	None
Third degree	Severe	Moderate	None to mild

ATFL = anterior talofibular ligament; CFL = calcaneofibular ligament; PTFL = posterior talofibular ligament.

TABLE 8.2 Most common positions that place the ankle ligaments at risk for injury

LIGAMENT	MOST COMMON MOI POSITION
Anterior talofibular	Plantar flexion/inversion
Calcaneal fibular	Neutral (anatomical position)/inversion
Posterior talofibular	Dorsiflexion/inversion
Deltoid	Eversion (plantar flexion, neutral, dorsiflexion)

MOI = mechanism-of-injury.

report hearing a "pop" or feeling the soft tissues "crunch" during the incident. Patients also report pain and swelling around the lateral malleolus, with the greatest amount of discomfort localized over the injured ligament(s).[1–3,9]

For people with a first degree inversion sprain, pain and swelling are minimal while strength and ROM are normal. The gait of these patients is only mildly affected. These symptoms are more pronounced in people with a second degree sprain, because motion and strength decreases are noticeable, causing the patient to walk with an obvious limp. The swelling associated with this injury is localized initially but becomes more diffuse as time passes. Indeed, after the first few days, swelling and ecchymosis appear around the fibula malleolus and lateral portion of the heel (Fig. 8.15). Because patients with a third degree ankle sprain have sustained a three-ligament injury, these people experience extreme pain and swelling and cannot walk without assistance. Because of the condition's severity, ROM and strength of the patient's affected ankle cannot be assessed in instances of a third degree inversion ankle sprain.[1–3,9]

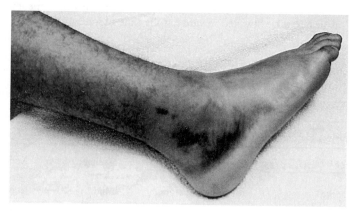

FIGURE 8.15 Swelling and ecchymosis appearing around the heel, distal to the malleolus, after a lateral ankle sprain.
From Starkey and Ryan: *Evaluation of Orthopedic Injuries and Athletic Injuries*, 2nd ed. 2002. Philadelphia: F.A. Davis Company, Fig. 5-15A, pg 149, with permission.

A lateral ankle sprain can be confirmed by performing the **anterior drawer**, **posterior drawer**, and **inversion talar tilt**, or *inversion stress*, **tests**. To perform the anterior drawer test (Fig. 8.16):[1-3,9]

- Instruct the patient to sit on the edge of a table with his or her knees flexed to 90°.
- With one of your hands, stabilize the leg by grasping the distal portions of the tibia and fibula just above the level of the malleoli. Cup your other hand around the posterior aspect of the calcaneus.
- With the ankle relaxed and in 10° of plantar flexion, perform the anterior drawer test by pulling the foot forward with the hand cupped around the calcaneus. Watch and feel for the presence of excessive anterior movement.

A first degree inversion sprain probably exists in cases where movement does not occur with the anterior drawer test, but other parts of the evaluation, such as a reported history of an inversion MOI and the presence of pain over the ATFL, indicate ligament damage. If, however, the anterior drawer test produces excessive movement, note the type of end-feel present. A hard end-feel is indicative of a second degree lateral ankle sprain, whereas a soft end-feel confirms the presence of a third degree injury.

To perform the posterior drawer test, position the patient with their ankle in the same position as for the anterior drawer test. However, instead of pulling the foot forward with the hand cupped around the calcaneus, push the foot backward with this hand. Watch and feel for the presence of excessive posterior movement. If movement occurs, note the type of end-feel present and document that the posterior drawer test is positive for injury to the PTFL.

To perform the inversion talar tilt test[1,3] (Fig. 8.17):

- Instruct the patient to sit on a table, knees straight, with his or her ankle situated just off the table's end.
- Cradle the plantar aspect of the patient's calcaneus.
- Tilt the talus by inverting it.
- Watch and feel for gapping on the ankle's lateral side.
- If gapping occurs, note the type of end-feel present and document that the inversion talar tilt test is positive for CFL injury.

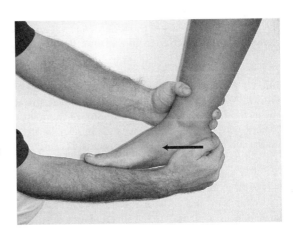

FIGURE 8.16 The anterior drawer test is used to check the integrity of the anterior talofibular ligament. To test for the integrity of the posterior talofibular ligament, perform the posterior drawer test by pushing back on the patient's foot.
From Starkey and Ryan: *Evaluation of Orthopedic and Athletic Injuries,* 2nd ed. 2002. Philadelphia: F.A. Davis Company, Box 5-4A, pg 158, with permission.

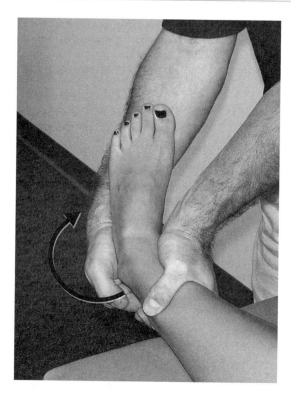

FIGURE 8.17 The inversion talar tilt test is used to check the integrity of the calcaneofibular ligament. From Starkey and Ryan: *Evaluation of Orthopedic and Athletic Injuries,* 2nd ed. 2002. Philadelphia: F.A. Davis Company, Box 5-5A, pg 159, with permission.

PEARL

Use the anterior drawer, posterior drawer, and inversion talar tilt tests to determine the integrity of the lateral ankle ligaments.

Be sure to perform both the bump and squeeze tests (described earlier in this chapter) to help rule out fracture in this region. Also, do not forget to closely inspect the base and tuberosity of the fifth metatarsal and the distal shaft of the fibula, because these bones can fracture from a plantar flexed/inverted mechanism.[9]

Management

Initially manage a lateral ankle sprain by deciding whether x-rays are needed. Use the Ottawa Ankle Rules (Fig. 8.11) to help make this determination. For patients with a suspected first degree sprain, immobilize the joint and prescribe crutches only if the patient walks with a limp, because unnecessarily limiting activity for this degree of injury can impede the recovery process. If crutches are needed, instruct the patient to use a four-point, pain-free touchdown crutch gait as described in PTH 6.1.[6,7]

For patients with a second or third degree lateral sprain, immobilize the ankle in a dorsiflexed/everted position. Doing so aids the healing process by shortening and approximating the ends of the injured ligaments and by preventing the ankle from stiffening in a plantar flexed/inverted position. Prescribe non-weight-bearing crutch use and, if indicated by the Ottawa Ankle Rules, obtain both standard ankle radiographs and anterior drawer and inversion talar tilt stress x-rays, because these help determine the extent of injury. Be sure this radiograph series include a view of the fifth metatarsal's base.[8,9,29]

Once a fracture has been ruled out, progress the patient to a four-point, pain-free touchdown crutch gait as pain allows. Slowly wean the patient from crutch use, because prolonged rest and immobilization for an ankle sprain are contraindicated. Implement the rehabilitation exercises outlined in PTH 8.1. Return the patient to activity when pain-free ROM and full muscle strength have been restored. Remember that full ligamentous strength, though impossible to measure clinically, may take months or years to achieve. Consider recommending that the patient use an external ankle support, such as an ankle brace, during activity. These can be purchased at a pharmacy or sporting goods store. Using an ankle brace does not guarantee that reinjury will not occur, and the use of such devices should not be substituted for properly rehabilitating the joint. If chronic instability develops, refer the patient to an orthopedist, because surgical intervention may be warranted in certain cases.[3,9,29]

PEARL

Progress patients with a second or third degree ankle sprain from a three-point, non-weight-bearing crutch gait to walking without crutches as quickly as pain and disability allow.

Medial Ankle Sprain

The deltoid ligament is usually injured as a result of an eversion mechanism combined with either plantar flexion or dorsiflexion (Table 8.2). Whereas injury to the lateral ankle ligaments is extremely common, injury to the deltoid ligament occurs infrequently. In fact, because forceful eversion causes the talus to collide with the distal end of the fibula, instead of causing an isolated deltoid sprain, this MOI usually results in either a distal fibula fracture or a combination deltoid ligament sprain and fibula fracture. When combined with extreme dorsiflexion, an eversion mechanism also causes a syndesmosis sprain, a condition discussed later in this chapter.[1,3]

PEARL

In addition to traumatizing the deltoid ligament, an eversion MOI may also fracture the distal end of the fibula.

History and Physical Examination

The patient with an eversion ankle sprain commonly reports that his or her ankle "twisted outward" at the time of injury. The patient reports pain around the area of the medial malleolus, with the greatest amount of discomfort localized over the deltoid ligament. As with a lateral ankle sprain, the patient's pain, swelling, and disability increase with the degree of injury, though when these conditions are compared, swelling is usually not as great with a deltoid ligament sprain.[1,3]

Assessing a patient for an eversion ankle injury begins with observing around the medial malleolus and the distal end of the fibula. As with the lateral ankle sprain, strength and ROM are affected relevant to the degree of injury. Be sure to test clinically for fracture by performing the bump and squeeze tests. Perform the **eversion talar tilt test** to confirm a deltoid ligament sprain. To perform this test, use the same patient and examiner positioning described for the inversion talar tilt test shown in Figure 8.17. However, instead of inverting the foot as shown in this figure, use the hand cradling the calcaneus to evert the foot. This tests the integrity of the deltoid ligament. Document the presence of gapping and note the type of end-feel present to determine the extent of injury.

Use the eversion talar tilt test to determine the integrity of the deltoid ligament.

Management
Manage the medial ankle ligament sprain as you would a lateral ligament sprain. However, because the incidence of fracture is greater with an eversion mechanism, order x-rays for all suspected deltoid ligament sprains. Make sure the radiograph evaluation includes the distal end of the fibula. Stress x-rays for eversion injuries are not normally ordered. Because the deltoid is a relatively large structure and is responsible for providing the ankle with most of its medial joint stability, a sprain to the deltoid usually takes much longer to heal than does a sprain to the lateral ankle ligaments.

Conditions of the Leg

Though acute musculoskeletal trauma can injure any leg structure, three of the more common areas injured are the syndesmotic complex, anterior compartment, and calcaneal tendon. Conversely, the most common overuse conditions in this region are classified under the umbrella term **medial tibial stress syndrome** (MTSS).

Syndesmosis Sprain
The syndesmosis sprain is one of the most disabling, and misunderstood, leg injuries. Though this injury is technically a leg condition, most people working in the clinical setting consider it to be an ankle injury. Indeed, this injury is commonly referred to as a *high ankle sprain*. Challenging to diagnose, the syndesmosis sprain is often overlooked when assessing acute ankle and leg trauma, because these injuries occur less frequently than ankle sprains. This is probably because a significant amount of force is needed to produce this injury. Thus, syndesmosis sprains tend to occur more in collision and contact sports than in limited-contact and non-contact sports. When a patient does incur this injury, in many instances it occurs in conjunction with other ankle ligament injuries, most commonly a deltoid ligament sprain. It is also subtle in appearance, making its diagnosis that much more difficult. However, by always evaluating for its presence when assessing any acute trauma to the ankle and leg regions, you can increase the chance of accurately identifying this injury.[30–32]

The syndesmosis sprain occurs less frequently than ankle sprains,
is subtle in appearance, and often occurs in conjunction with
other ankle ligament injuries.

Any action that forces the talus into the syndesmotic complex can cause a syndesmosis injury. Typically, this occurs when the ankle is forced into dorsiflexion because, as discussed previously, it is in this position that the wide portion of the talus fits snugly between the malleoli. This results in a separation of the DTF joint and injury to the AITFL. In severe cases, the interosseous membrane is also affected. This dorsiflexion MOI is usually accompanied with external rotation of the talus, but forceful eversion, inversion, plantar flexion, internal talar rotation, or any combination of these motions can cause this injury.[9,30–32]

Forced dorsiflexion and external talar rotation are the primary causes
of a syndesmosis sprain.

History and Physical Examination

The patient with a syndesmosis sprain describes an MOI consistent with that of forced dorsiflexion. The patient states, or you notice, that he or she cannot bear weight on the affected extremity. The distal leg is also often swollen, albeit much less than what occurs in a lateral ankle sprain. However, several days after the date of injury, ecchymosis may be present over the DTF joint. When palpated, the area over the AITFL is tender. Depending on the severity of injury, pain may extend proximally to the interosseous membrane. Patients with this condition are unable to actively dorsiflex the ankle and rise on their toes, and the squeeze test (Fig. 8.10) almost always causes pain in the area of the DTF joint, all telltale signs of a syndesmosis sprain. Injury to the AITFL and syndesmotic complex can be confirmed clinically by performing the **external rotation**, or *Kleiger*, **test** (Fig. 8.18). To perform this test[1,9,31,32]:

- Instruct the patient to sit on the edge of a table with his or her knees flexed to 90°.
- Stabilize the proximal leg with one hand, and grasp the foot with the other.
- Using your distal hand, force the talus into the syndesmotic complex by dorsiflexing and everting the foot in one continuous motion.
- The external rotation test is positive if pain occurs in the area of the DTF joint.

Use the external rotation test to determine whether injury to the
syndesmotic complex has occurred.

Management

Manage a syndesmosis sprain as you would a lateral ankle sprain, including using the Ottawa Ankle Rules (Fig. 8.11) to determine when to order x-rays. Most, if not all,

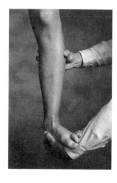

FIGURE 8.18 The external rotation, or Kleiger, test, is used to check the integrity of the anterior inferior tibiofibular ligament and syndesmotic complex.
From Gulick: *Ortho Notes: Clinical Examination Pocket Guide.* 2005. Philadelphia: F.A. Davis Company, pg 215, with permission.

suspected syndesmosis sprains require x-ray evaluation as fractures, particularly those to the distal tibia, which commonly occur with this injury. In addition to obtaining a standard x-ray series, order abduction stress radiographs to confirm widening of the space between the distal tibia and fibula. The amount of space widening can help determine the severity of injury. First and second degree injuries have no separation of the tibia and fibula, whereas widening is present in third degree injuries.[31,32]

Initially treat first and second degree sprains with a four-point, pain-free touch-down crutch gait, as described in PTH 6.1. The patient should progress to full weight-bearing without crutch use as soon as he or she can ambulate without a limp. Implement the rehabilitation exercises outlined in PTH 8.1 and return the patient to activity when pain-free ROM and full muscle strength have been restored. Syndesmosis sprains have a recovery period usually twice that of ankle sprains, which can be very frustrating for those who want to return to sports quickly.[31,32]

PEARL

Syndesmosis sprains have a recovery period usually twice as long as that of ankle sprains.

Prescribe non-weight-bearing crutch use, and refer all patients with third degree injuries, or first and second degree injuries with other remarkable x-ray findings, to an orthopedist. The treatment goal of a third degree syndesmosis sprain is to stabilize the talus within the mortise. This is usually accomplished by cast immobilization and/or screw fixation.[32]

Medial Tibial Stress Syndrome

Commonly referred to as *shin splints*, MTSS accounts for the majority of overuse exercise-induced leg injuries. Although the terms *shin splints* and *MTSS* are used interchangeably in the clinical setting, doing so is incorrect because *shin splints* is a term used to describe any pain in the leg region, whereas *MTSS* refers to specific conditions of the leg. The term *MTSS* is used here because it is a more accurate and a medically accepted term to describe nondescript pain in the leg region.[10,11]

Although pain caused by MTSS can occur anywhere along the medial shaft of the tibia, the most frequently affected area is the tibia's distal two-thirds. This can be a difficult condition to manage, because many soft tissue pathologies, such as strains to the muscles in the leg's posterior compartment, chronic compartment syndrome, entrapments of arteries or nerves, muscle herniations, tendonitis, and myositis, can be the cause of medial tibial pain. However, it is believed the most common cause of MTSS is an irritation of the soleus muscle at its insertion point on the medial tibia and surrounding fascia. This produces fasciitis, periostitis, and/or soleus strain. Regardless, the types of pain produced by any soft tissue injury in this region are similar, as are the treatment plans used to manage the pain.[4,10,11]

When evaluating a patient presenting with pain in this region, it is extremely important to differentiate a soft tissue injury from a tibial stress fracture, which is another common cause of medial tibial pain. This can be challenging, because a stress fracture produces symptoms similar to those of a soft tissue injury. This means that distal leg pain experienced by one patient may be caused by a stress fracture, a potentially serious condition, whereas the same pain in a second patient might be caused by a less serious soft tissue condition. To complicate matters, two or more of these conditions can occur at the same time.[4,10,21] Strategies to clinically determine whether shin pain is caused by a stress fracture or by soft tissue injury are presented later in this chapter.

PEARL

Soft and hard tissue pathologies can cause similar medial tibial pain symptoms.

The reasons for MTSS development, as listed in Box 8.2, are varied and, in some cases, contradictory. For example, one patient may experience distal leg pain due to exercising on too soft a surface, such as a grass field, whereas the same pain in a second person may be due to exercising on too hard a surface, such as running on pavement. It does appear, however, that those involved in running and jumping activities maintain the highest risk of development of MTSS. Also, patients with this condition usually report some change in exercise routine immediately preceding the onset of symptoms. In the high school and collegiate settings, for example, the change of playing seasons, such as what happens when a person stops playing football on a Saturday and starts to compete in basketball on the following Monday, places the leg at great risk for MTSS. Other common changes associated with the development of MTSS include increasing the intensity of exercise bouts and decreasing the amount of rest time between exercise sessions. Regardless of the events leading up to its development, the underlying factor that causes MTSS pain is the inability of the many tissues in the area, including muscles, tendons, and fascia, to quickly adapt to changes in a person's exercise routine.[5,10,11]

BOX 8.2
CAUSES OF MEDIAL TIBIAL STRESS SYNDROME

Exercising on a hard surface	Use of worn-out footwear
Exercising on a soft surface	Exercising while fatigued
Abrupt change in exercise surfaces	Foot pronation
Abrupt change in exercise intensity	Pes planus
Abrupt change in exercise frequency	

PEARL

Patients with MTSS usually report some change in exercise routine immediately preceding the onset of symptoms.

History and Physical Examination

The most important aspect of differentiating among the many conditions that cause MTSS is determining the relation of the patient's pain to exercise. In the early stages of MTSS, the patient reports that dull aching occurs along the distal posteromedial tibia during exercise and subsides with rest. As the condition worsens, the patient reports that pain becomes sharper and more consistent during exercise and is present both before and after exercise. Even after trying periodic trials of complete rest, the patient reports a return of symptoms with a resumption of the offending activity. These patients are point tender on the tibia's posteromedial edge, and pain occurs when they perform one or more of the maneuvers listed in Box 8.3.[4,10,11]

Once you document its existence, determine whether the pain the patient is experiencing is of soft tissue or bone origin. This can be difficult to do, because the initial symptom of a stress fracture, the gradual onset of activity-related pain, is similar to that produced by MTSS. In both instances, this pain starts as an ache that, in its early stages, usually does not affect the patient's ability to exercise. As the condition progresses, pain increases with continued activity, is present at rest, and ultimately continuously stays with the patient, even during the nighttime hours. In this latter injury stage, the pain associated with a stress fracture becomes very focal and intensifies with continued exercise. The developing stress fracture may become palpable in the form of an elevated mass over the tender area, with the posteromedial border of the lower two-thirds of the tibia being the most common place of occurrence. Redness, warmth, and swelling may also be present at the site of fracture. The bump test may be positive if a fracture is present. Ultimately, the pain associated with either a stress fracture or MTSS progresses to the point that the patient has to limit the quantity and quality of exercise and, at times, causes the patient to cease all activity for a period of time.[4,5,10,11,33]

PEARL

Clinical findings of a tibial stress fracture include focal pain, a positive bump test, warmth, redness, and a palpable mass at the injury site.

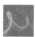

BOX 8.3
FUNCTIONAL TESTS FOR MEDIAL TIBIAL STRESS SYNDROME*

Active plantar flexion with resistance	One-leg stance toe raise
Passive dorsiflexion	(10 repetitions)
Two-leg stance toe raise	Two-leg standing jump
(10 repetitions)	

*Pain produced by any of these maneuvers is a positive sign for medial tibial stress syndrome.

Management

If the results of the clinical assessment indicate the presence of MTSS without stress fracture, treat the condition conservatively by modifying the patient's participation in the offending activity. For example, the patient may have to decrease the intensity and frequency of exercise while the injury heals. In the case of the high school or collegiate athlete, doing this may allow the person to be able to conclude the playing season before you prescribe a more aggressive treatment program of complete rest for the involved area. If indicated, correct for pronation and/or pes planus as previously described. Instruct the patient to treat the area with ice massage, because MTSS responds well to this form of cryotherapy. After pain disappears, prescribe stretching exercises for the calcaneal tendon as presented in PTH 8.1, because performing these exercises too early in the treatment process may aggravate the condition. As symptoms of MTSS lessen, gradually increase the amount of time the person spends, and intensity with which the person participates, in the offending activity. Because of the complexities surrounding this condition, managing MTSS takes some trial and error.[10,11]

For those patients who do not respond to the above treatment plan and for those whose clinical assessment leads to the conclusion that a stress fracture is present, begin managing the condition by obtaining plain-film radiographs. In an MTSS injury, x-ray findings will be normal, but in cases of a stress fracture, callous formation around the painful area may be seen if the condition has been present for 2 or more weeks. Follow-up negative x-ray findings with a bone scan, because this definitively differentiates MTSS from a stress fracture. Once a stress fracture is documented, remove the patient from the offending activity until the fracture is fully healed. Apply a short leg cast, or use a tibial walking boot, and prescribe a four-point, pain-free touchdown crutch gait as described in PTH 6.1 for patients who cannot walk without a limp and for those you suspect will not follow your advice regarding nonparticipation. After the stress fracture has fully healed, gradually return the person to the offending activity. Conservative treatment usually allows a gradual return to participation 6 to 12 weeks after the initiation of treatment.[4,5,10,11]

PEARL

Once a stress fracture is documented, remove the patient from the offending activity until the fracture is fully healed.

Anterior Compartment Syndrome

As reviewed in Chapter 1, compartment syndrome can occur in any of the body's fascial compartments. In the leg, the anterior compartment is most commonly affected because it is most exposed to direct trauma and the amount of space within this compartment is limited, making it vulnerable to pressure increases. Both chronic exertional compartment syndrome (CECS) and acute compartment syndrome (ACS) occur in the leg's anterior compartment. Though it happens less frequently in the leg, ACS has a greater potential for causing permanent tissue damage because of the rapid increases in intracompartmental pressure associated with this injury. Regardless, each condition requires prompt diagnosis and treatment.[34]

History and Physical Examination

The patient presenting with ACS usually relates a history of receiving a direct blow to the leg. This commonly occurs in the sport of soccer, which, because of its nature, places the anterior compartment at risk for such injury. In these instances, the patient usually states that he or she was "kicked in the shin," causing pain beyond what normally occurs in a simple shin bruise. In severe cases, the patient may report an inability to dorsiflex the ankle, a symptom related to the affect the rising intracompartmental pressure has on the muscles within the compartment.[34]

Patients with CECS of the anterior compartment report being involved in an activity that requires them to repetitively dorsiflex the ankle. Thus, this condition occurs in long-distance runners and is also seen in baseball and softball catchers because of the constant squatting demands of these positions. The person with this condition relates a bilateral feeling of tightness, cramping, burning, and aching pain of the anterior compartment muscles during and immediately after exercise. The patient also reports numbness and a "pins and needles" feeling in the foot. A key sign of CECS is that these symptoms usually subside within a few minutes after exercise. However, in many instances, the amount of exercise the person can do the day after a CECS episode is less than it was the day before.[4,10,11,33,34]

PEARL

A bilateral feeling of tightness, cramping, and burning and an aching pain of the anterior compartment during exercise are indicative of CECS.

When observed, the patient with ACS presents the hallmark findings of redness, swelling, and extremely tight skin over the site of the injury. In these cases, the area is usually hot and stiff when palpated. Passive plantar flexion also causes pain because it stretches the structures located in the anterior compartment. In some instances, distal circulation and sensation are compromised; these signs can be confirmed by checking the patient's dorsalis pedis pulse and capillary refill and by feeling in the web space located between the heads of the first and second metatarsals.[34,35]

PEARL

Redness, swelling, heat, and stiffness over the anterior compartment are hallmark signs of ACS.

Whereas the physical examination of the person with ACS produces remarkable findings, the anterior compartment of patient's with CECS usually appears normal because CECS symptoms subside quickly after activity has been stopped. In these instances, try to reproduce symptoms by having the patient perform the offending activity before you perform the physical examination. If this is not possible, rely on the information gleaned in the history portion of the examination to make a diagnosis of CECS.[10,11,34]

Management

Initially, treat those with ACS and CECS with protection, rest, ice, and elevation. Do not apply a compression wrap, because this may increase intracompartmental pressure. Instruct the patient to use ice massage on the area, because applying an ice bag to the region, even without using an elastic wrap to secure the bag, may increase intracompartmental pressure.

Immediately refer the patient with ACS to an orthopedist. If symptoms are worsening and/or if distal circulation and sensation are compromised, an orthopedist should assess the condition the same day of your evaluation. If this is not possible, arrange for hospital admission, because this condition is a true medical emergency. If possible, transport the patient in a supine position with the leg elevated. If the patient has to ambulate under his or her own power, prescribe non-weight-bearing crutch use as described in PTH 6.1. Depending on the level of intracompartmental pressure and the swiftness with which the pressure is building, the patient either will be monitored to ensure that the tissues within the anterior compartment do not become necrotic or will undergo an immediate surgical decompression through a **fasciotomy**. If left untreated, this condition can lead to a loss of ankle dorsiflexion, otherwise known as **drop foot**. Patients with drop foot are unable to dorsiflex the ankle when walking, making them incapable of maintaining a normal heel-to-toe walking gait. This results in the plantar aspect of the foot "slapping" on the ground when the person strides. Depending on the extent of tissue damage, this can be either a transient or a permanent condition.[34,35]

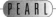

PEARL

Immediately refer patients with **ACS** to an orthopedist or admit them to a hospital, especially in cases in which distal circulation and sensation have been compromised.

Initially, treat the patient with CECS conservatively by limiting the involvement in the offending activity. Once symptoms subside, gradually return the person to full activity. If the results of the initial evaluation question the health of the tibia or fibula, obtain plain-film radiographs and/or bone scan to rule out a fracture. Other imaging techniques, such as MRI, are not overly useful in the early treatment stages for CECS. Refer the patient to an orthopedist if he or she does not respond to conservative treatment or if symptoms increase to the point that distal circulation or sensation is compromised. Fortunately, the complications associated with ACS (foot drop, necrosis) rarely occur in instances of CECS.[34]

Calcaneal Tendon and Retrocalcaneal Bursa Overuse Pathologies

The calcaneal tendon, the body's largest and strongest tendon, and the retrocalcaneal bursa are prone to overuse injury when they are exposed to repeated or sustained episodes of ankle joint dorsiflexion. This MOI causes an array of chronic musculoskeletal conditions, such as tendonitis, tendinosis, tenosynovitis, and bursitis. Although tendonitis is thought to be the most common result of calcaneal tendon irritation, as discussed in Chapter 1, most cases of tendonitis are, in reality, tendinosis conditions. However, because the term *tendonitis* is most commonly used to describe overuse trauma to this tendon, this term is used here.

PEARL

The calcaneal tendon and retrocalcaneal bursa are prone to overuse injury any time they are exposed to repeated or sustained episodes of ankle joint dorsiflexion.

The symptoms produced by the many overuse conditions in this region are similar at times, making it difficult to arrive at a specific diagnosis. Fortunately, in the primary care setting these symptoms, regardless of underlying pathology, are managed very similarly. This makes recognizing that the tendon, the bursa, or both have been injured and implementing a proper treatment plan more important than making an exact diagnosis.

History and Physical Examination

Calcaneal tendon pathology most commonly occurs in long-distance runners and is usually associated with some type of training error. For example, during the history portion of the evaluation, patients may report that they recently increased the number of miles they run per day (or week), that they increased the intensity of their exercise sessions, or that they made a sudden change in surfaces on which they train. In addition, poor calf flexibility, faulty footwear, pronation and pes planus, and the aging process have all been identified as contributing to these conditions.[1,36-38]

As with calcaneal tendon pathologies, retrocalcaneal bursitis can be associated with an error in training, poor footwear, and structural abnormalities. However, this condition usually results from the posterior aspect of the person's shoe rubbing against the calcaneus at the calcaneal tendon's attachment site. This puts people who participate in sports such as ice hockey and figure skating at high risk for development of this condition because the firm boot of an ice skate commonly rubs against the person's heel. This condition also occurs in young females as they begin to wear high-heeled shoes.[4,27]

When evaluating this region, patients with calcaneal tendon pathology relate a history of pain and stiffness 2 to 6 cm above the tendon's insertion on the calcaneus. This corresponds to an area of decreased blood supply, which becomes more and more avascular as a person ages. Initially, this discomfort occurs upon arising in the morning, only to disappear as the day goes on. As the injury progresses, these symptoms reappear at the start and toward the end of the patient's exercise session. By the time the patient comes to see you, pain and stiffness are usually present throughout the day and intensify as the person's exercise session progresses, when the person ascends and descends hills while running, and when the person walks up and down stairs. Symptoms that are continuously present and intensify with activity indicate that the injury is most likely in an advanced stage. In many instances, the only physical finding relating to overuse calcaneal tendon pathology is the presence of swelling on either side of the tendon. If the injury is severe and/or if the area is particularly irritated, the region may also be red and warm to the touch. The presence of crepitus, which can be felt as the patient plantar flexes and dorsiflexes the ankle, is indicative of calcaneal tendon tendonitis. In some cases, passive ankle dorsiflexion may cause pain and be limited. A plantar flexion manual muscle test may also be painful.[1,36-38]

Crepitus occurring while the patient actively dorsiflexes and plantar flexes the ankle is indicative of calcaneal tendon tendonitis.

In contrast to calcaneal tendon pathology, people with retrocalcaneal bursitis report posterior heel tenderness when they wear shoes, a symptom that goes away when the shoes are removed. Though other symptoms, such as swelling, redness, and warmth, similar to what is seen in calcaneal tendon pathology, may also exist, patients with bursitis usually do not experience the crepitus and limited dorsiflexion ROM commonly associated with tendon pathology. If left untreated, the bursa can become thickened, and the calcaneus, in response to the irritation, may attempt to protect itself by developing an exostosis. Ultimately, this process results in **Haglund's deformity**, otherwise known as a *pump bump*, a condition characterized by a thickened retrocalcaneal bursa on the lateral side of the heel with or without an underlying calcaneal exostosis. If present, this thickened bursa is clearly evident on the lateral side of the heel and matches up with a rounded, worn area on the inside of the patient's shoe.[3,27]

Management

Treat patients with overuse calcaneal tendon pathology with complete rest, or at least a decrease in the amount of time they spend participating in the offending activity. Correct for pronation and pes planus if needed, and advise overweight and obese patients to lose weight. Prescribe calcaneal tendon stretches and calf-strengthening exercises as outlined in PTH 8.1. Instruct patients to perform these activities without causing pain, and have them slowly increase the time they spend stretching and the amount resistance used for strengthening as pain and discomfort allow. Advise patients to place a heel cup in their shoes to take pressure off the tendon. A heel cup can be purchased at a pharmacy store. However, using a heel cup causes the triceps surae to shorten, which predisposes this structure to injury. Thus, any use of a heel cup must occur in conjunction with a calcaneal tendon stretching routine. Gradually return the patient to activity as pain and stiffness subside, but avoid too rapid a return, because doing so is a prime cause of tendon reinjury. Refer all who do not respond to conservative treatment for orthopedic consultation.[36–38]

In addition to treating patients with retrocalcaneal bursitis with rest, advise these patients to relieve the friction imposed by their shoes. Do this by discouraging the use of high heels and by encouraging the use of shoes with good heel padding. Increasing shoe size by one-half may also relieve symptoms. Padding the shoes for those who have a pump bump deformity and encouraging these people to use a heel lift, which relieves pressure by raising the hind foot out of the shoe counter, may alleviate symptoms. If these measures do not remedy the situation, refer the patient to an orthopedist for an aggressive treatment approach. Surgical intervention includes excising the soft tissue deformity and, if necessary, the calcaneal prominence. Unless excised, the thickened bursa will always be present to some extent.[3,27]

Calcaneal Tendon Rupture

Although acute injury to the calcaneal tendon occurs less frequently than overuse injury, it is important to distinguish an acute tear, or rupture, from a chronic injury. Indeed, this injury is misdiagnosed fairly often in the primary care setting.

Whereas episodes of repeated dorsiflexion cause overuse injury to the calcaneal tendon, a tendon rupture is usually the result of a forced, rapid dorsiflexion mechanism, particularly when this action occurs at the same time the triceps surae undergoes an eccentric contraction. This commonly happens when a person returns to the ground after completing a jump, because the triceps surae is partially responsible for absorbing the landing forces produced by this return to earth. A calcaneal tendon rupture can also be the result of one massive concentric contraction of the triceps surae. This commonly happens when a person initiates a jump, because the triceps surae, by powerfully plantar flexing the ankle, is responsible for propelling the body upward. Thus, it should come as no surprise that calcaneal tendon ruptures commonly occur in those who participate in jumping sports, such as basketball and volleyball. It is also seen in those who participate in racket sports, such as tennis and racquetball, because these require participants to constantly perform quick changes of direction during play, placing great stress on the calcaneal tendon. Although anyone who participates in the above activities is at an increased risk for a calcaneal tendon rupture, it most commonly occurs in men aged 30 to 50 years, in those just starting out in a sporting activity, and in those increasing their physical activity level. It is also seen more in recreational athletes than in professional athletes.[1,36,38]

PEARL

Calcaneal tendon ruptures occur most commonly in men aged 30 to 50 years, in those just starting out in a sporting activity, and in those increasing their physical activity level.

History and Physical Examination

Patients presenting with a calcaneal tendon rupture report that they felt and heard a "pop" coming from the back of the ankle at the time of injury. Patients typically state that they felt as if they were struck in the area of the calcaneal tendon at the time of injury, only to find this was not the case. For example, a basketball player may relate that she thought she was kicked by an opposing player, or a racquetball player may relate that he felt as if he was hit with the ball during play. Patients with a ruptured calcaneal tendon may or may not be in substantial pain, because a complete tendon rupture also tears the nerves in the area. This prevents free nerve endings in the injured area from sending pain impulses to the brain. Some report a history of a painful tendon before the incidence of injury, because it is common for those with tendinosis to experience acute calcaneal tendon trauma.[1,36,38]

Patients with a calcaneal tendon rupture present with swelling and a palpable gap in the tendon's avascular zone 2 to 6 cm above its calcaneal insertion (Fig. 8.19). If a gap is present, the calcaneal tendon has ruptured, or separated from its musculotendinous junction with the triceps surae. Noticeable weakness occurs during a plantar flexion manual muscle test, but some strength still exists because other muscles of the posterior compartment also perform the action of plantar flexion. These patients are unable to stand on tiptoe because doing so is virtually impossible due to muscle weakness and instability. The **Thompson test** is also positive when performed on those with a complete calcaneal tendon tear. To perform this test[1,36,38] (Fig. 8.20):

- Instruct the patient to lie prone, with his or her feet dangling off the end of the table.
- Position yourself at the side of the patient.
- Squeeze the belly of the triceps surae.
- A positive test occurs when the ankle does not plantar flex.

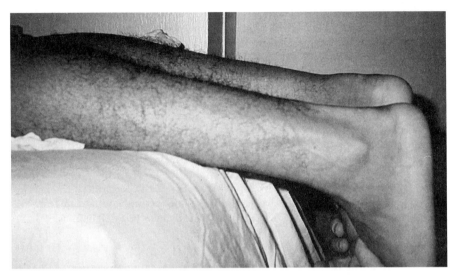

FIGURE 8.19 Ruptured calcaneal tendon. The patient's right (far) tendon has been ruptured. Note the depression proximal to the calcaneus and the involved swelling.
From Starkey and Ryan: *Evaluation of Orthopedic and Athletic Injuries*, 2nd ed. 2002. Philadelphia: F.A. Davis Company, Fig. 5-29, pg 175, with permission.

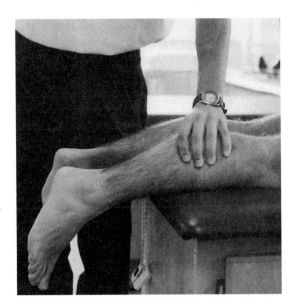

FIGURE 8.20 The Thompson test is used to check the integrity of the calcaneal tendon.
From Starkey and Ryan: *Evaluation of Orthopedic and Athletic Injuries,* 2nd ed. 2002. Philadelphia: F.A. Davis Company, Box 5-10, pg 177, with permission.

A positive Thompson test is indicative of a complete calcaneal
tendon rupture.

Management

Although imaging techniques, such as MRI, may aid in diagnosing this condition, a ruptured calcaneal tendon can easily be made clinically. Thus, for all suspected tendon ruptures, prescribe three-point gait, non-weight-bearing crutch use, as described in PTH 6.1, and refer the patient to an orthopedist. Most patients are able to ambulate without trouble, because pain is usually minimal and other posterior compartment muscles are able to substitute for the actions performed by the triceps surae. It is best, however, to recommend that patients use crutches, because this helps protect the body part from further injury while the patient arranges for an evaluation from an orthopedist.

Partial calcaneal tendon tears are almost always treated conservatively. Depending on certain factors, including the patient's age and future desired activity level, complete tendon ruptures are treated either conservatively or surgically. Regardless, an extensive period of functional bracing and rehabilitation follow a complete tendon tear. Full recovery and a return to sports after this injury usually take 12 to 18 months.[1,38]

Refer all patients with suspected calcaneal tendon ruptures
to an orthopedist.

Lifespan Considerations

Although the symptoms produced by a specific musculoskeletal condition of the foot, ankle, or leg are, for the most part, similar across age groups, when reported by younger patients, these symptoms may be caused by a different pathology. For example, the adult who reports morning plantar heel pain that subsides as the day progresses most likely has plantar fasciitis. However, the same heel pain reported by a child may indicate an apophyseal injury. Thus, it is important to be aware of the more common musculoskeletal conditions germane to younger age groups so these can be considered when arriving at a differential diagnosis for this population.

Sever's Disease

Sever's disease, or *calcaneal apophysitis*, is a traction-type injury caused by the calcaneal tendon pulling so strongly on its distal attachment site that microavulsion of the secondary ossification center of the calcaneus occurs. Most commonly seen in boys aged 8 to 10 and girls aged 10 to 12 years, Sever's disease is the number one cause of heel pain in active children. It is primarily associated with those who participate in activities requiring repetitive contractions of the triceps surae, such as running and jumping, and commonly occurs at the beginning of a new sport or playing season. Conditions that present as Sever's disease include plantar fasciitis, calcaneal tendon tendonitis, and retrocalcaneal bursitis.[3,27,39,40]

Sever's disease is the number one cause of heel pain in active children.

Children with Sever's disease usually report a history of growth spurt immediately before symptom development. A growth spurt causes the long bones of the leg to exceed increases in muscle and tendon length, resulting in a lack of flexibility of the triceps surae. This lack of flexibility is the ultimate cause of the calcaneal tendon pulling on the calcaneus's secondary ossification center. The patient also reports intermittent or continuous heel pain with weight-bearing. The patient usually states that pain is absent in the morning, increases as the day progresses and as activity increases, and subsides at night. Upon evaluation, the patient's foot is tender along the medial and lateral portions of the calcaneus and just anterior to the insertion of the calcaneal tendon. Passive dorsiflexion is limited, and performing this action increases pain. Pain elicited when the patient stands on tiptoe is a positive sign for Sever's disease. Plain-film radiographs are not helpful in evaluating this condition, so rely on clinical findings to make the diagnosis.[3,27,39,40]

Rely on clinical findings, rather than the results of radiographs, to make a diagnosis of Sever's disease.

Sever's disease is managed symptomatically by modifying the offending activity and by stretching and strengthening the triceps surae and the calcaneal tendon as out-lined in PTH 8.1. Patients with this condition should avoid walking barefoot and should use shoes that maintain good heel support. Placing heel lifts in the person's shoes also offers some relief of symptoms. Partial weight-bearing or no weight-bearing is helpful in instances in which the patient cannot walk without a limp. Most cases of Sever's disease resolve within a few weeks if managed properly. If not, the patient should be referred to an orthopedist. More aggressive treatment includes the use of a short leg cast for 3 to 6 weeks. Regardless of the treatment plan, symptoms ultimately subside when the heel's ossification center joins the main calcaneal body. This occurs around the age of 12 in most patients.[3,39,40]

Freiberg's Infraction

Freiberg's infraction is avascular necrosis of a metatarsal epiphysis, located at the metatarsal's head. Although any metatarsal can be affected, this condition most commonly occurs in the second. Usually caused by repetitive foot trauma associated with excessive pressure on the metatarsal head associated with foot pronation, this infraction can also be caused by a macrotrauma event, such as when a person stubs his or her toe. The average age of the affected person is 13 years, and 75% of those affected are active, young females.[27,41,42]

Active, young adolescent females are most at risk of development of a Freiberg's infraction.

The patient with a Freiberg's infraction reports unilateral pain over the head of the affected metatarsal. Initially, the person has trouble identifying an area of point tenderness but does relate that it worsens with impact activities, such as running and jumping. When palpated, the MTP joint formed by the affected metatarsal head is tender, and moving this joint causes pain and crepitation. When these symptoms are present, a Freiberg's infraction is sometimes mistaken for other forefoot conditions, such as metatarsalgia, a phalangeal and/or metatarsal fracture, or an MTP joint sprain.[27,42]

PEARL

A Freiberg's infraction is sometimes mistaken for other forefoot conditions, such as metatarsalgia, a phalangeal and/or metatarsal fracture, or an MTP joint sprain.

A Freiberg's infraction is initially managed by obtaining plain-film radiographic images to document the infraction's existence and to rule out other pathologies. If an x-ray fails to reveal the defect, which occurs if the condition is in its early stages of development, a bone scan or MRI can confirm the infraction. Early stage infractions, defined as those identified by minimal joint irregularity and no loose body formations, are treated conservatively with a short leg cast and a four-point, pain-free touchdown crutch gait as described in PTH 6.1. These patients can progress to full weight-bearing and have the cast removed when symptoms subside enough to allow for pain-free walking. At this time, patients should use stiff-soled shoes because these decrease pain by limiting MTP motion. The patient's activity level is then increased as tolerated. During this time, periodic radiographs are used to monitor the health of the MTP joint. It may take as long as 4 months for these patients to become asymptomatic.[41,42]

If any imaging technique reveals that a Freiberg's infraction has affected the MTP joint in the form of extensive irregularity and a flattening of the metatarsal head, the patient should be referred to an orthopedist. In these instances, the person is treated surgically with joint débridement and removal of loose bodies.[41]

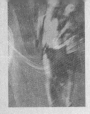

CASE STUDY
Conditions Involving the Foot, Ankle, and Leg

SCENARIO
A 21-year-old male college junior comes to your campus university health service after injuring his left ankle 3 days ago while playing intramural flag football. He states that after jumping to catch the ball, he came down and "twisted" his ankle. He reports hearing and feeling at the time of injury a "crunching" on the outside of the ankle. He reports feeling immediate pain, and although he walked off the field and returned to his dorm room under his own power, he limped the entire way. After icing the ankle for 20 minutes, he noticed that the joint was swollen, and after the effects of the cold treatment wore off, the pain worsened and the ankle started to throb. For the past 2 days, he has been periodically icing the injury and has been walking from his dorm room to class and the dining hall. Although he reports that the ankle is painful and still throbs, these symptoms have greatly improved.

PERTINENT HISTORY
Medications: Currently taking ibuprofen 200 mg qid. No other medications.

Family History: No significant family illnesses reported.

PERSONAL HEALTH HISTORY
Tobacco Use: Smokes on occasion, usually on the weekends when "partying" with his friends.

Recreational Drugs: Denies use.

Alcohol Intake: 5 to 6 drinks on both Friday and Saturday nights. Denies drinking during the school week.

Caffeinated Beverages: 1 cola per day.

Exercise: In addition to playing flag football, the patient also plays pickup basketball games at the student recreation center 2 or 3 days per week.

Past Medical History: Generally healthy. Chicken pox at age 10; mumps at age 4.

PERTINENT PHYSICAL EXAMINATION*
On physical examination, his left ankle is severely swollen around the area of the lateral malleolus, and ecchymosis has started to develop distal to the malleolus. He cannot bear full weight on the affected ankle. ROM is decreased in all planes, with plantar flexion and inversion being most affected. He has tenderness over the lateral malleolus, distal end of the fibula, base of the fifth metatarsal, ATFL, and CFL. The anterior drawer and inversion talar tilt tests are positive, with a hard end-feel. The eversion talar tilt, external rotation, bump, and squeeze tests are all negative.

*Focused examination limited to key points for this case.

(case study continues on page 224)

CASE STUDY
Conditions Involving the Foot, Ankle, and Leg (continued)

RED FLAGS FOR THE PRIMARY HEALTH CARE PROFESSIONAL TO CONSIDER

- A history of a "twisted" ankle almost always means an inversion ankle sprain and injury to the lateral ankle ligaments.
- Positive anterior drawer and inversion talar tilt tests are indicative of sprains to the ATFL and CFL.
- Bony tenderness and an inability to bear weight immediately after the injury and/or in the office indicate the need for radiograph evaluation (Ottawa Ankle Rules).
- Tenderness over the base of the fifth metatarsal indicates a possible fracture (Jones fracture) and justifies the need for x-ray evaluation.

RECOMMENDED PLAN

- Treat with the PRICE acronym by doing the following:
  - Immobilize in a dorsiflexed, everted position.
  - Prescribe non-weight-bearing crutch use.
  - Advise use of ice bag treatment with elevation and compression.
- Change medication to acetaminophen 1000 mg qid.
- Obtain standard and stress x-rays.
- Refer to an orthopedist if a fracture is identified.
- If x-ray findings are negative, provide the patient with a written home management care plan to include ankle ROM and strengthening exercises.
- Refer for physical therapy.
- Encourage the patient to progress to four-point, pain-free touchdown crutch gait as pain and discomfort allow.
- Instruct the patient to stop using the crutches as soon as he can walk without a limp.
- Reevaluate the patient in 2 weeks.

REFERENCES

1. Rubin A, Sallis R. Evaluation and diagnosis of ankle injuries. *Am Fam Physician* 1996;58:1609.
2. Safran MR, Benedetti RS, Bartolozzi AR III, et al. Lateral ankle sprains: a comprehensive review, part I: etiology, pathoanatomy, histopathogenesis, and diagnosis. *Med Sci Sports Exerc* 1999;31(7 suppl):S429.
3. Manusov EG, Lillegard WA, Raspa RF, et al. Evaluation of pediatric foot problems, part II: the hindfoot and the ankle. *Am Fam Physician* 1996;54:1012.
4. Schon LC, Baxter DE, Clanton TO. Chronic exercise-induced leg pain in active people: more than just shin splints. *Phys Sportsmed* 1992;20(1):100.
5. Brunker P. Exercise-related lower leg pain: bone. *Med Sci Sports Exerc* 2000; 32(3 suppl):S15.
6. Bachmann LM, Kolb E, Koller MT, et al. Accuracy of Ottawa ankle rules to exclude fractures of the ankle and mid-foot: systematic review. *BMJ* 2003;326:417.
7. Plint AC, Bulloch B, Osmond MH, et al. Validation of the Ottawa ankle rules in children with ankle injuries. *Acad Emerg Med* 1999;6:1005.
8. Lazarus ML. Imaging of the foot and ankle in the injured athlete. *Med Sci Sports Exerc* 1999;31(7 suppl):S412.
9. Wolfe MW, Uhl TL, Mattacola CG, et al. Management of ankle sprains. *Am Fam Physician* 2001;63(1):93.
10. Couture CJ, Darlson KA. Tibial stress injuries: decisive diagnosis and treatment of shin splints. *Phys Sportsmed* 2002;30(6):29.
11. Kortenbein PM, Kaufman KR, Basford JR, et al. Medial tibial stress syndrome. *Med Sci Sports Exerc* 2000; 32(3 suppl):S27
12. Simons SM. Foot injuries of the recreational athlete. *Phys Sportsmed* 1999;27(1):57.
13. Ganzhorn R, Toy BJ. Fractures to the fifth metatarsal: speedy conservative treatment for hockey players. *Phys Sportsmed* 1990;18(12):67.
14. Torg JS, Balduini FC, Zelko RR, et al. Fractures of the base of the fifth metatarsal distal to the tuberosity: classification and guidelines for non-surgical and surgical management. *J Bone Joint Surg Am* 1984;66:209.
15. Zelko RR, Torg JS, Rachun A. Proximal diaphyseal fractures of the fifth metatarsal: treatment of the fractures and their complications in athletes. *Am J Sports Med* 1979;7:95.
16. Mindrebo N, Shelbourne KD, Van Meter CD, et al. Outpatient percutaneous screw fixation of the acute Jones fracture. *Am J Sports Med* 1993;21:720.
17. Hockenbury RT. Forefoot problems in athletes. *Med Sci Sports Exerc* 1999;31 (7 suppl):S448.
18. Rodeo SA, O'Brien SJ, Warren RF, et al. Turf toe: diagnosis and treatment. *Phys Sportsmed* 1989;17(4):132.
19. Perron AD. Metatarsal stress fracture. *eMedicine*. Retrieved from: http://www.emedicine.com/sports/topic81.htm. Accessed 7/29/08.
20. Perron AD, Brady WJ, Kats TA. Management of common stress fractures: when to apply conservative therapy, when to take an aggressive approach. *Postgrad Med* 2002;111(2):95.
21. Brunkner P, Bradshaw C, Bennell K. Managing common stress fractures. *Phys Sportsmed* 1998;26(8):39.
22. Protzman PR. Physiologic performance of women compared to men at the U.S. Military Academy. *Am J Sports Med* 1979;7:191.
23. Kadel NJ, Teitz CC, Kronmal RA. Stress fractures in ballet dancers. *Am J Sports Med* 1992;20:445.
24. Shea M, Fields KB. Plantar fasciitis: prescribing effective treatments. *Phys Sportsmed* 2002;30(7):21.
25. Cornwall MW, McPoil TG. Plantar fasciitis: etiology and treatment. *J Orthop Sports Phys Ther* 1999;29:756.
26. Kibler WB, Goldberg C, Chandler TJ. Functional biomechanical deficits in running athletes with plantar fasciitis. *Am J Sports Med* 1991;19:66.
27. Omey ML, Micheli LJ. Foot and ankle problems in the young athlete. *Med Sci Sports Exerc* 1999;31(7 suppl):S470.
28. Garrick JG. The frequency of injury, mechanism of injury, and epidemiology of ankle sprains. *Am J Sports Med* 1977;5:241.

29. Safran MR, Zachazewski JE, Benedetti, et al. Lateral ankle sprains: a comprehensive review, part 2: treatment and rehabilitation with an emphasis on the athlete. *Med Sci Sports Exerc* 1999;31(7 suppl):S438.
30. Norkus SA. The anatomy and mechanics of syndesmotic ankle sprains. *J Athl Train* 2001;36:68.
31. Boytim MJ, Fischer DA, Neuman L. Syndesmotic ankle sprains. *Am J Sports Med* 1991;19:294.
32. Taylor DC, Bassett FH. Syndesmosis ankle sprains: diagnosing the injury and aiding recovery. *Phys Sportsmed* 1993;21(12):39.
33. Brukner P. Exercise-related lower leg pain: an overview. *Med Sci Sports Exerc* 2000; 32(3 suppl):S1.
34. Swain R. Lower extremity compartment syndrome: when to suspect acute or chronic pressure buildup. *Postgrad Med* 1999;105(3):159.
35. Stuart MJ, Karaharju TK. Acute compartment syndrome: recognizing the progressive signs and symptoms. *Phys Sportsmed* 1994;22(3):91.
36. Clement DB, Taunton JE, Smart GW. Achilles tendinitis and peritendinitis: etiology and treatment. *Am J Sports Med* 1984;12:179.
37. Leach RE, Schepsis AA, Takai H. Achilles tendinitis: don't let it be an athlete's downfall. *Phys Sportsmed* 1991;19(8):87.
38. Mazzone MF, McCue T. Common conditions of the Achilles tendon. *Am Fam Physician* 2002;69:1805.
39. Madden CC, Mellon MB. Sever's disease and other causes of heel pain in adolescents. *Am Fam Physician* 1996;54:1995.
40. Adirim TA, Cheng TL. Overview of injuries in the young athlete. *Sports Med* 2003;33:75.
41. Sproul J, Klaaren H, Mannarino F. Surgical treatment of Freiberg's infraction in athletes. *Am J Sports Med* 1993;21:381.
42. Veenema KR. Forefoot pain in a young girl. *Phys Sportsmed* 1999;27(1):91.

SUGGESTED READINGS

Ganley TJ. Ankle injury in the young athlete: fracture or sprain? *J Musculoskeletal Med* 2000;17:311.
Judd D, Kim D. Foot fractures frequently misdiagnosed as ankle sprains. *Am Fam Physician* 2002;66:785.
Walgenbach AW. The ankle joint: the evaluation and treatment of sprains. *Nurse Pract Forum* 1996;7(3):120.

WEB LINKS

http://www.nlm.nih.gov/medlineplus/footinjuriesanddisorders.html. Accessed 7/29/08.
    Excellent resource for diagnosing, treating, and managing foot injuries and disorders.
http://www.nismat.org/ptcor/ankle_sprain. Accessed 7/29/08.
    Presents methods to grade, treat, and rehabilitate ankle sprains.
http://www.nlm.nih.gov/medlineplus/leginjuriesanddisorders.html. Accessed 7/29/08.
    Excellent resource for diagnosing, treating, and managing leg injuries and disorders.

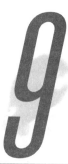

Conditions Involving the Knee and Thigh

● Brian J. Toy, PhD, ATC

The knee consists of two joints: the **tibiofemoral** (TFJ) and the **patellofemoral** (PFJ). Together these joints form the largest and most complex freely moveable structure in the body. Frequently injured during sports participation, knee trauma results from intrinsic factors, such as poor bony alignment, and from extrinsic factors, such as when an external force is applied to the body. Structures commonly injured include ligaments, tendons, cartilage, and bone. While these tissues help to stabilize and protect the joint, they also provide the knee with significant mobility. The fact that the knee is both stable and mobile points to its importance in enabling the body to partake in a wide variety of athletic activities.

Anatomy of the Knee

Anatomical structures important when evaluating musculoskeletal injury to the knee include bones, ligaments, muscles, tendons, cartilage, bursae, and retinacula. These structures, as well as the motions allowed by the TFJ and PFJ, are discussed here.

Bones and Joints (Fig. 9.1)

Bones that compose the knee include the femur, tibia, and patella. Although the fibula acts as an attachment point for many soft tissues, it is not involved in the knee's bony

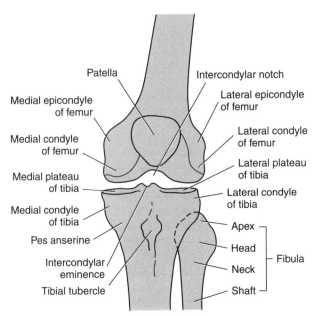

FIGURE 9.1 Bony and articular structures of the knee: anterior view. Adapted from McKinnis: *Fundamentals of Musculoskeletal Imaging*, 2nd ed. 2005. Philadelphia: F.A. Davis Company, Fig. 10-1, pg 330, with permission.

makeup. Thus, the discussion here is limited to the contribution the fibula plays as an attachment point for surrounding soft tissues.

The largest long bone in the body, the femur is a major weight-bearing structure that also acts as an attachment point for numerous muscles and ligaments. Its distal portion flares to form convex medial and lateral condyles, with medial and lateral epicondyles rising off these structures. Anteriorly, the medial and lateral condyles meet to form a shallow depression termed the patellar, or *femoral*, groove. Posteriorly, the condyles diverge and are separated by an intercondylar notch.

Like the femur, the tibia is a major weight-bearing structure and acts as an attachment point for numerous muscles and ligaments. Its proximal end consists of concave medial and lateral condyles with medial and lateral plateaus. These are separated by the intercondylar eminence, situated on top of these condyles. The menisci of the knee, discussed later in this chapter, are situated on these plateaus. It is these plateaus that articulate with the femoral condyles to form the TFJ. Other tibial bony landmarks include the tibial tubercle, also known as the *tibial tuberosity*, located on the anterior surface of the tibia just distal to the patella, and the pes anserinus, located on the anteromedial aspect of the tibia just distal to the medial condyle. Finally, the inverted triangle–shaped patella, the largest **sesamoid bone** in the body, rides within the femoral groove to form the PFJ.

Motions

Classified as a modified hinge joint, TFJ allows for the primary motions of flexion, extension, internal rotation, and external rotation (Figs. 9.2 and 9.3). The average ranges of motion (ROMs) for each of these movements are listed in Box 9.1. Accessory motions that accompany these primary motions include anterior, posterior, medial, and lateral translation of the tibia's plateaus on the femur's condyles. That is, the tibia glides forward, backward, and side to side during normal knee motion. Although the amount of tibial translation is usually quite small, the movement is necessary for the knee to function properly. As explained later in this chapter, a knee examination that produces excessive amounts of tibial translation, particularly in the anterior/posterior plane, is an indication of knee pathology.

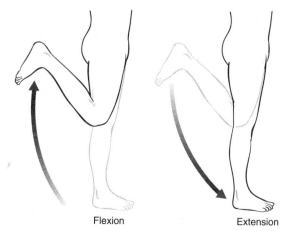

FIGURE 9.2 Flexion and extension of the knee.
From Lippert: *Clinical Kinesiology and Anatomy*, 4th ed. 2006. Philadelphia: F.A. Davis Company, Fig. 18-2, pg 252, with permission.

Flexion   Extension

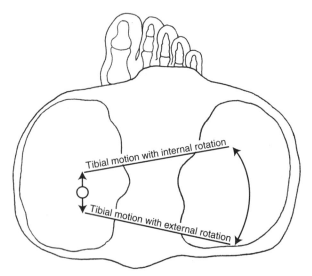

FIGURE 9.3 Internal and external rotation of the knee. From Levangie and Norkin: *Joint Structure and Function: A Comprehensive Analysis,* 4th ed. 2005. Philadelphia: F.A. Davis Company, Fig. 11-31, pg 412, with permission.

BOX 9.1
ACTIVE RANGES OF MOTION OF THE TIBIOFEMORAL JOINT

135° Flexion	10°–20° Internal rotation
0° Extension	20°–30° External rotation

The motions of the PFJ are defined by the direction the patella moves within the femoral groove when the knee flexes and extends. During flexion, the patella moves distally, whereas during extension, it moves proximally. The patella can also move medially and laterally during TFJ motion. As with the TFJ's accessory motions, the amount the patella moves is relatively small, but a normally functioning PFJ is important in maintaining overall knee health.

Ligaments

The knee's bony makeup does not contribute greatly to its strength. Instead, the primary knee ligaments provide the knee with much of its stability. These include the collaterals and cruciates of the TFJ (Fig. 9.4). The **patellar ligament** provides stability for the PFJ (Fig. 9.5).

Collateral Ligaments (Fig. 9.4)

As stated in Chapter 1, all hinge joints have collateral ligaments that provide medial and lateral joint stability. In the knee, the medial collateral ligament (MCL) is also known as the *tibial collateral ligament* (TCL), and the lateral collateral ligament (LCL) is referred to as the *fibular collateral ligament* (FCL). These structures are named this

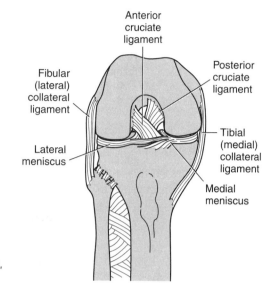

FIGURE 9.4 Collateral and cruciate ligaments and menisci of the tibiofemoral joint: anterior view.
Adapted from McKinnis: *Fundamentals of Musculoskeletal Imaging*, 2nd ed. 2005. Philadelphia: F.A. Davis Company, Fig. 10-3, pg 331, with permission.

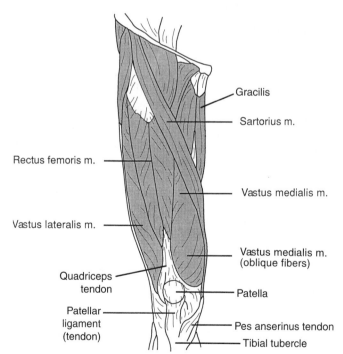

FIGURE 9.5 The patella ligament, quadriceps tendon, pes anserinus tendon, and anterior and medial muscles of the thigh.
Adapted from Starkey and Ryan: *Evaluation of Orthopedic and Athletic Injuries*, 2nd ed. 2002. Philadelphia: F.A. Davis Company, Fig. 6-11, pg 191, with permission.

way because of their respective distal attachments on the tibia and fibula. In the clinical setting, most providers commonly refer to the knee collaterals by using the MCL and LCL designations. Because there are numerous MCLs and LCLs in the body (e.g., the MCLs of the right and left elbows, the LCLs of the distal interphalangeal joints of the right and left third toes), identifying knee collaterals by the generic terms *MCL* and *LCL* can cause confusion. It is for this reason that the terms *TCL* and *FCL* should be used to identify these structures. These are the terms used throughout this chapter.

The broad, flat TCL consists of deep and superficial layers. The deep portion is located within the joint capsule, whereas the superficial portion lies outside the joint capsule. Proximally, both portions attach to the medial femoral epicondyle. Distally, the deep portion attaches to the medial tibial plateau, whereas the superficial portion attaches to the medial aspect of the tibia just below the pes anserinus. The primary function of the TCL is to limit valgus motion of the knee. It also acts as a secondary restraint to external rotational and to anterior translation forces.

Unlike the TCL, the FCL is a relatively thin, cord-like structure that runs from the femur's lateral epicondyle to the head of the fibula. Whereas the TCL maintains deep and superficial portions, the FCL is one structure that lies entirely outside the joint capsule. It limits varus motion and provides a secondary restraint to rotational forces.

Cruciate Ligaments (Fig. 9.4)

Though all hinge joints in the body are supported by collateral ligaments, the knee is the only one that has cruciate ligaments. This is because the articular surfaces of the tibia and femur have little to offer by way of rotary stability. Rather, it is the anterior cruciate (ACL) and posterior cruciate (PCL) ligaments, working in concert with other soft tissues, that provide this stability. These ligaments cross each other within the TFJ's joint cavity (the term *cruciate* is derived from the Latin "to cross"). This makes the cruciates intraarticular structures. Although these structures are intracapsular (located within the joint's capsule), they are extrasynovial because they lie outside the joint's synovial cavity. Although portions of the ligament are taut throughout the knee's ROM, the ACL is most taut in a position of full extension and most lax in a position of 40° to 70° flexion. Its primary function is to limit anterior translation of the tibia on the femur. Others functions include resisting hyperextension, internal rotation, external rotation, and valgus and varus forces.

PEARL

The primary functions of the ACL include limiting anterior translation of the tibia on the femur and resisting hyperextension, internal rotation, external rotation, and valgus and varus forces.

When compared with the ACL, the PCL is shorter and stronger, making it a primary stabilizer of the knee. As with the ACL, portions of this ligament are taut throughout the knee's ROM. In contrast with the ACL, the PCL is most taut in full flexion and most lax in extension. Its primary function is preventing posterior translation of the tibia on the femur. Secondary functions include resisting medial rotation, valgus, varus, and hyperextension forces.

Patellar Ligament (Fig. 9.5)

The patellar ligament arises from the distal pole as well as the medial and lateral borders of the patella, terminating at the tibial tubercle. In reality, its fibers are merely a continuation of the quadriceps femoris tendon, discussed later in this chapter. For this reason, in the clinical setting the patellar ligament is commonly referred to as the *patellar tendon*.

Muscles and Tendons

Two major muscle groups, the quadriceps femoris and hamstrings, are primary movers and protectors of the knee joint. Other muscles and tendons that act on the knee include the gastrocnemius, sartorius, and gracilis.

Quadriceps Femoris (Fig. 9.5)

As its name implies, the quadriceps femoris muscle group, or *quads*, consists of four muscles: the vastus medialis oblique (VMO), vastus lateralis oblique (VLO), vastus intermedius, and rectus femoris. Located anteriorly on the thigh, the proximal attachment of these muscles is from either the upper femur or the pelvis. Distally, these muscles combine to form the common quadriceps tendon, which inserts into the superior, lateral, and medial portions of the patella. The strands of this tendon pass over and encase the patella (classifying the patella as a sesamoid bone) and continue distally as the patellar ligament. The large and powerful quadriceps provides the knee with excellent protection, extends the TFJ, and is responsible for tracking the patella within the femoral groove.

Hamstrings (Fig. 9.6)

The hamstring muscle group is made up of the semitendinosus, semimembranosus, and biceps femoris muscles. As a group, these posterior thigh muscles originate from the ischial tuberosity (discussed in Chapter 10), insert on the tibia or fibula, and act to flex the knee. The medial hamstrings (semitendinosus and semimembranosus) also internally rotate the knee, whereas the biceps femoris, positioned laterally, externally rotates the knee. These muscles also form the superior portion of the popliteal fossa, a diamond-shaped depression located on the knee's posterior aspect.

Related Muscles and Landmarks

Described more fully in Chapter 8, the gastrocnemius is a knee flexor and serves as the distal boundaries of the popliteal fossa (Fig. 9.6). The distal tendons of the sartorius and gracilis muscles, described more fully in Chapter 10, combine with the tendon of the semitendinosus to form the common pes anserinus (goose's foot) tendon before attaching to the tibia (Fig. 9.5). These muscles act as knee flexors and internal rotators.

Menisci

The menisci of the knee (Fig. 9.4) are specialized semicircular, fibrocartilaginous disks that aid in the stability of the TFJ by deepening the joint's socket. They also help cushion the joint by absorbing and dispersing forces applied to the lower extremity. Do not confuse these menisci with the layer of articular cartilage found on the joint surfaces of bones. In the clinical setting, when providers discuss sports-related injuries to knee cartilage, they are usually referring to damage of a meniscus and not the articular cartilage.

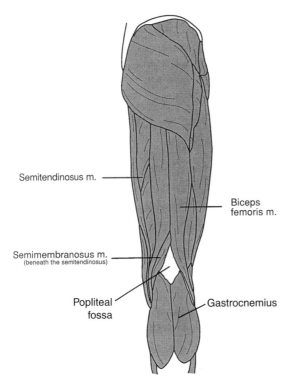

Semitendinosus m.

Biceps
femoris m.

Semimembranosus m.
(beneath the semitendinosus)

Popliteal
fossa

Gastrocnemius

FIGURE 9.6 The hamstring and gastrocnemius muscles and the popliteal fossa.
Adapted from Starkey and Ryan: *Evaluation of Orthopedic and Athletic Injuries*, 2nd ed. 2002. Philadelphia: F.A. Davis Company, Fig. 6-12, pg 194, with permission.

The peripheries of the menisci attach to their corresponding medial and lateral tibial plateaus via many small **coronary ligaments**. This means that the blood supply and subsequent healing properties of the outer-third of each meniscus are very good. However, the inner two-thirds of the menisci are relatively avascular, with nourishment to these meniscal portions coming primarily from the joint's synovial fluid. This makes the healing properties of the inner two-thirds of the menisci very poor.

The medial meniscus is shaped like the letter *C*, with its open portion facing toward the tibia's intercondylar eminence. The outer portion of this meniscus is directly attached to the deep portion of the TCL, making it vulnerable to injury when the TCL is traumatized. In contrast, the lateral meniscus is shaped like the letter *O* and is not attached to its corresponding FCL. This helps prevent the lateral meniscus from becoming injured.

Related Structures

Though many bursae surround the knee, the one most often injured in sport is the prepatellar. Located between the skin and the patella, this structure helps prevent the patella from being traumatized. Attached to the medial and lateral borders of the patella and to either side of the patellar ligament are the medial and lateral patellar retinacula (Fig. 9.7). These structures are continuations of the VMO and VLO muscles. Along with the medial and lateral patellofemoral ligaments, the retinacula function to hold the patella within the femoral groove.

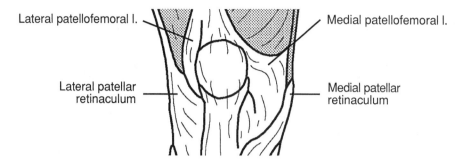

Lateral patellofemoral l.

Medial patellofemoral l.

Lateral patellar retinaculum

Medial patellar retinaculum

FIGURE 9.7 Patellar retinacula and patellofemoral ligaments.
From Starkey and Ryan: *Evaluation of Orthopedic and Athletic Injuries*, 2nd ed. 2002. Philadelphia: F.A. Davis Company, Fig. 7-3, pg 245, with permission.

Examination of the Knee

As shown by the review of anatomy, the knee is an extremely complicated structure, and its evaluation can overwhelm even the most seasoned health care provider. Combine the below with what is presented in Chapter 7 to ensure that all essential aspects of the evaluation are covered when assessing macrotrauma and microtrauma conditions of the knee.

History

To obtain a history, ask the patient the relevant questions from Box 7.1 on page 165. Focus questions about acute knee trauma on what position the lower extremity was in when the injury occurred (e.g., foot planted on the ground or not planted, knee extended or flexed) and whether the injury was caused by contact or noncontact means. In cases of chronic injury, include questions such as, "Are you experiencing locking, clicking, or giving way of the knee when you squat, walk, run, or ascend and descend stairs?" These symptoms indicate internal knee derangement such as a torn meniscus. Also, be sure to ask questions related to the ankle, hip, pelvis, and lumbar spine, because problems in these areas can affect the knee joint. Even though patients will most likely present with either a TFJ or a PFJ problem, be sure to collect information on both joints, because doing so helps prevent vital information from being missed.[1-3]

Obtain a detailed history of both the TFJ and PFJ joints as part of your comprehensive knee evaluation.

Physical Examination

Begin the physical examination with observation and palpation, followed by ROM testing and strength testing. Complete the examination by applying knee-specific stress and special tests.

Observation

After a thorough history has been completed, observe the patient's knees in the following fashion. With the patient standing, note the alignments of the TFJs. Normal and abnormal alignments are presented in Figure 9.8. Note that the incidences of genu valgum and genu recurvatum are increased in females. Next, have the patient sit with his or her legs hanging off the edge of a table. Evaluate the patellae for the malalignments presented in Figure 9.9. In most cases, documenting the alignment of the patient's TFJs and PFJs occurs in response to subacute and chronic conditions, because these structural abnormalities are not normally associated with acute injury.[1,2,4]

Follow observing the TFJ and PFJ by inspecting both extremities for any signs of swelling, discoloration, or erythema. Do this by instructing the patient to sit relaxed on a table, with his or her knees extended. If swelling is observed, measure the circumference of the knee to document the amount present. Compare the size of the quadriceps of the involved knee to that of the uninvolved knee, because this is the first muscle group to atrophy in response to knee injury. Measure thigh circumference in cases where there appears to be a visual difference, and record the findings. This documents the amount of atrophy and helps track patient progress during treatment and rehabilitation.[1,2,4]

PEARL

The quadriceps femoris muscle group is the first to atrophy in response to knee injury.

Palpation

Systematically palpate the region with the patient in the seated position. Although all anatomical structures should be palpated, pay particular attention to the quadriceps, patella, patellar ligament, collateral ligaments, and joint line.

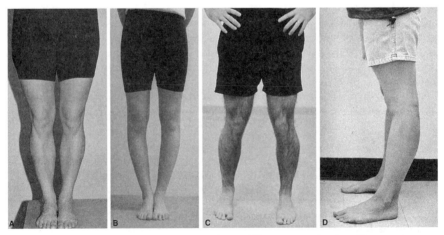

FIGURE 9.8 Alignment of the tibiofemoral joint. Normal (A), genu varum (bowlegs; B), genu valgum (knock-knees; C), and genu recurvatum (hyperextension; D).
From Starkey and Ryan: *Evaluation of Orthopedic and Athletic Injuries*, 2nd ed. 2002. Philadelphia: F.A. Davis Company, Fig. 6-16, pg 200, with permission.

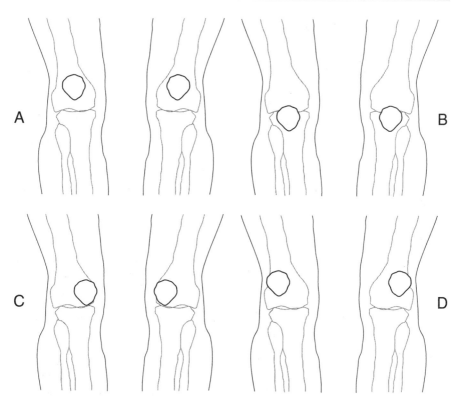

FIGURE 9.9 Malaligned patellae positions: (A) alta (high riding), (B) baja (low riding), (C) squinting (pointing medially), and (D) frog-eyed (pointing laterally).
From Starkey and Ryan: *Evaluation of Orthopedic and Athletic Injuries,* 2nd ed. 2002. Philadelphia: F.A. Davis Company, Box 7-2, pg 248, with permission.

Find the joint line by internally and externally rotating the tibia on the femur. Doing so causes the tibial plateaus to press against the skin during the extreme ranges of these motions. Palpate the joint line for pain and swelling, which is indicative of meniscal injury. Though its borders cannot be easily identified, palpate the length of the TCL by pressing on the area between the ligament's attachment sites. To palpate the FCL, instruct the patient to place the foot of the involved extremity on the contralateral quadriceps muscle group. This puts the extremity in a figure-four position. From this position, palpate the lateral aspect of the knee for the cord-like FCL as it runs from the lateral femoral epicondyle to the head of the fibula. Understand that because they are intra-articular structures, you cannot palpate the cruciate ligaments. Check the integrity of the patella and patellar ligament by palpating the entire surface areas of these structures. Continue the assessment by palpating the pes anserinus and popliteal fossa. Check for muscle spasm by palpating the distal portions of the quadriceps and hamstring muscle groups.[1,2,4]

The cruciate ligaments cannot be palpated because they are intra-articular structures.

Range-of-Motion and Strength Testing

To check the knee's active ROM, have the patient flex and extend each knee from a seated position. If decreased motion on the injured side occurs, measure the difference between sides with a goniometer. Move the knee through these ranges to test passive flexion and extension. With the patient in the same seated position, apply resistance to the distal portion of the leg just superior to the ankle as the patient extends his or her knee. This tests the strength of the quadriceps. To test the strength of the hamstrings, have the patient flex his or her knee against resistance from the extended position.[1,2]

Stress and Special Testing

The most accurate and commonly used stress and special tests for each musculoskeletal condition of the knee are covered in this chapter. All are performed with the patient either supine or prone and many require the patient's lower extremity to be supported by the examiner's upper extremities. When performing these tests, tell the patient to completely relax the extremity being tested until the body part feels like "dead weight" in your grasp. If this does not happen, the quadriceps muscle group is probably contracted, prohibiting full relaxation from occurring. In these cases, instruct the patient to avoid looking at the knee during the examination, because doing so may cause tension and apprehension. As all examiners quickly discover, a fully relaxed lower extremity can be quite heavy regardless of patient size. Thus, though most providers can perform knee stress tests safely, to protect yourself from injury be sure to follow the guidelines presented with regard to examiner and patient positioning.

Musculoskeletal Imaging

Although most knee injuries are soft tissue in nature, fractures, dislocations, avulsions, and loose bodies within the joint must be considered as part of the differential diagnosis. However, determining whether the knee should be x-rayed can be challenging, because standards regarding when to obtain an x-ray are limited. In these instances, use the Ottawa Knee Rules, presented in Box 9.2, to help make this decision.[5]

If it is determined that x-rays are needed, obtain standard plain-film radiographic projections, which consist of anteroposterior, lateral, and oblique views of the TFJ. Include with these views a posteroanterior axial "tunnel" view (x-ray with the patient's knee in 40° flexion), because this evaluates the intercondylar fossa. To ensure that the patella is accurately assessed, obtain a tangential view of the PFJ (patient lies supine, knee flexed to 90°) as part of the standard knee x-ray series. Though commonly used to evaluate the health of the ankle, stress x-rays of the knee are not typically obtained. If needed, magnetic resonance imaging (MRI) can be used to evaluate the health of soft tissue structures such as the collateral and cruciate ligaments and the menisci.[2,4,6–8]

Use the Ottawa Knee Rules to determine whether an x-ray is needed in response to knee trauma.

BOX 9.2
OTTAWA KNEE RULES. OBTAIN KNEE RADIOGRAPHS IF ANY OF THE LISTED ITEMS ARE PRESENT

Patient aged >55 years	Inability to walk four steps
Isolated patella tenderness	• after the injury
Head of the fibula tenderness	• in the emergency room
<90° active knee flexion	• in the office

Stiell IG, Greenberg GH, Wells GA, et al. Derivation of a decision rule for the use of radiography in acute knee injuries. *Ann Emerg Med* 1995;26:405.

Conditions of the Tibiofemoral Joint

Macrotrauma injuries of the TFJ are some of the most common injuries resulting from sports participation. These usually occur when the knee is exposed to one of the following:

• an external force, as when a person makes contact with another person's knee;
• a twisting force, as when a person pivots on one leg in an attempt to change direction quickly; or
• an external force applied at the same time a twisting force occurs.

In most instances, the potential for injury is worse if the foot is planted firmly on the ground than if it is dangling in the air at the time an external force is applied to the body. It is also easier for an opposing player to strike the outside than the inside of the knee. This makes the knee more likely to be injured from valgus forces than from varus forces. Although it may seem that an external force has the potential to cause greater damage than a twisting force, this is not always the case.[1,9]

The knee is more likely to be injured from valgus forces than from varus forces.

Collateral Ligament Sprains

The collateral ligaments are injured from either a varus or a valgus force mechanism of injury (MOI), which usually occurs in combination with some type of rotational component. The FCL is at risk from varus forces applied to the knee, whereas the TCL is commonly injured from valgus forces (Fig. 1.5 on page 11). This means the FCL is not injured nearly as often as the TCL. Furthermore, because the TCL is attached to other structures, such as the medical meniscus, a multiple structure injury commonly occurs when this ligament is traumatized. However, if the injury force is great enough, a multiple structure injury may occur regardless of the injury mechanism.[1,6,9,10]

History and Physical Examination

A patient with a collateral ligament sprain relates that the knee "bent" the wrong way at the time of injury. In the case of a TCL sprain, the person states that the knee bent "inward," whereas for a FCL sprain, the patient states that the knee bent "outward." As with most cases of lower extremity injury, the gait of those with a first degree collateral sprain is only mildly affected, whereas a patient with a second or third degree injury walks with a distinctive limp.[1,4,6,10]

Regardless of severity, a patient with a collateral ligament sprain reports pain at the site of the tear, which hurts when it is palpated. If the area is painful over a ligament's attachment site (e.g., medial epicondyle of the femur for the TCL), an avulsion fracture may exist. If the amount of pain is greatest over the medial joint line, the medial meniscus, as well as the TCL, may be injured. Be aware that those who sprain the collateral ligaments usually do not have much swelling, though the knee of a person with a TCL injury swells more than that of someone with an FCL sprain. This is because the TCL is directly attached to the joint capsule, making swelling more common when this structure is injured, particularly in second degree sprains involving the TCL's deep portion and in all third degree injuries. Knee strength and ROM are normal in those with a first degree collateral ligament sprain, whereas people with a second degree injury experience motion and strength decreases. It is usually impossible to test knee ROM and strength of those with a third degree injury because of the pain associated with an injury this severe.[1,4,6,9,10]

Confirm the presence of a collateral ligament sprain by applying the **valgus** (TCL) and **varus** (FCL) **stress tests.**[1,4,9,10] To perform the valgus stress test (Fig. 9.10):

• Instruct the patient to lie supine, with the involved extremity positioned close to the table's edge.
• Grab the distal leg with one hand and the lateral portion of the knee and thigh with your other hand.
• Cradle the popliteal fossa with your fingers, place your palm on the lateral side of the joint, and situate your thumb over the distal portion of the quadriceps. If needed, support the knee against your body.
• From this position, flex the knee 25° to 30°.
• With your proximal hand, apply a valgus force to the knee while abducting the leg with your distal hand.
• Watch the medial joint line for the presence of excessive motion, or joint "opening," between distal femur and proximal tibia.
• Repeat this test with the knee fully extended.

To perform the varus stress test (Fig. 9.11):

• Instruct the patient to lie supine, with the involved extremity positioned close to the table's edge.

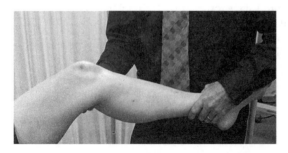

FIGURE 9.10 Valgus stress test with the left knee flexed 25°.

- Abduct the patient's hip to 45°, and position your body between the table and the patient's abducted lower extremity.
- Grab the distal leg with one hand and the medial portion of the knee and thigh with your other hand.
- Cradle the popliteal fossa with your fingers, and place your palm on the medial side of the joint. If needed, support the knee against your body.
- From this position, flex the knee 25° to 30°.
- With your proximal hand, apply a varus force to the knee, and adduct the leg with your distal hand.
- Watch the lateral joint line for the presence of excessive motion, or joint "opening," between the distal femur and proximal tibia.
- Repeat this test with the knee fully extended.

In cases where minimal movement occurs with either of these tests while the knee is flexed, a first degree sprain probably exists. If, however, the valgus or varus stress test produces excessive movement, note the type of end-feel present. A hard end-feel is indicative of a second degree collateral sprain, whereas a soft end-feel confirms the presence of a third degree injury. When applying these tests on a healthy patient with the knee flexed, no laxity exists on the medial side of the joint, whereas some lateral laxity is normally present. Thus, so as not to confuse this normal laxity with an injury, be sure to compare varus stress test findings with those of the patient's uninjured knee.[1,9,10]

If a first degree sprain exists, performing valgus and varus stress tests with the knee extended almost always produces a negative response, indicating that other structures, such as the ACL, have not been damaged. However, in cases of a second or third degree injury, performing these tests with the knee extended may produce a positive finding. Thus, knee joint laxity produced by either a valgus or a varus stress test indicates that other soft tissues, such as the ACL, have also been injured.[1,4]

(P E A R L)

A positive valgus or varus stress test performed with the knee in an extended position indicates that other soft tissues, such as the ACL, have been injured.

Management

Treat all those with an isolated first degree collateral ligament sprain symptomatically. Prescribe a four-point, touchdown crutch gait as described in Patient Teaching

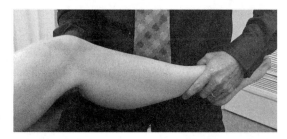

FIGURE 9.11 Varus stress test with the right knee flexed 25°.

Handout (PTH) 6.1 in cases where the patient's gait is hampered. Obtain plain-film radiographs for those who have tenderness over a ligament attachment site. If a fracture exists, refer the patient to an orthopedist. Wean all others from crutch use as soon as pain and discomfort subside. Prescribe ROM and strengthening exercises as presented in PTH 9.1.[1,9,10]

Apply a splint, prescribe a non-weight-bearing (NWB) crutch gait, and refer all patients with second and third degree injuries, and those with sprains complicated by injury to other structures, to an orthopedist. After x-rays rule out fracture, the orthopedist may order an MRI to confirm the injury. People with these conditions are usually treated conservatively because the collateral ligament's blood supply is more than adequate to promote healing. Surgical intervention is usually necessary if the ligament avulses from one of its attachment sites and/or the sprain is associated with other pathology. In some instances, the time needed for the FCL to heal is longer than for a TCL injury of the same severity.[1,9,10]

Refer all patients with suspected second and third degree collateral ligament sprains to an orthopedist for evaluation and treatment.

Cruciate Ligament Sprains

An ACL sprain is the most common knee ligament injury sustained during sports activities. Caused by contact and noncontact mechanisms, the ACL sprain usually results when the following occur simultaneously:

• Foot firmly planted.
• Slightly flexed knee moving into full extension.
• Knee externally rotated.
• Valgus force.

Noncontact ACL injuries happen when a sudden deceleration force is applied to the knee. This typically occurs when a person who is running tries to stop and change direction suddenly, as when a basketball player quickly stops and pivots on one leg in an attempt to move in a different direction. These noncontact injuries account for most ACL sprains and occur more in females than in males. Although explanations of females' higher rate of noncontact ACL injury are not definitive, some current theories are listed in Box 9.3. A contact ACL injury commonly occurs when an external valgus force is applied to the knee at the exact moment the person stops and attempts to change direction as described above. This injury is mostly associated with collision sports, such as football and lacrosse, in which it is legal for participants to make bodily contact during the course of play.[6,10–12]

The ACL is the most commonly injured ligament in the knee.

Fortunately, the PCL is injured much less frequently than the ACL. This is because the PCL is most vulnerable when the knee is in a hyperflexed, versus hyperextended, position. Although not unheard of, it is rare for the knee to be in a hyperflexed position during most sports activities. When PCL injury does occur, the patient usually reports receiving

BOX 9.3
POSSIBLE REASONS FOR INCREASED NONCONTACT ANTERIOR CRUCIATE LIGAMENT INJURIES
IN FEMALES

Small tibial intercondylar notch	Increased ligament laxity
Hormonal influences	Increased dependency on ACL for
Increased incidence of normal genu	knee stability
valgus	
Genu valgus increases during the	
landing phase of a jump	

ACL = anterior cruciate ligament

blunt-force trauma to the front of the tibia with the knee in a flexed position. Though not common in sports, PCL injury is quite common in front-end automobile accidents that force the car's dashboard into the legs of the passengers sitting in the front seat.[1,10]

History and Physical Examination

Patients with an acute cruciate ligament sprain usually report hearing a loud "pop" and experience a "giving way" of the knee at the time of injury. This is particularly true in cases of a third degree ACL injury. Those with this condition report experiencing immediate disability, and, within the first few hours after the traumatic event, massive swelling occurs as a result of the developing **hemarthrosis** that is so common with an ACL injury. In these instances, swelling can be so extensive that the outline of the patella may be unrecognizable during the evaluation. The patient is also unable to walk without a limp or move the knee through its full range. At times, the combination of massive hemarthrosis, pain, and decreased ROM makes a complete assessment difficult to perform. In these cases, wait a few days to allow pain and swelling to subside before performing a complete examination. Although it is a serious condition, recognize that the swelling, pain, and disability resulting from PCL injury are usually less than with an ACL sprain of the same severity. Thus, whereas the ACL-injured patient usually seeks medical attention soon after the trauma occurs, it is not uncommon for the PCL-injured patient to wait days, weeks, or even months before having the knee evaluated.[6,10-12]

Two classic signs of ACL injury include the patient hearing a loud "pop"
at the time of injury and the presence of massive swelling soon after
injury occurrence.

Stress tests used to evaluate the integrity of the cruciate ligaments include the anterior drawer test and **Lachman test** for the ACL and the posterior drawer test and **sag test** for the PCL.[1,4,7,10-13] To perform the anterior drawer test (Fig. 9.12):

• Instruct the patient to lie supine on an examination table with the knee flexed to 90° and the hip flexed to 45°.
• With the knee in the neutral position, (that is, the knee is neither internally nor externally rotated), sit on the patient's foot.
• Place the fingers of both hands in the popliteal fossa behind the proximal portion of the leg. Place your thumbs on either side of the patellar ligament.

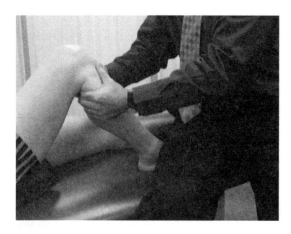

FIGURE 9.12 Anterior drawer test.

- Encourage the patient to relax the hamstring muscles, because tight or contracting hamstrings pull posteriorly on the tibia, resulting in a false-negative finding.
- Focus your eyes on the knee's joint line as you pull forward on the tibia. This causes the tibia to anteriorly translate on the femur. Although some anterior translation is normal, injury to the ACL may produce an excessive amount.
- Repeat this test with the knee in an internally, and then externally, rotated position.

PEARL

To avoid a false-negative finding, make sure the patient's hamstring muscles are relaxed before performing the anterior drawer test.

If the anterior drawer test reveals excessive anterior translation of the tibia on the femur, ACL injury is indicated. Indeed, for years this test was the definitive clinical diagnostic tool used to determine the integrity of the ACL. Although still used in the clinical setting, we now know this is not the best test to diagnose acute ACL injury because, even when performed correctly, it produces a false-negative finding 60% of the time in acute ACL injuries. This is primarily because the test examines the ACL with the knee flexed. Because the ACL is usually injured when the knee is extended, testing in a flexed position violates the premise that a stress test is performed in a position that commonly injures the ligament. Also, this is a very difficult test to perform on an acutely injured knee, because the massive hemarthrosis and loss of ROM associated with ACL injury makes it difficult to place the knee in the test position of 90° flexion. However, this test is useful for detecting knee instability due to an old ACL injury, so be sure to perform it on patients who are experiencing chronic knee laxity and/or report a history of previous traumatic knee injury.[12,13]

In recent years, the Lachman test has supplanted the anterior drawer test as the definitive clinical diagnostic tool for evaluating ACL integrity.[1,4,11–13] To perform this test (Fig. 9.13):

- Instruct the patient to lie supine, with the knee in a position of 20° to 30° flexion.

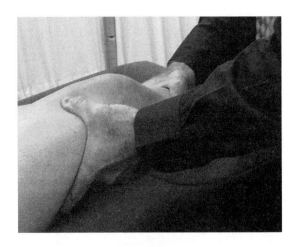

FIGURE 9.13 Lachman test (traditional) performed on the right knee.

• With your proximal hand, grab the distal end of the femur by placing your fingers posteriorly in the popliteal fossa and your thumb across the distal portion of the quadriceps.
• Place your distal hand around the proximal portion of the tibia, with the thumb positioned over the patellar ligament and the fingers cradling the posterior leg.
• While visualizing the joint line, pull forward on the tibia and push back on the femur. In an ACL-deficient knee, you will feel and see the tibia translating anteriorly on the femur. If the test is positive, note the type of end-feel present.

(PEARL)

The Lachman test is the definitive clinical diagnostic tool for evaluating ACL integrity.

Although the traditional Lachman examination is the preferred method to evaluate ACL integrity, this test can be difficult to perform if you have small hands and/or if the patient has large thighs. When it is difficult for you to get your entire hand around the distal end of the patient's thigh, test the integrity of the ACL by using the modified Lachman test.[12]

(PEARL)

Use the modified Lachman test to evaluate the integrity of the ACL when the size of your hands and/or the patient's thigh precludes you from performing the traditional test.

To perform a modified Lachman test (Fig. 9.14):

• Instruct the patient to lie prone, with the dorsal aspect of the patient's foot on your shoulder. This places the knee in a position of 30° flexion.
• Place the index and middle fingers of your hand closest to the knee on the medial and lateral sides of the patellar ligament.

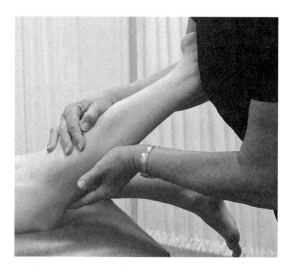

FIGURE 9.14 Lachman test (modified) performed on the left knee.

• Place your other hand over the proximal aspect of the gastrocnemius muscle.
• Push the leg toward the table. This causes anterior translation of the tibia on the femur.
• Feel the amount of translation present, compare the amount of movement with that of the opposite side, and note the type of end-feel present.

Unlike the anterior drawer test for ACL insufficiency, the posterior drawer test is highly sensitive for both acute and chronic PCL injury. To perform this test, position yourself and the patient the same way as for the anterior drawer test (Fig. 9.12). As you focus on the knee's joint line from this position, push the tibia backward. An excessive amount of posterior translation of the tibia on the femur indicates PCL involvement.[1,4,7]

Complete your evaluation of the cruciates by performing the sag test. Do this by positioning the patient as you would to perform the anterior and posterior drawer tests. With the patient in this position, observe his or her knees from the side of the involved extremity. If the PCL is injured, the patellar ligament and tibial tubercle of the involved extremity will sag lower when compared with the same structures on the contralateral side.[1]

Management

Determining the proper course of treatment for the patient with an ACL injury depends on a number of factors, including the severity of injury, the age of the patient, and whether the injury is acute or chronic. One factor that greatly influences the treatment decision is the patient's future planned activity level. For example, a conservative, non-surgical treatment plan may be recommended if the patient is most concerned about being able to perform activities of daily living and participating in general fitness programs versus returning to competitive sports. Surgical intervention may be the preferred course of treatment for those interested in returning to high-intensity athletics.[10]

Refer all patients with a suspected ACL injury to an orthopedist. Prescribe an NWB crutch gait as described in PTH 6.1. Diagnostic techniques the physician uses to confirm ACL injury include aspirating the knee joint to determine the source of swelling and performing an MRI. If the physician and patient decide surgery is the best course of action, the patient will most likely undergo any one of a number of procedures used to reconstruct the ACL with either **allograft** or **autograft** tissues. Regardless of treatment protocol, a period of prolonged rehabilitation, which can approach up to a year in length, awaits the ACL-injured patient.[1,10]

PEARL

Refer all patients with a suspected ACL injury to an orthopedist for evaluation and treatment.

As with the ACL-injured patient, refer all people with a suspected PCL-deficient knee for orthopedic evaluation. The use of crutches is not indicated unless the patient cannot bear weight without a limp or does not feel confident in the knee's ability to support his or her body weight. Typically, the PCL-deficient patient does quite well with nonsurgical treatment unless it is determined that other structures are also injured.

Meniscal Tears

As with the cruciates, the menisci of the knee are injured as a result of both contact and noncontact mechanisms. Because the medial meniscus is directly attached to the TCL, it is vulnerable to any externally applied valgus knee force. Noncontact injuries, which occur in both menisci, are usually caused by rotational forces, as when a person plants the foot firmly on the ground and changes direction quickly. This pivoting action can cause the meniscus to tear as it becomes pinched between the femur and tibia. Because the medial meniscus is less mobile than the lateral, it has a higher rate of noncontact injury. Females aged 11 to 20 years and males aged 21 to 40 years are most susceptible to meniscal injury.[1,14,15]

PEARL

The medial meniscus is injured more frequently than the lateral.

History and Physical Examination

Patients with an acute, isolated tear of a meniscus typically report that they felt pain after they "twisted" their knee. They may also report hearing a "pop" at the time of injury, followed by a gradual loss of ROM and strength. This progressive decline in function is usually due to increases in both pain and swelling along the joint line around the area of the damaged meniscus. In many instances, the patient experiences minor discomfort before going to sleep for the night, only to wake with a painful and swollen joint. However, an acutely torn meniscus will not swell as fast or as much as a recently injured ACL. Indeed, this is a key way to distinguish between these two conditions in the clinical setting.[1,14,15]

PEARL

The swelling associated with an acute meniscal injury develops more slowly and is less significant than the swelling associated with a recent ACL sprain.

Sometimes the pain and swelling of a torn meniscus subside so quickly that the patient does not seek immediate medial attention. In these cases, additional symptoms, including sensations of clicking, popping, and snapping within the joint, often develop over time. As the condition degenerates, the knee starts to buckle for no apparent reason. Transient swelling may develop whenever the patient is physically active, and the knee may "lock up" from time to time. This is a sign that a torn piece of meniscus is becoming lodged between the tibial plateau and femur during movement. In many instances, it is the combination of transient swelling, locking, and buckling of the joint that convinces the patient to seek medical attention. In these cases, be sure to measure the patient's thigh girth bilaterally, because quadriceps atrophy is indicative of internal knee derangement.[1,14,15]

Use **Apley's compression**, **Apley's distraction**, and McMurray's tests to verify meniscal injury.[1,14,15] To perform Apley's compression test (Fig. 9.15):

• Instruct the patient to lie prone, with the involved knee in a position of 90° flexion.
• Grab the patient's foot, and apply downward pressure as you internally and externally rotate the tibia. This test is positive if the patient feels pain, popping, or crepitus with this maneuver.

Be aware that the twisting that results from performing Apley's compression test also stresses the collateral ligaments. Thus, in instances where Apley's compression test is positive, use Apley's distraction test to differentiate between meniscal and ligament injury. Do this by pulling up on the patient's ankle as he or she lies in the Apley's compression test position. You may have to place one hand on the distal aspect of the patient's hamstrings to stabilize the lower extremity while performing this test. If Apley's distraction test relieves symptoms, the patient most likely has meniscal damage, because this test reduces pressure on the menisci. However, if the Apley's distraction test produces pain (a positive sign), the patient has probably experienced a collateral ligament injury, because distracting the joint in this fashion elongates these ligaments.

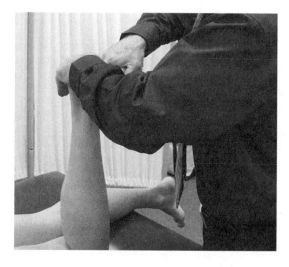

FIGURE 9.15 Apley's compression test.

McMurray's test, commonly perceived as the definitive clinical diagnostic tool for evaluating meniscal injury, is challenging to perform. Also, its ability to diagnose a meniscal tear is directly related to the examiner's experience in performing this test. To perform this test:

- Stand lateral and just distal to the supine-lying patient.
- Flex the patient's knee by placing your distal hand on the person's foot and your proximal hand on the knee. Place the index finger of your proximal hand on the medial joint line and your thumb of this hand on the lateral joint line.
- To test the medial meniscus, externally rotate the tibia, apply a varus force, and extend the knee.
- To test the lateral meniscus, return to the flexed position, internally rotate the tibia, apply a valgus force, and extend the knee.
- A positive test occurs if you feel or hear abnormalities such as popping, snapping, or cracking or if the patient reports pain during these maneuvers.

Management

Refer all patients with a suspected meniscal tear to an orthopedist for a definitive diagnosis. In acute cases, prescribe an NWB crutch gait as described in PTH 6.1, but most patients with a chronic meniscal condition do not need an ambulatory aid. Diagnostic techniques used to confirm meniscal injury include MRI and arthroscopic evaluation.[14,15]

Treatment for a torn meniscus includes both surgical and nonsurgical measures and depends largely on the type and location of the tear. Smaller injuries, which occur in the outer third of the meniscus, are treated conservatively, whereas larger tears in this region are repaired surgically. Regardless, both require periods of immobilization and NWB to allow for full healing, which takes 8 to 12 weeks for the conservatively treated patient and up to 3 months for postoperative patients. Surgical intervention in the form of a partial meniscectomy is the treatment of choice for tears in the inner two-thirds, because healing in this portion of the meniscus is poor. Although a partial meniscectomy requires removal of meniscal tissue, recovery only takes a few weeks. This quicker recovery time sometimes influences patients to choose a partial meniscectomy for outer-third tears. This is particularly true of athletes, who may view a 2- or 3-month recovery period as too long to be excluded from participation. If you are advising patients with regard to treatment options, strongly advise those with tears that may potentially heal to chose either surgical repair or conservative treatment options, because removal of any portion of the meniscus creates increased potential for development of degenerative joint disease (DJD). This is why a total meniscectomy procedure, commonly used in years past, is rarely performed anymore. However, patients who have DJD after having a meniscus removed years ago are still seen in the clinical setting.[14,15]

Unhappy Triad

An unhappy, or *terrible*, triad is a knee injury that involves the TCL, ACL, and medial meniscus. It results when a combination of valgus, rotational, and hyperextension forces act on the knee at the same time. Include an unhappy triad as part of the differential diagnosis if a valgus stress test in full extension and the Lachman test are positive. Refer all patients with a suspected unhappy triad to an orthopedist for treatment, which usually includes surgical intervention.

Conditions of the Patellofemoral Joint

Patellofemoral (PF) *syndrome*, *PF pain syndrome*, and *PF compression syndrome* are just a few of the terms used to describe the same clinical entity of pain and dysfunction of the PFJ. Irrespective of the term used, PF pathology associated with sports participation can be caused by both macrotrauma and microtrauma events. Microtrauma conditions develop from a repetitive overloading of the joint and are associated with factors such as malalignment of the patella within the femoral groove. Indeed, it is these "mechanical factors" that greatly contribute to the development of PFJ pathology.

Mechanical Factors Associated With Patellofemoral Pathology

As previously mentioned, malalignment of the patella within the femoral groove is the primary cause of PF pain and dysfunction. Mechanical factors that contribute to this malalignment are listed in Box 9.4. Most of these factors force the patella to track laterally in the groove. Of note is the quadriceps, or *Q*, angle, because patients with a larger angle maintain an increased risk of development of PF pathology. This angle is formed as a line drawn from the anterior superior iliac spine of the pelvis to the mid patella bisects with a line drawn from the tibial tubercle to the mid patella (Fig. 9.16). Females have a naturally larger Q angle than males do because of the increased anatomical width of the female's pelvis. This is the primary reason why females are more prone to chronic PF pathology than males are.[1,16,17]

PEARL

Patellofemoral pathology is more common in females than in males.

Chondromalacia Patella

Chondromalacia patella, or *patella malacia*, is a softening of the cartilage that lines the undersurface of the patella. Of all PF conditions, this is the most nondescript with regard to etiology and symptoms reported by the patient. It is most commonly caused

BOX 9.4
MECHANICAL FACTORS THAT CONTRIBUTE TO PATELLOFEMORAL PATHOLOGY

Weak VMO muscle
Pes planus or pes cavus
Increased size of the quadriceps (Q) angle
 • >10° in males = pathologic
 • >15° in females = pathologic
Abnormal patella position (alta, baja, squinting, frog-eyed)
Genu valgus
Tight lateral patella retinaculum

VMO = vastus medialis oblique.

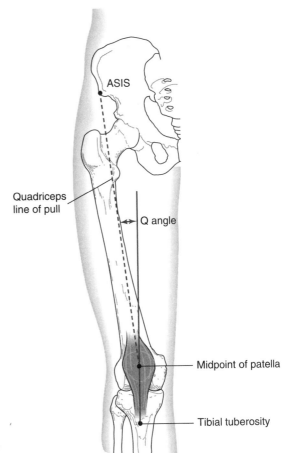

FIGURE 9.16 Measuring the Q angle. ASIS = anterior superior iliac spine.
From Lippert: *Clinical Kinesiology and Anatomy*, 4th ed. 2006. Philadelphia: F.A. Davis Company, Fig. 18-7, pg 253, with permission.

by repetitive stress acting on a PFJ during activities such as running. It also occurs as a result of performing repeated squatting maneuvers over an extended period of time.[1,3,16,17]

History and Physical Examination

A patient with chondromalacia patella reports general anterior knee pain that increases with activity. Pain also increases as a result of placing the knee in a continuous flexed position such as when sitting in a movie theater seat for an extended period (**theater sign**). Some patients report increasing their level of physical activity just before the onset of symptoms. In other cases, symptoms occur after the patient has been participating in an activity for an extended period of time, such as toward the end of an athletic season. Regardless, as this condition worsens, the patient reports a grating, or grinding, sandpaper-like feeling on the undersurface of the patella. This condition also commonly develops with age, especially in active people. Confirm the presence of the condition by performing the **patellar grind test**, also called *Clarke's sign*.[1,3,16,17] To check for Clarke's sign (Fig. 9.17):

- Have the patient lie supine, with the knee extended.
- Place the index finger and thumb of one hand around the superior aspect of the patella.
- Gently force the patella distally, and then ask the patient to contract the quadriceps muscles.
- Force the patella into the femoral groove by maintaining pressure as the patella attempts to migrate proximally.
- Any increase in pain; a grating, grinding, or crunching feeling; or the patient not being able to maintain the contraction is a positive sign for chondromalacia patella.

Management

Manage chondromalacia patella conservatively by modifying the patient's activity level. Prescribe straight leg raise (SLR) and short-arc quadriceps (SAQ) strengthening exercises presented in PTH 9.1. Have the patient try a patellar-stabilizing knee sleeve, because these braces sometimes help to decrease symptoms (Fig. 9.18). These can be purchased at most pharmacy, surgical supply, or sporting goods stores. If symptoms do not subside, refer the patient to an orthopedist for further evaluation.

Patellar Tendonitis and Rupture

In **patellar tendonitis** and rupture, the patellar ligament either becomes inflamed or ruptures from its attachment site on the patella. Because tendonitis cannot occur in a ligament, the term patellar tendonitis is a misnomer, as is the term **patellar tendon rupture**. In addition, as discussed in Chapter 1, it is questionable whether tendons experience inflammation in response to irritation. Nevertheless, currently the terms *patellar tendonitis* and *patellar tendon rupture* are well accepted in the medical community, so these are the terms used when evaluating and treating these conditions.

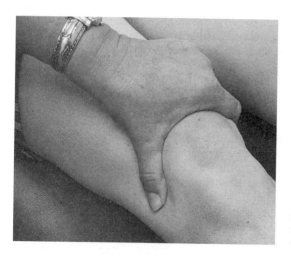

FIGURE 9.17 The patellar grind test, or Clarke's sign, for chondromalacia patella.

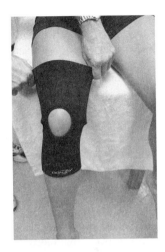

FIGURE 9.18 Patellar stabilizing knee sleeve.
From Beam: *Orthopedic Taping, Wrapping, Bracing and Padding.*
2006. Philadelphia: F.A. Davis Company, Fig. 6–16, pg 185, with
permission.

Commonly referred to as *jumper's knee*, patellar tendonitis most often occurs in people who perform repetitive jumping activities for extended periods of time. It is usually caused by the landing, versus takeoff, phase of the jump because, over time, the eccentric contractions performed by the quadriceps during the landing phase place tremendous amounts of stress on the ligament's patellar attachment point. This condition usually occurs unilaterally, because most people are one-leg dominant, causing them to perform most jumping activities off the same leg. It is also associated with participating on hard playing surfaces and with increases in training sessions. Athletes in sports such as basketball and volleyball, or in the track-and-field events of long jump, triple jump, and high jump, maintain an increased risk of development of this condition.[1,4,10,18]

As with patellar tendonitis, the eccentric contraction forces produced during the landing phase of jumping activities can cause the patellar ligament to rupture from its attachment point on the patella. However, unlike patellar tendonitis, a patellar tendon rupture is a macrotrauma event, caused by one massive eccentric force of the quadriceps. Although this injury rarely happens to people involved in general physical activity programs, it is seen frequently in patients involved in high-intensity athletic endeavors. In addition, those who have a history of patellar tendonitis maintain an increased risk of a patellar tendon rupture.[1,4,10,18]

Those who have a history of patellar tendonitis maintain an increased
risk of a patellar tendon rupture.

History and Physical Examination

Use the history portion of the examination to differentiate between patellar tendonitis and a patellar tendon rupture. Patients with patellar tendonitis report chronic anterior knee pain when jumping and with ascending and descending stairs, whereas those with a patellar tendon rupture report a singular episode of feeling immediate anterior knee pain upon landing from a jump. These people often also state they heard a "pop" at the time of injury. This is followed by immediate disability, which results from the injury's effect on the knee's extensor mechanism (quadriceps tendon, patella, patellar ligament). During physical examination, both patellar tendonitis patients and those with a patellar tendon rupture have extreme tenderness at the ligament's patellar attachment site. However, those with a rupture maintain a palpable defect in this region. These people are also unable to actively extend the knee with any great force.[1,4,10,18]

Management

Obtain x-rays of the patella to rule out patellar ligament rupture for all patients who you suspect may have this injury. Also, secure radiographs to rule out **Sinding-Larsen-Johansson disease** (discussed later in this chapter) for all adolescents who report pain in this region regardless of cause. Prescribe an NWB crutch gait as described in PTH 6.1, and refer patients with positive radiograph findings to an orthopedist. In cases of a patellar tendon rupture, surgical reattachment of the ligament is indicated if the rupture is complete. Treat all patients with patellar tendonitis conservatively by modifying the patient's activity and by increasing the strength of the person's quadriceps and surrounding musculature. Do this by prescribing the SLR and SAQ exercises presented in PTH 9.1. As with chondromalacia, a patellar-stabilizing brace, as shown in Figure 9.18, may help to decrease the patient's symptoms.[1,18]

Acute Dislocation/Subluxation and Chronic Subluxation of the Patella

For some patients, the mechanical factors related to PF pathology as outlined in Box 9.4 lead to an insidious onset of a chronic subluxating patella, in which the patella subluxates from its femoral groove during knee motion. Obese patients are at particular risk for this condition because they usually exhibit greater Q angles and extreme genu valgus. Because the patella is forced laterally, it almost always subluxates in this direction. A chronic subluxating patella can also develop after an episode of an acute patellar subluxation or dislocation. Underlying pathology includes a stretching or tearing of the medial soft tissues, particularly the medial retinaculum and PF ligament, to the point that they cannot stop the patella from moving laterally.

If a patella dislocates, is usually does so as the result of a macrotrauma event. As in the case of a chronic subluxation, the patella usually moves laterally out of its femoral groove, with the underlying pathology being a stretching or tearing of the medial retinaculum and PF ligament. This injury is caused by both contact and noncontact mechanisms. In cases where the patella remains dislocated, it must be actively relocated. This usually occurs through emergency medical means. However, in some instances, an acute patellar dislocation reduces spontaneously, otherwise known as an *acute patellar subluxation*. It is more common in the primary care setting to see patients with a history consistent with an episode of an acute subluxation versus dislocation.[4,10]

History and Physical Examination

Patients who experience an episode of acute patellar subluxation report a singular event that caused their knee to "dislocate." They may state that they saw their kneecap "sticking out of the side of the knee" before "going back into joint." After the incident, most report a functional knee to some degree, but with an inability to continue the activity that caused the injury. If present, swelling is localized to the medial side of the patella. Palpation reveals tenderness over the areas of the medial retinaculum and PF ligament and lateral femoral condyle. Pain over the condyle is a direct result of the patella striking this area when the dislocation occurred.[4,10]

In contrast to those relating a history of an acute subluxation, patients who present with a chronic subluxing patella report a knee that "dislocates" as they walk. When patients relate such a history, they are certainly referring to pathology of the PFJ and not the TFJ. The subluxation may be visible when the patient flexes and extends the affected knee in the NWB position. Because there is no direct injury to the knee with this condition, the patient may not initially report pain or discomfort beyond the fact that the knee feels unstable. As the condition progresses, however, the undersurface of the patella deteriorates from constantly rolling over the lateral femoral condyle. This increases the patient's level of pain and discomfort.[1]

Use the **patellar apprehension test** to assess the stability of the patella within the femoral groove. To perform the apprehension test (Fig. 9.19):

- Instruct the patient to lie supine, with the knees extended.
- Place your thumbs on the medial side of the patella.
- Gently force the patella laterally.
- Because this action has the potential for causing the patella to subluxate, look at the patient's face for an apprehensive reaction as the patella migrates laterally. Do not be surprised if the patient physically tries to stop you from completing the test. Any sign of apprehension when you perform this test is a positive sign for a subluxating patella.

Management

Refer the patient with a subluxating patella to an orthopedist. If the patient cannot fully bear weight without discomfort or reports that the knee "gives way" while walking, prescribe an NWB crutch gait as described in PTH 6.1. After obtaining an x-ray to rule out fracture, the orthopedist will treat the condition either conservatively, by trying to build strength of the quadriceps muscle group, or through surgical intervention, via a lateral retinaculum release. Long-term management includes the use of a patellar-stabilizing brace as shown in Figure 9.18.

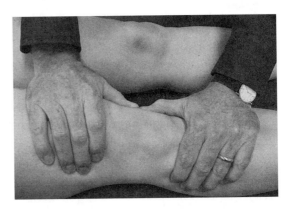

FIGURE 9.19 The patellar apprehension test assesses the stability of the patella within the femoral groove.

Prepatellar Bursitis

Because of its location, the prepatellar bursa is highly vulnerable to injury. Acute bursitis occurs when the patella receives a direct blow, whereas chronic bursitis develops when the patella is exposed to continual direct pressure, such as what happens when someone kneels for an extended period of time.

History and Physical Examination

Swelling over the anterior surface of the patella, ranging from golf ball to softball size, is a hallmark sign of prepatellar bursitis. Although this is a painful condition, the patient may be able to maintain normal knee function as long as the swelling does not affect knee motion. Because the swelling associated with this condition can be extensive, it must be differentiated from the swelling caused by injury to the TFJ. Do this by determining the swelling's origin and location. Swelling caused by prepatellar bursitis is situated anterior to the patella, whereas swelling caused by cruciate and menisci injury is located within the joint cavity.

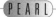

PEARL

Swelling caused by prepatellar bursitis is situated anterior to the patella, whereas swelling caused by cruciate and menisci injury is located within the joint cavity.

Management

Treat mild swelling conservatively with a compression wrap, elevation, and cryotherapy. Patients with excessive swelling or mild swelling that does not subside should be referred to an orthopedist. In most instances, the physician will drain the bursa and administer a corticosteroid injection. In severe cases, the bursa is removed. For all cases, monitor for infection, particularly if an open wound accompanies a case of acute bursitis.

Conditions of the Thigh

The most common conditions of the thigh include strains and contusions. The hamstrings are most likely to be strained, whereas the quadriceps sustain both strains and contusions.

Quadriceps Strain and Contusion

Because of its anterior location on the thigh, the quadriceps of those who participate in collision and contact sports is vulnerable to being contused. Because these injuries result from blunt-force trauma to the anterior, medial, or lateral thigh, it is mandatory for those who participate in activities such as football, ice hockey, and lacrosse to wear thigh padding to protect from this injury. When the quadriceps is strained, the injury is primarily in its middle or proximal third and usually results in an incomplete muscle tear.[19,20]

History and Physical Examination

It is important to differentiate between a quadriceps strain and a contusion, because a person with a strain usually takes longer to heal than a person with a contusion of the same severity. This is best done by taking a thorough history of the injury. Those with a quadriceps strain typically report a "pulled" muscle, whereas those with a contusion state that they were struck by another player or object, such as a football helmet. Although both cause the patient pain and swelling, a strain tends to be more superficial and is generally isolated to the rectus femoris muscle, whereas a contusion usually affects a deeper part of the entire muscle group. As with all second and third degree strains, these injuries produce a palpable defect caused by a bulge in the belly of the rectus femoris, particularly when a knee extension manual muscle test is performed. Occasionally, there is a palpable mass associated with a contusion, owing to the development of an underlying hematoma. The pain associated with both of these injuries increases when the patient's knee is actively or passively flexed. Indeed, those with a strain or contusion experience a decrease in knee flexion, because the quadriceps must stretch for this joint to realize full ROM.[19,20]

As discussed in Chapter 1, muscle strains and contusion are graded by their severity. A person with a first degree strain usually presents with little, if any, functional deficits, whereas those with a second or third degree strain maintain significant strength and ROM losses, causing these patients to walk with a significant limp. They also present with a palpable deformity as previously mentioned. Though those with a quadriceps contusion present similarly with regard to functional deficits, grading the severity for a person with this injury is based on how much the patient can flex the knee 24 to 48 hours after injury. For example, patients with a first degree contusion can achieve knee flexion greater than 90°, whereas those with a second degree injury can flex the knee 45° to 90°. People who cannot perform knee flexion beyond 45° have sustained a third degree contusion.[19,20]

Management

Treat those with either a first or second degree quadriceps strain conservatively. Prescribe NWB crutch use, as described in PTH 6.1, for patients who cannot walk without a limp. Instruct the patient to apply ice massage to the quadriceps with the muscle group in a stretched position, because this treatment works well for this injury. Have the patient initiate quadriceps stretching exercises, shown in PTH 9.1, as early as possible in the treatment process. Add strengthening exercises shown in PTH 9.1 once the patient can successfully perform resistance exercises without pain. Prescribe NWB crutch use, and refer to an orthopedist all patients with a suspected third degree injury.[20]

Regardless of injury severity, the proper initial treatment of a quadriceps contusion includes applying ice and compression with the patient's knee flexed as far as pain allows. Doing so helps maintain normal knee ROM and decreases the probability that the patient will have development of myositis ossificans, discussed later in this section. Hopefully, this is the course of action the patient pursued immediately after the injury incident. In any case, prescribe NWB crutch use, as described in PTH 6.1, for people who cannot walk without a limp. Rule out the development of compartment syndrome, though rare, in instances of second and third degree injury. Pain that continues with rest or mild passive stretching and a thigh that becomes tense as a result of excessive swelling in the region are signs of pending compartment syndrome. Confirm this condition's presence by measuring the patient's thigh circumference. Excessive swelling in the region that causes the girth of the injured extremity to be 4 cm greater than the contralateral side is indicative of compartment syndrome in this area. Initiate passive ROM and strengthening exercises, shown in PTHs 3.1 and 9.1, respectively, as soon as pain and disability allow.[19,20]

Even if treated properly, the patient with a quadriceps contusion may have development of myositis ossificans (Fig. 9.20). This happens when the body begins to lay down bone within the muscle as a result of either a very severe quadriceps contusion or repeated episodes of blunt-force trauma to the quadriceps. This latter cause commonly occurs when people with a mild contusion continue to participate in collision and contact activities before allowing an initial quadriceps contusion to properly heal. Others at risk for development of myositis ossificans include those with less than 120° of active knee flexion from an initial contusion, those who experience a 3-day delay in treating a contusion, those with a previous history of a quadriceps injury, and those who have development of ipsilateral knee swelling in the absence of a knee injury.[19]

Hamstring Strain

Though any number of conditions can occur in the hamstrings, strains of this muscle group are among the most common injuries in sport. These injuries occur in activities such as soccer, track and field, football, and rugby, which require the knee to extend rapidly and involve bursts of rapid acceleration and deceleration forces. This results in the hamstrings contracting eccentrically, increasing the potential for injury. Hamstring strains also occur in sports such as martial arts and dance, where the muscle group is constantly placed in a position of maximal extension. Realize

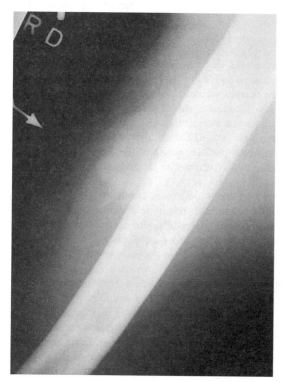

FIGURE 9.20 Myositis ossificans resulting from a quadriceps contusion.
From Starkey and Ryan: *Evaluation of Orthopedic and Athletic Injuries,* 2nd ed. 2002. Philadelphia: F.A. Davis Company, Fig. 8-25, pg 300, with permission.

that because the hamstrings span two joints, they are subject to stretching at more than one point.[21,22]

As with all muscle strains, a number of factors are believed to contribute to the cause of hamstring strains. These include improper warm-up, fatigue, strength imbalance between the quadriceps and the hamstrings, and poor flexibility. However, as discussed in Chapter 1, research supporting a cause-and-effect relationship between any of these reported predisposing risk factors and muscle strains does not exist. What is known is that a history of previous hamstring injury is a chief risk factor for reinjury, because these strains tend to reoccur. Reinjury is also related to returning the patient to activity before the initial injury is totally healed and not correcting errors in how a patient performs a psychomotor skill. These errors in training technique place great stresses on soft tissues. Ultimately, the patient who experiences multiple instances of hamstring injury is classified as having a chronic hamstring strain.[21-23]

History and Physical Examination

People with an acute hamstring strain report a feeling of pain in the posterior thigh. In instances of a second or third degree injury, most report that they felt and heard a painful "pop" at the time of injury. In these cases the patient presents with a limp, whereas the gait of the person with a first degree strain is usually not affected. Ecchymosis is usually present if the patient is evaluated a few days after the date of injury. Irrespective of injury severity, palpable tenderness is present over the site of injury, which, in most cases, occurs at the proximal muscle-tendon junction. In cases of a second or third degree injury, the strength of the patient's hamstring is decreased. In these instances, a noticeable indentation, or gapping, occurs at the site of injury when the muscle group is contracted (Fig. 9.21). Because the hamstrings also extend the hip (see Chapter 10), passive hip flexion is decreased because of the pain caused when the hamstrings are stretched. Recognize that when a patient injures the proximal hamstring, what initially appears to be a strain may actually be an avulsion fracture of the ischial tuberosity. These patients often have a palpable defect extending from the retracted muscle belly proximally to the ischium.[21,22]

As previously mentioned, if not treated properly, an acute hamstring strain can develop into a chronic condition. These patients present with a palpable defect due to distal retraction of the muscle belly and obvious asymmetry of the hamstring muscles. Do not be surprised if people with a chronic hamstring strain wait weeks, if not months, to seek medical attention.[21]

Management

The vast majority of hamstring strains are treated nonsurgically. In addition, imaging studies, such as x-rays, are not routinely ordered for these injuries. Also, universally accepted treatment and rehabilitation programs for hamstring strains have yet to be developed. For this reason, providing management feedback to patients with this condition can be frustrating.[21,23]

Treat those with either a first or second degree hamstring strain conservatively. Prescribe NWB crutch use, as described in PTH 6.1, for those who cannot walk without a limp. Have the patient initiate stretching exercises as early as possible in the treatment process, as shown in PTH 9.1. Add strengthening exercises, shown in PTH 9.1, once the patient can successfully perform resistance exercises without pain. Prescribe NWB

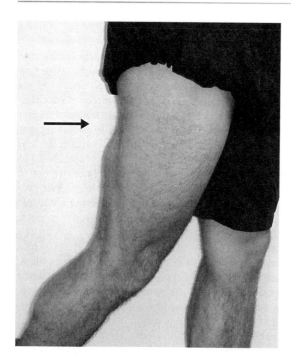

FIGURE 9.21 A tear of the hamstrings. Note the indentation and associated bulging of the muscle. From Starkey and Ryan: *Evaluation of Orthopedic and Athletic Injuries,* 2nd ed. 2002. Philadelphia: F.A. Davis Company, Fig. 8-15, pg 283, with permission.

crutch use, and refer to an orthopedist all patients who you suspect may have a third degree strain or an avulsion fracture of the ischial tuberosity. Surgery is usually indicated in cases of avulsion fracture, whereas it may or may not be recommended in cases of even the most severe strain.[21,23]

Lifespan Considerations

Usually, an injury mechanism that causes soft tissue damage in adults will do the same in adolescents. However, certain stresses are more likely to injure bone in this population because the adolescent skeletal system is still developing and may not be strong enough to resist the force being applied. For example, a valgus force applied externally to the adolescent knee may cause a fracture without injuring the TCL or ACL. In these cases, injury usually involves a bone's epiphysis. Always consider this possibility when establishing a differential diagnosis for the injured adolescent knee.

Sinding-Larsen-Johansson Disease

Sinding-Larsen-Johansson disease is a traction apophysitis condition that occurs when the patellar ligament pulls excessively on the inferior pole of the patella (Fig. 9.22A). Whereas this type of stress causes patellar tendonitis in the adult, the immature adolescent patella fragments at its lower pole. This causes bone fragments to become embedded in the ligament. Within a month from symptom onset, x-ray evaluation confirms the condition.[24]

Consider a diagnosis of Sinding-Larsen-Johansson disease for any adolescent who reports point tenderness where the patellar ligament attaches to the patella. Be particularly suspicious when this occurs in males aged 10 to 12 years who are involved in jumping and running activities, such as basketball, volleyball, and soccer. If symptoms have been present for at least 1 month, order x-rays, because the lateral view may confirm calcification and ossification in the ligament. Treat the condition by limiting the patient's activity, clearing the adolescent for return to participation only when the patella has matured enough to stand the stresses of physical activity. The use of a patellar-stabilizing knee sleeve, as shown in Figure 9.18, may help relieve symptoms.[24]

Osgood-Schlatter Disease (Tibial Tubercle Apophysitis)

Osgood-Schlatter disease, or *tibial tubercle apophysitis*, develops in adolescents whose patellar ligament is stronger than the tubercle's apophysis. It most commonly affects active adolescents who participate in jumping and running activities, because these activities cause a repetitive traction-type injury in which the ligament separates from the tubercle's apophysis (Fig. 9.22B). Not surprisingly, it is common for Osgood-Schlatter disease to develop in conjunction with Sinding-Larsen-Johansson disease.[17,25,26]

Osgood-Schlatter disease typically develops at the beginning of an adolescent's growth spurt and is most commonly seen in males aged 10 to 15 years. Thus, if an active young male reports with an insidious onset of tenderness, swelling, and prominence of the tibial tubercle, consider a diagnosis of Osgood-Schlatter disease. Order plain-film radiographs, but be aware that x-rays may not reveal the inflammation. In these cases, rely on your clinical findings to make the diagnosis. Place the patient with Osgood-Schlatter disease on a course of self-restricted activity for a period of a few years until symptoms subside. Symptom resolution indicates that the tibial apophysis is mature enough to support the demands of physical activity.[17,25,26]

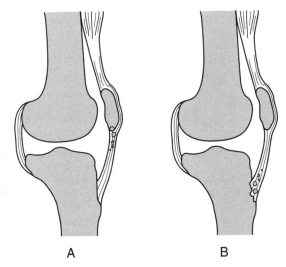

FIGURE 9.22 Traction apophysitis. Sinding-Larsen-Johansson disease (A) and Osgood-Schlatter disease (B). From McKinnis: *Fundamentals of Musculoskeletal Imaging*, 2nd ed. 2005. Philadelphia: F.A. Davis Company, Fig. 10-44, pg 353, with permission.

A   B

Limiting activity level is the treatment of choice for pediatric patients with traction apophysitis conditions.

Salter-Harris Fracture

A Salter-Harris fracture of the knee typically occurs at the adolescent's medial femoral condyle's growth plate in response to valgus and/or rotational forces. Thus, consider this condition any time you suspect a TCL or ACL injury in this population, because a positive valgus stress test and/or Lachman test may indicate that these ligaments have avulsed from their femoral attachments. Other signs of a Salter-Harris fracture include angular deformity and crepitus in the area of the medial femoral epicondyle.[27–29]

PEARL

Consider the possibility of a Salter-Harris fracture in those adolescents who present with positive signs for TCL or ACL injury.

Order standard knee x-rays for patients with a suspected Salter-Harris fracture. Also obtain a valgus stress x-ray, because this view may reveal the defect. Obtain an MRI if radiograph findings are negative and your clinical examination still suggests a fracture. Immobilize, prescribe NWB crutch gait as described in PTH 6.1, and refer any patient with a suspected or documented Salter-Harris fracture to an orthopedist. Treatment consists of NWB and long-cast immobilization until the fracture heals.[27–29]

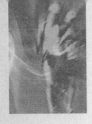

CASE STUDY
Conditions Involving the Knee

SCENARIO

A 16-year-old female high school sophomore comes to your practice reporting ongoing right knee pain after an injury that occurred 5 days ago during basketball practice. While running down the court, she tried to change direction by planting and pushing off her right foot in an attempt to quickly move to the left. She denies making contact with another player at the time of injury. She reports hearing a loud "pop" and feeling severe pain just before falling to the gymnasium floor. She was helped off the court by her teammates, and the injury was treated with protection, rest, ice, compression, and elevation (PRICE) by the team's coach. She was able to walk to the bus for her ride home, but her knee felt "sloppy" and she feared it would "give out" when she walked. After a restless night's sleep, she awoke with the knee extremely swollen and painful. She could not bend the knee or walk without a major limp. Findings of x-rays taken 4 days ago, as part of an orthopedic evaluation at the local hospital emergency department, were negative. She was fitted for crutches, was advised to continue with the PRICE treatments, and was told to take ibuprofen 600 mg tid and to make a follow-up appointment with her primary care provider.

PERTINENT HISTORY

Medications: Currently taking ibuprofen 600 mg tid. No other medications except for a daily multivitamin.

Family History: No significant family illnesses reported.

PERSONAL HEALTH HISTORY

Tobacco Use: Denies smoking cigarettes.

Recreational Drugs: Denies use.

Alcohol Intake: None.

Caffeinated Beverages: 2 to 3 diet sodas per day.

Exercise: In addition to playing basketball, the patient also plays soccer in the fall and participates in track and field in the spring.

Past Medical History: Generally healthy. Mumps at age 6 and chicken pox at age 4. Tonsils and adenoids removed at age 8.

PERTINENT PHYSICAL EXAMINATION*

On physical examination, the patient's right knee is severely swollen and warm to the touch. Can only flex about 30° and lacks the last 10° of full extension. You cannot check the strength of the quadriceps and hamstrings because of the amount of pain (6 on a scale of 1 to 10). Modified Lachman test is positive, with a soft end-feel. All other knee stress and special tests are negative. Patient is using crutches to ambulate, unable to bear any weight.

---

*Focused examination limited to key points for this case.

(case study continues on page 264)

CASE STUDY
Conditions Involving the Knee (continued)

RED FLAGS FOR THE PRIMARY HEALTH CARE PROFESSIONAL TO CONSIDER
- Basketball is commonly associated with noncontact ACL sprains.
- Females are at a high risk for noncontact ACL injury.
- A popping sound, the development of massive edema, and calor are prime indicators that an acute ACL sprain has occurred.
- The Lachman test is the definitive clinical diagnostic tool to diagnose ACL injury.

RECOMMENDED PLAN
- Refer the patient to an orthopedist for evaluation and further treatment.
- Continue with the present plan of non–weight-bearing and PRICE treatments until the appointment with the orthopedist.
- Change medications to acetaminophen 1000 mg qid.
- Advise the patient to have copies of the x-rays taken at the hospital forwarded to the orthopedist's office.
- Provide the patient with a written home management care plan.

REFERENCES

1. Austermuehle PD. Common knee injuries in primary care. *Nurse Pract* 2001;26(10):26.
2. Walgenbach AW. The knee joint: evaluation and treatment. *Nurse Pract Forum* 1996;7(3):1112.
3. Randolph CL. Considerations for the orthopedic nurse in diagnosis and treatment of adolescent sports injuries. *Nurs Clin North Am* 1998;33:615.
4. Altchek DW. Diagnosing acute knee injuries: the office exam. *Phys Sportsmed* 1993;21(7):85.
5. Stiell IG, Greenberg GH, Wells GA, et al. Derivation of a decision rule for the use of radiography in acute knee injuries. *Ann Emerg Med* 1995;26:405.
6. Onieal ME. Knee injuries: collateral ligament sprains. *J Am Acad Nurse Pract* 1993;5(6):271.
7. Onieal ME. Injuries to the anterior and posterior cruciate ligaments of the knee. *J Am Acad Nurse Pract* 1994;6(1):37.
8. Calkins C, Sartoris DJ. Imaging acute knee injuries: direct diagnostic approaches. *Phys Sportsmed* 1992;20(6):91.
9. Meislin RJ. Managing collateral ligament tears of the knee. *Phys Sportsmed* 1996;24(3):67.
10. Bach BR. Acute knee injuries: when to refer. *Phys Sportsmed* 1997;25(5):39.
11. Moeller JL, Lamb MM. Anterior cruciate ligament injuries in female athletes. *Phys Sportsmed* 1997;25(4):31.
12. Draper DO. A comparison of stress test used to evaluate the anterior cruciate ligament. *Phys Sportsmed* 1990;18(1):89.
13. Toy BJ, Morse DE, Yeasting RA, et al. Anatomy of the ACL: influence on the anterior drawer and Lachman tests. *Athl Ther Today* 1999;4(2):54.
14. Levy M, Smith AD. Diagnosing meniscus injuries: focus on the office exam. *Phys Sportsmed* 1994;22(5):47.
15. Brindle T, Nyland J, Johnson DL. The meniscus: review of basic principles with application to surgery and rehabilitation. *J Athl Train* 2001;36:160.
16. Galea AM, Albers JM. Patellofemoral pain: beyond empirical diagnosis. *Phys Sportsmed* 1994;22(4):48.
17. Adirim TA, Cheng TL. Overview of injuries in the young athlete. *Sports Med* 2003;33:75.
18. Colosimo AJ, Bassett FH. Jumper's knee: diagnosis and treatment. *Orthop Rev* 1990;19:139.
19. Ryan JB, Wheeler JH, Hopkinson WJ, et al. Quadriceps contusions: West Point update. *Am J Sports Med* 1991;19:299.
20. Keading CC, Sanko WA, Fischer RA. Quadriceps strains and contusions: decisions that promote rapid recovery *Phys Sportsmed.* 1995;23(1):59.
21. Best TM, Garret WE. Hamstring strains: expediting return to play. *Phys Sportsmed* 1996;24(8):37.
22. Garrett WE. Muscle strain injuries. *Am J Sports Med* 1996;24:S2.
23. Croisier JL. Factors associated with recurrent hamstring injuries. *Sports Med* 2004;34:681.
24. Medlar RC, Lyne D. Sinding-Larsen-Johansson disease: its etiology and natural history. *J Bone Joint Surg Am* 1978;60A:1113.
25. Wall EJ. Osgood-Schlatter disease: practical treatment for a self-limiting condition. *Phys Sportsmed* 1998;26(3):29.
26. Traverso A, Baldari A, Catalani F. The coexistence of Osgood-Schlatter's disease with Sinding-Larsen-Johansson's disease. *J Sports Med Phys Fitness* 1990;30:331.
27. Veenema KR. Valgus knee instability in an adolescent: ligament sprain or physeal fracture. *Phys Sportsmed* 1999;27(8):62.
28. Bertin KC, Goble EM. Ligament injuries associated with physeal fractures about the knee. *Clin Orthop Relat Res* 1983;177:188.
29. Decoster LC, Vailas JC. Fracture through the distal femoral epiphysis. *J Athl Train* 1995;30:154.

SUGGESTED READINGS

Adams N. Knee injuries. *Emerg Nurs* 2004;11(10):19.
Larson CM, Almekinders LC, Karas SG, et al. Evaluating and managing muscle contusions and myositis ossificans. *Phys Sportsmed* 2002;30(2):41.
Szucs PA, Richman PB, Mandell M. Triage nurse application of the Ottawa knee rule. *Acad Emerg Med* 2001;8:112.

WEB LINKS

http://www.niams.nih.gov/Health_Info/Knee_Problems/default.asp. Accessed 8/4/08.
  Provides questions and answers for common knee problems.

http://www.nlm.nih.gov/medlineplus/kneeinjuriesanddisorders.html. Accessed 8/4/08.
  Describes various knee injuries and disorders. Provides prevention, screening, and rehabilitation information. Video resources and links to relevant peer-reviewed journal articles are available.

http://www.medicineonline.com/healthtopics/topics/Knee_Injuries_and_Disorders. Accessed 8/4/08.
  Describes various knee injuries and disorders. Includes sections specific to children, teenagers, and women.

Conditions Involving the Hip, Pelvis, and Sacral and Lumbar Spines

● **Tina L. Claiborne, PhD, ATC, and Brian J. Toy, PhD, ATC**

W hen combined with the thigh, knee, leg, and foot, the hip and pelvis complete the lower extremity. Along with the lumbar spine, these structures form the center of the body's motion, transfer and dissipate external forces entering the body, and provide the body with its primary support for posture. They also coordinate and synchronize movement between the lower portion of the axial skeleton and the rest of the lower extremity. Consequently, injury to any of these structures may lead to debilitating pain and dysfunction. Not only can this limit a person's ability to participate in sports, it can also interfere with the completion of activities of daily living (ADLs) such as sitting, standing, walking, and climbing stairs.

Anatomy of the Hip, Pelvis, and Sacral and Lumbar Spines

The anatomy of these regions is extremely complex. Consequently, this review is limited to those structures health care professionals need to know to evaluate traumatic and nontraumatic conditions that typically occur in patients seen in the primary care setting.

Bones and Joints

Bones in this region include the femur; pelvic, or *innominates*; and vertebrae. Joints include the hip, sacroiliac, intervertebral, and facet (Figs. 10.1 and 10.2).

As discussed in Chapter 9, the femur, in addition to being the largest long bone in the body, is a major weight-bearing structure. Its proximal bony landmarks include the head, neck, and lesser and greater trochanters. The pelvis is composed of three separate bones: the ilium, ischium, and pubis. These bones fuse together shortly after birth in the acetabulum. It is the cup-shaped acetabulum that accepts the head of the femur to form the hip, or *coxofemoral*, joint.

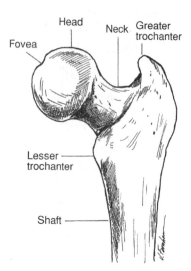

FIGURE 10.1 Bony anatomy of the proximal femur. From Levangie and Norkin: *Joint Structure and Function: A Comprehensive Analysis*, 4th ed. 2005. Philadelphia: F.A. Davis Company, Fig. 10-4, pg 358, with permission.

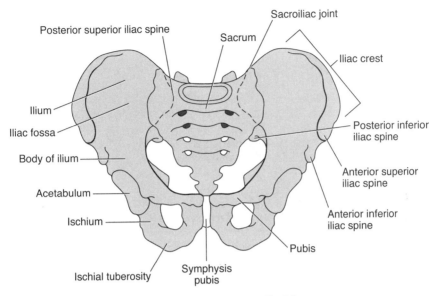

FIGURE 10.2 Bony anatomy of the pelvis, sacrum, and sacroiliac joints. Adapted from McKinnis: *Fundamentals of Musculoskeletal Imaging*, 2nd ed. 2005. Philadelphia: F.A. Davis Company, Fig. 9-1, pg 292, with permission.

Bony landmarks associated with the ilium, the largest of the three pelvic bones, include the iliac fossa and the iliac crest. This crest terminates anteriorly as the anterior superior iliac spine (ASIS) and posteriorly as the posterior superior iliac spine (PSIS). Just distal to these are the anterior inferior iliac spine (AIIS) and posterior inferior iliac spine (PIIS), respectively. Running medially from each acetabulum, the pubic bones join at the pubic symphysis. The ischium, which extends posteriorly from the pubis and acetabulum, maintains the large ischial tuberosity, also called the *sit bone* because it is the prominence on which we put pressure when we sit.

The spinal column is composed of 33 vertebrae, which are arranged as follows: 7 cervical, 12 thoracic, 5 lumbar, 5 sacral, and 4 coccyx (Fig. 10.3). Each of these areas maintains its own natural curvature, adding to the overall health of the spine. The lumbar curve is concave, whereas the sacral is convex. The five lumbar vertebrae consist of the following bony landmarks: spinous process, lamina, transverse processes, pedicle, body, and superior and inferior articular processes (Fig. 10.4). These vertebrae, as all others above this level, serve to protect the spinal cord as it runs in the vertebral, or *spinal*, canal, a channel formed by the vertebral foramen of each vertebra. Because the spinal cord typically ends at the level of L1/L2, the foramina of the lower lumbar vertebrae house the cauda equina (Fig. 10.5), a bundle of nerves that arise from the terminal end of the spinal cord. Articulations in this region include the intervertebral joints (IVJs) and the facet joints (FJs) (Fig. 10.3). The IVJs are formed between the bodies of the vertebrae, and the FJs are formed as the articulation between the inferior articular process of the superior vertebrae articulates with the superior articular process of the inferior vertebrae. The FJs also help form

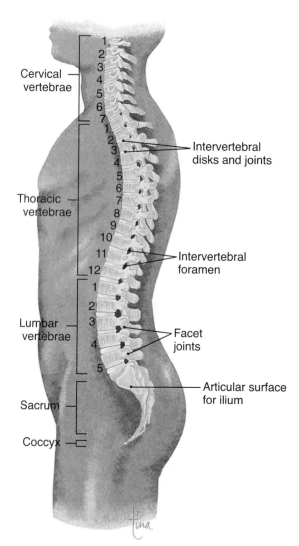

Cervical vertebrae

1
2
3
4
5
6
7

Thoracic vertebrae

1
2
3
4
5
6
7
8
9
10
11
12

Lumbar vertebrae

1
2
3
4
5

Sacrum

Coccyx

Intervertebral disks and joints

Intervertebral foramen

Facet joints

Articular surface for ilium

FIGURE 10.3 The vertebral column, intervertebral disks, intervertebral foramen, and facet joints. The figure also shows where the ilium articulates with the sacrum to form the sacroiliac joint. ASIS = anterior superior iliac spine. Adapted from Scanlon: *Essentials of Anatomy and Physiology*, 5th ed. 2007. Philadelphia: F.A. Davis Company, Fig. 6–10A, pg 120, with permission.

a separate intervertebral foramen (Fig. 10.3), which, as expanded on later in this chapter, allows for the passage of individual nerve roots exiting the spinal cord. The region between the superior and inferior facets of a vertebra is termed the *pars interarticularis,* a common area of injury.

Unlike those in the lumbar region, the vertebrae that compose the sacrum and coccyx are fused. Though this makes these structures fairly immobile, the sacrum does articulate with the fifth lumbar vertebrae to form an IVJ and FJs. The sacrum also articulates with the posterior aspect of each ilium to form the sacroiliac joints (SIJs) (Fig. 10.2). These joints serve as the union between the axial skeleton and the lower extremity.

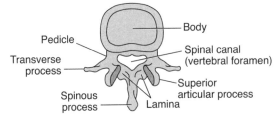

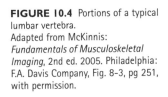

FIGURE 10.4 Portions of a typical lumbar vertebra.
Adapted from McKinnis: *Fundamentals of Musculoskeletal Imaging,* 2nd ed. 2005. Philadelphia: F.A. Davis Company, Fig. 8-3, pg 251, with permission.

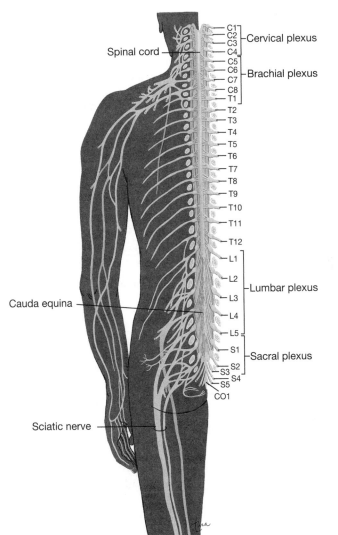

FIGURE 10.5 The spinal nerves, plexuses, and sciatic nerve.
Adapted from Scanlon: *Essentials of Anatomy and Physiology,* 5th ed. 2007. Philadelphia: F.A. Davis Company, Fig. 8-4, pg 173, with permission.

Motions

The hip is a true ball-and-socket joint, allowing the actions of flexion, hyperextension, abduction, adduction, and internal (medial) and external (lateral) rotation (Fig. 10.6). Average ranges of motion (ROMs) for each hip movement are listed in Box 10.1. Although it is one of the most freely moveable joints in the body, the hip sacrifices ROM for strength, making it one of the most stable diarthrodial joints in the body.

(PEARL)

The hip sacrifices ROM for strength, making it one of the most stable diarthrodial joints in the body.

Although not classified as such, the lumbar spine acts like a ball-and-socket joint, because the motions produced by this region are similar to those produced by such a joint (Figs. 10.7). This is because the total amount of motion achieved by this area is derived from a combination of the small amounts of movement occurring between each IVJ and FJ.

Though the SIJs do move, a significant amount of controversy surrounds the amount and type of motion associated with these joints. There is general agreement,

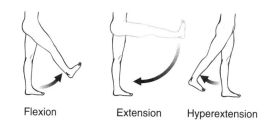

Flexion   Extension   Hyperextension

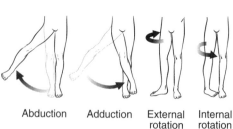

Abduction   Adduction   External   Internal
                           rotation   rotation

FIGURE 10.6 Motions of the hip. Adapted from Lippert: *Clinical Kinesiology and Anatomy*, 4th ed. 2006. Philadelphia: F.A. Davis Company, Fig. 17–3, pg 232, with permission.

BOX 10.1
ACTIVE RANGES OF MOTION OF THE HIP JOINT

<140° Flexion (knee extended)	45° Abduction
140° Flexion (knee flexed)	20° Adduction
30° Extension (knee extended)	40° Internal rotation
<30° Extension (knee flexed)	50° External rotation

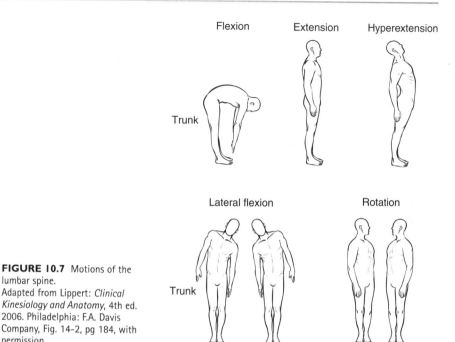

Flexion   Extension   Hyperextension

Trunk

Lateral flexion   Rotation

Trunk

FIGURE 10.7 Motions of the lumbar spine.
Adapted from Lippert: *Clinical Kinesiology and Anatomy*, 4th ed. 2006. Philadelphia: F.A. Davis Company, Fig. 14-2, pg 184, with permission.

however, that the SIJs afford small amounts of anterior and posterior sacral tilt and cephalic and caudal translation. A more detailed discussion of SIJ motion is discussed latter in this chapter.

Ligaments, Bursae, Nerves, and Intervertebral Disks

In addition to the joint's capsule, the hip is further supported by strong ligamentous tissue, adding to its status as a very stable joint. The SIJ is primarily supported by the ventral and dorsal sacroiliac (SI) ligaments and, as their names suggest, they resist anterior and posterior sacral motions (Fig. 10.8). Accessory SI ligaments include the sacrotuberous and sacrospinous, which, under load, resist anterior sacral motion. Finally, the joints of the spinal column are supported by numerous ligaments that run between vertebrae.

Of the several bursae that surround the hip and pelvis, one of the most clinically significant is the trochanteric. Located between the greater trochanter and the tendons of the gluteus medius, tensor fasciae latae, and iliotibial tract (all discussed later in this chapter), it functions to reduce friction in this area when the hip moves.

The spinal column maintains 31 pairs of spinal nerves (Fig. 10.5). As previously mentioned, in the lumbar region, these nerve roots exit the spinal column through individual intervertebral foramina (Fig. 10.3). In the sacrum, these nerves exit through sacral foramina. Some of these nerve roots are grouped in what is known as a *plexus*. The sciatic nerve, the largest of the body, is formed as the L4–S3 nerve roots join (Fig. 10.5). This nerve passes from the lumbosacral region to the posterior thigh, ultimately terminating in the popliteal fossa (discussed in Chapter 9). This nerve, or one of its many branches, provides motor function to the hamstrings and

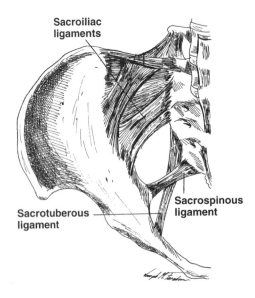

Sacroiliac ligaments

Sacrotuberous ligament

Sacrospinous ligament

FIGURE 10.8 The sacroiliac ligaments.
From Levangie and Norkin: *Joint Structure and Function: A Comprehensive Analysis*, 4th ed. 2005. Philadelphia: F.A. Davis Company, Fig. 4-48, pg 173, with permission.

to the muscles of the leg and foot. It also sends sensory information from these areas back to the spinal cord.

Separating the bodies of adjacent vertebrae throughout the lumbar spine, as well as the junction between L5 and the first sacral vertebra, are the intervertebral disks (Fig. 10.3). These structures act as shock absorbers by cushioning forces applied to the spinal column. They are composed of a tough, outer ring called the *annulus fibrosis*, which is charged with keeping the gel-like inner portion, otherwise known as the *nucleus pulposus*, from protruding outward. As people age, the thickness of these intervertebral disks decreases as a result of constant gravitational forces and a progressive loss of water content of the nucleus pulposus. This predisposes the disk to injury and for most people results in a loss of height due to the aging process.

Muscles and Tendons

The muscles of this region are divided into those which move the hip and those which move the lumbar spine. Normal muscle function in this region plays a critical role in maintaining postural control and lower extremity function. Refer to Figures 9.5 and 9.6 on pages 231 and 234, respectively, and Figures 10.9, 10.10, and 10.11 as the hip muscles are reviewed.

Muscles of the Hip

Muscles that surround and act on the hip are divided into two layers: superficial and deep. Superficial muscles are those which are easily palpated and include the hamstrings, sartorius, rectus femoris, gluteus maximus, tensor fasciae latae, and the adductor group, composed of the gracilis, pectineus, and adductor longus, brevis, and magnus. Deep muscles include the iliacus, psoas major, gluteus medius and minimus, and the external rotator group. Though all of these muscles move the hip in multiple directions, for the purposes of this discussion only the primary movers within each action classification are reviewed.

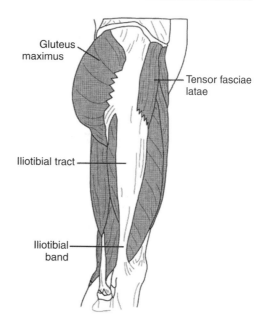

FIGURE 10.9 Superficial, lateral, and posterior hip muscles. The gluteus medius and minimus lie deep to the gluteus maximus. The iliotibial tract and iliotibial band are also presented.
Adapted from Starkey and Ryan: *Evaluation of Orthopedic and Athletic Injuries*, 2nd ed. 2002. Philadelphia: F.A. Davis Company, Fig. 8-10, pg 278, with permission.

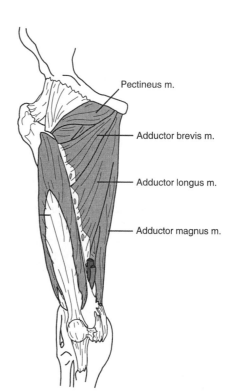

FIGURE 10.10 Adductors of the hip.
Adapted from Starkey and Ryan: *Evaluation of Orthopedic and Athletic Injuries*, 2nd ed. 2002. Philadelphia: F.A. Davis Company, Fig. 8-9, pg 278, with permission.

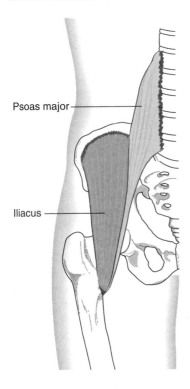

FIGURE 10.11 The iliopsoas muscle complex is made up of the psoas major and iliacus.
From Lippert: *Clinical Kinesiology and Anatomy*, 4th ed. 2006. Philadelphia: F.A. Davis Company, Fig. 17-16, pg 239, with permission.

The hamstrings, which originate from the ischial tuberosity, work in conjunction with the gluteus maximus to extend the hip. Originating from the sacrum and coccyx and inserting on the proximal femur and iliotibial tract, the gluteus maximus primarily extends the hip when the knee is flexed, whereas the hamstrings extend the hip when the knee is extended. The gluteus maximus is also responsible for externally rotating the hip, as are the external rotators, a group of six muscles that lie deep to the gluteus maximus.

As with hip extension, the action of hip flexion is produced by two distinct entities. The rectus femoris, part of the quadriceps muscle group, and the sartorius flex the hip when the knee is flexed. These muscles originate from the AIIS and ASIS, respectively. In contrast, the deep psoas major and iliacus muscles primary flex the hip when the knee is extended. The psoas major arises from the lower thoracic and upper lumbar vertebrae, whereas the iliacus originates from the iliac fossa. Because these muscles attach at a common site on the lesser trochanter of the femur, together they are frequently referred to as the *iliopsoas complex*.

Situated laterally, the gluteus medius, tensor fasciae latae, and gluteus minimus, all of which originate from the ilium, are primarily responsible for abducting the hip. The gluteus medius and minimus insert on the greater trochanter of the femur, whereas the tensor fascia latae continues distal to form the iliotibial tract. This structure ultimately ends as the iliotibial band (ITB), a structure that passes lateral to the knee joint to insert on the tibia. The gluteus medius and minimus are also responsible for internally rotating the hip. Medially the hip adductors all originate from the pubis and, except for the gracilis, insert along the shaft of the femur. As discussed in Chapter 9, the gracilis inserts in the pes anserine along with the sartorius and the semitendinosus hamstring muscle.

Muscles of the Lumbar Spine

The anterior muscles of the lumbar spine are those muscles that make up the abdominal wall. Refer to Chapter 14 for a detailed description of these muscles. Posteriorly, the muscles that extend the spine run parallel on either side of the spinous processes from the lumbar to the cervical region. They are also responsible for keeping the trunk erect when a person is standing or sitting, giving rise to their name, the *erector spinae* (Fig. 10.12). In the low back, this muscle group is referred to as the *lumbar erector spinae*.

Examination of the Hip, Pelvis, and Sacral and Lumbar Spines

Most patients who report to the primary care setting for musculoskeletal injuries of the hip, pelvis, and sacral and lumbar spines do so for conditions that are typically classified as chronic. This makes evaluation of these regions challenging for any health care provider. To complicate matters, any pathology of the lower extremity may affect the health of these regions. Consequently, always be sure to include a thorough evaluation of the lower extremity when assessing hip, pelvis, or sacral or lumbar spine injury.[1-3]

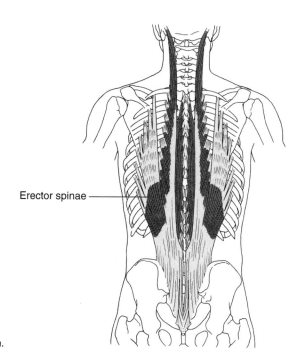

Erector spinae

FIGURE 10.12 The erector spinae muscle group. Adapted from Levangie and Norkin: *Joint Structure and Function: A Comprehensive Analysis*, 4th ed. 2005. Philadelphia: F.A. Davis Company, Fig. 4-60, pg 181, with permission.

History

In addition to asking the patient relevant questions listed in Box 7.1 on page 165, inquire about the location and type of pain the person is experiencing and whether the injury is the result of a traumatic or atraumatic event. Though traumatic conditions that occur in these regions are easily recognized, such as a contusion of the iliac crest (discussed later in this chapter), atraumatic conditions are more subtle to detect. For example, patients presenting with chronic groin or hip pain may have any number of conditions, such as a **sports hernia** (discussed in Chapter 14) or osteoarthritis (discussed in Chapter 1). Obtaining a detailed history also helps differentiate extra-articular from intra-articular hip pain. Some patients with extra-articular pain are able to point with one finger to the site of pain, such as in the case of **snapping hip syndrome** (discussed later in this chapter), whereas others with intra-articular pain report a more diffuse sensation of pain. In these instances, be sure to consider the age of the patient. Idiopathic diffuse hip pain in the young may be a sign of a growth-related condition such as **Legg-Calvé-Perthes disease** (discussed later in this chapter), whereas this same pain in the older patient is most likely due to degenerative changes, such as avascular necrosis.[2,4–7]

When taking a history, consider the location and type of pain, when the pain occurs, how long the pain has persisted, and the age and activity level of the patient.

One of the most challenging aspects of evaluating injury to these regions is to differentiate between pain originating from the SIJ and pain coming from the lumbar spine. Typically, patients who have injured the SIJ report discomfort below the level of L5 while performing ADLs. In contrast, those with a lumbar spine condition state that their pain remains at, or above, this level. In some instances, these patients experience radiating pain into the lower extremity, often following the path of the sciatic nerve.[3,8]

Physical Examination

As part of the physical examination process, observe, palpate, and test the ROM and strength of the hip, pelvis, and low back. Apply the special tests presented in this section every time a patient reports with pain in these regions. Doing so helps ensure that common features associated with hip, pelvis, and sacral and lumbar spines conditions are not overlooked.

Observation

Begin the observation portion of the physical examination as soon as the patient enters the office. Note abnormal gait patterns, posturing, and facial expressions that indicate the person's level of discomfort. A limp in the absence of other lower extremity pathology is a sign of hip, pelvis, or low back pain. A Trendelenburg gait, characterized by a pelvis tilting toward the non-weight-bearing side when the patient walks, is indicative of hip abductor weakness often associated with hip pathology. Next, with the patient standing, get a general sense of the person's posture by looking at him or her from the front, side, and back. Compare the height of the patient's greater trochanters, iliac crests, ASISs, and PSISs. Normal alignment of the ASISs is shown in Figure 10.13. An uneven alignment, otherwise known as *pelvic tilt*, is indicative of a structural abnormality. For example, a lateral pelvic tilt, which occurs when the ASIS, PSIS, and iliac crests on one side of the body are lower than the same structures on the contralateral side (Fig. 10.14), is typically associated with a leg length discrepancy (LLD) (discussed later in this chapter). In contrast, an anterior pelvic tilt, which occurs when both ASISs move anteriorly and inferiorly, is associated with hyperlordosis, a condition caused by a drooping abdomen, as in those who are obese or pregnant. In these instances, the person needs to hyperextend, or arch, their lumbar spine to support the additional abdominal weight. Hyperlordosis is also prevalent in athletes who are involved in activities such as gymnastics, which require the person to hyperextend the lumbar spine during activity. Hyperextending the lumbar spine for prolonged periods causes

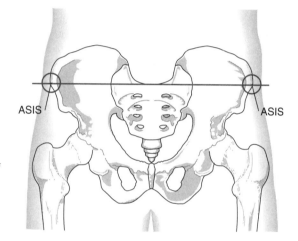

FIGURE 10.13 Normal position of the pelvis.
From Lippert: *Clinical Kinesiology and Anatomy*, 4th ed. 2006. Philadelphia: F.A. Davis Company, Fig. 16-14, pg 224, with permission.

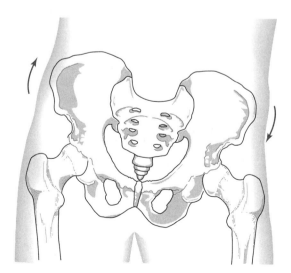

FIGURE 10.14 Lateral tilting of the pelvis.
From Lippert: *Clinical Kinesiology and Anatomy*, 4th ed. 2006. Philadelphia: F.A. Davis Company, Fig. 16-15, pg 225, with permission.

the hamstrings to stretch and the iliopsoas complex to shorten, ultimately resulting in a tilted pelvis. Such an imbalance in flexibility and strength eventually manifests in lumbar, SIJ, and/or hip pain.[1–3,6,8,9]

Continue the observation portion of the examination by inspecting all the areas for ecchymosis, lacerations, or obvious deformity, as well as for muscle atrophy or hypertrophy. Examine the patient's iliac crest and ASIS for swelling and bruising, indicating the presence of a contusion, and possible fracture. Look at the rotational position and shortening of the limbs relative to the trunk and pelvis. Such findings may indicate that the person has incurred an acute injury to the hip or pelvis. Indeed, patient's who present with the hip "stuck" in a position of flexion, internal rotation, and adduction almost surely have some degree of hip instability and should be referred immediately for an orthopedic consult.[2,4,10]

Palpation

Use the palpation portion of the examination to evaluate for soft and hard tissue pathologies. For you to complete this segment of the assessment, the patient must be moved so access can be gained to the entire region. Thus, palpate all available structures with the patient in one position before repositioning the patient. Doing so increases efficiency and minimizes patient discomfort.

Start by examining the hip and pelvis with the patient supine. Palpate the ASIS and pubis, because doing so assesses the integrity of these bony landmarks as well as the status of the underlying attachment points for the hip adductors and rectus abdominis (pubis) and sartorius (ASIS). Further assess the adductor muscle group by abducting the hip and discretely palpating for tenderness and deformity. Next, ask the patient to lie on his or her unaffected side and palpate the iliac crest for tenderness. Because this is the attachment site for many muscles, including the abdominal obliques (Fig. 14.2 on page 445), pain in this area may indicate a fracture, contusion, or muscle strain. Move inferiorly to palpate the ischial tuberosity, greater trochanter, tensor fasciae latae, iliotibial tract, trochanteric bursa, and gluteus medius. Swelling and tenderness in the area of the ischial tuberosity are indicative of a hamstring injury (discussed in Chapter 9), whereas lateral hip pain indicates bursitis, muscle strain, tendinosis, or underlying hip pathology. Conclude by palpating the length of the ITB distally to its insertion on the tibia.[2,9]

With the patient lying prone, palpate the gluteus maximus, checking for pain, spasm, or defect. Doing so may also cause irritation to an inflamed sciatic nerve running deep to this muscle. Move superiorly and palpate the PSISs and SIJs. Tenderness in these areas indicates SIJ pathology. Palpate over the spinous processes of the lumbar vertebrae and the lumbar erector spinae muscle group. When structures in this region have been injured, this muscle group is often in spasm. Recognize that as the erector spinae is palpated, the health of the underlying portions of the vertebrae, such as the facet joints and transverse processes, is also being assessed.[2,9]

Range-of-Motion and Strength Testing

Range-of-motion and strengthen testing in this area involves assessing the hip and lumbar spines. However, before performing these assessments, first check the hip's joint stability by "log rolling" the lower extremity. Do this by internally and externally rotating the joint with the patient lying supine on a table, with the knee fully extended. This causes extreme pain to patients with an intra-articular problem, such as fracture or infection. In these instances, do not attempt to further test the hip joint's ROM.[2]

For those who do not experience increased discomfort with the log rolling test, check the patient's hip ROM by having the patient perform the motions illustrated in Figure 10.6. Test active hip flexion, abduction and adduction with the patient supine, and internal and external rotation with the patient seated. Conclude the ROM portion of the examination by testing hip hyperextension with the patient prone. Remember that the hamstrings and rectus femoris are two joint muscles, so it is important to be aware that knee position affects hip flexion and extension. For example, testing these actions with a flexed knee increases the amount of hip flexion but decreases the amount of hip extension. Consequently, be sure to measure hip flexion and extension with the knee both flexed and extended. This helps differentiate between rectus femoris and hamstring tightness from other ROM issues caused by bony blocks or joint capsule tension.[2,9,11]

Continue this portion of the evaluation by manual muscle testing (MMT) all hip motions shown in Figure 10.6. Use the same patient positioning prescribed for ROM testing. Be sure to apply resistance above the level of the knee when performing an MMT for flexion and extension and with the knee extended for abduction and adduction. For seated internal and external rotation, apply resistance at the leg, just above the ankle. Test the strength of the hip flexors with the patient sitting and the strength of the extensors with the patient prone with the knee flexed, because doing this helps isolate the rectus femoris (hip flexion) and gluteus maximus (hip extension) muscles.

In the primary care setting, lumbar ROM and strength are typically evaluated simultaneously, because performing an MMT for this part of the body is extremely challenging and places both the practitioner and the patient at risk for injury. Thus, test the lumbar spine by asking the patient to do the following as shown in Figure 10.7:

- touch the toes (flexion);
- look at the ceiling while keeping the neck straight (hyperextension);
- lateral flex to each side, running the tip of the middle finger to the level of the knee's joint line;
- rotate the trunk 90° without moving the pelvis and hips.

Stress and Special Testing

There are a number of specific special tests that should always be used when evaluating injury to a patient's hip, pelvis, or sacral and lumbar spines, particularly when the person has a chronic condition. Use these tests in conjunction with those outlined for the specific musculoskeletal conditions covered in this chapter to help develop a differential diagnosis.

The **Thomas test** determines whether a patient's hip flexors are tight or inflexible. As already discussed, tight hip flexors place undue stress on the lumbar spine, ultimately contributing to hip, pelvic, and sacral and lumbar pathology.[2,9,12,13] To perform this test (Fig. 10.15):

- Instruct the patient to lie supine, with both knees flexed over the end of the table.
- Place one of your hands between the table and lumbar spine.
- Using your other hand, passively flex one hip to the patient's chest (or you can ask the patient to use his or her hands to bring this knee to the chest).

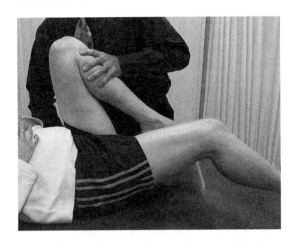

FIGURE 10.15 The Thomas test to assess for hip flexor tightness. (This figure illustrates a positive Thomas test for iliopsoas tightness.)

• A positive test occurs when the leg on the table moves into extension and the lumbar spine rises off the table (rectus femoris tightness) or when this leg rises off the table (iliopsoas tightness).

Similar to the Trendelenburg gait, the **Trendelenburg sign** tests for hip abductor weakness.[2,9] To perform this test (Fig. 10.16):

• Instruct the patient to stand with his or her weight evenly distributed between the feet.
• Ask the patient to stand on one leg.
• Note the position of the patient's ASISs, PSISs, and iliac crests.
• A positive test results when the pelvis drops, or tilts, laterally toward the non-weight-bearing side, indicating gluteus medius weakness on the weight-bearing side.

The **hip scouring test** is a general test that evaluates the health of the hip joint. To perform this test (Fig. 10.17):

• Instruct the patient to lie supine.
• Tell the patient to relax while you fully flex the hip and knee.
• Apply downward pressure on the knee along the shaft of the femur.
• Maintaining firm pressure, internally and externally rotate the hip.
• Pain produced by this test indicates the presence of hip degeneration, such as osteoarthritis.

The active **double straight leg test** is useful to distinguish SIJ pain from lumbar spine involvement. To perform this test:

• Instruct the patient to lie supine.
• Tell the patient to actively raise both feet off the table by flexing the hips while keeping the knees straight.
• Instruct the patient to raise both lower extremities to 90°.
• Pain occurring at the beginning of this test indicates SIJ involvement, whereas pain occurring toward the end of the maneuver is indicative of lumbar spine pathology.

As previously mentioned, an LLD is a structural abnormality that predisposes a patient to countless overuse conditions of the low back and lower extremity. Two types of LLD exist: true, otherwise known as *structural*, and apparent, or *functional*. When a

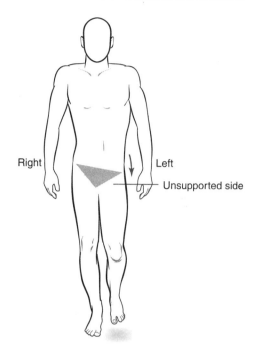

FIGURE 10.16 Trendelenburg sign for a weak gluteus medius muscle. From Lippert LS: *Clinical Kinesiology and Anatomy*, 4th ed. 2006. Philadelphia: F.A. Davis Company, Fig. 16-16, pg 225, with permission.

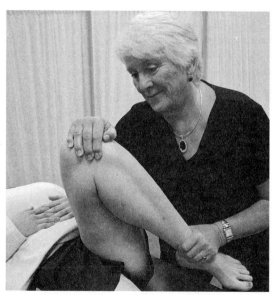

FIGURE 10.17 Hip scouring test for hip degeneration.

patient has a true LLD, an actual difference exists between the lengths of the person's tibias and/or femurs. In contrast, an apparent discrepancy is caused by deformities of the pelvis, such as what occurs if the pelvis is rotated, or by deformities of the spine, such as scoliosis. To determine whether a patient has an LLD, use a tape measure to measure the length of the person's lower extremities. Measure first for the presence of a true LLD. If this is present, there is no need to test for an apparent LLD. However, test for the presence of an apparent LLD if a true LLD does not exist.[1,2,9,14] To test for an LLD (Fig. 10.18):

• Ask the patient to lie supine.
• Measure from the patient's ASIS to the medial malleoli on the same side. A difference >5 mm between lower extremities is indicative of a true LLD.
• Measure from the umbilicus to each medial malleoli. A difference >5 mm between lower extremities is indicative of an apparent LLD.

Refer people with a true LLD and those with an apparent LLD >5 mm to an orthopedist so a decision can be made with regard to the best way to treat these patients. If an apparent LLD of <5 mm exists, treat the patient's deficit by placing an orthopedic "heel lift" in the shoe of the person's shorter extremity. These over-the-counter products can be purchased at most pharmacies, surgical supply stores, and sporting goods stores. Instruct the patient to perform the pelvic exercises outlined in Patient Teaching Handout (PTH) 10.1. Ultimately, people with an apparent LLD may have to be referred for orthopedic consult if these measures do not lessen the pain and discomfort.[15]

Neurological Examination

Assessing injury to these regions, particularly those occurring in the lumbar and sacral spines, should include a complete neurological examination of the lower extremity. Indeed, conditions involving the sacral and lumbar spines can easily affect the nerve roots exiting from the spinal cord at these levels. This neurological evaluation includes assessing the patient's motor and sensory functions, as well as performing reflex testing.[8]

Determining the health the patient's motor nerves occurs via the completion of the MMT portion of the examination. Realize, however, that lumbosacral nerve root pathology can affect any muscle group supplied by the nerve roots exiting the spinal cord at this level. Thus, in addition to testing the strength of the hip and low back muscles, be sure to MMT all muscle groups of the knee, ankle, and foot (described in Chapters 8 and 9). Evaluate for sensory deprivation by testing the patient's dermatomes, following the patterns shown in Figure 10.19. By comparing the patient's ability to normally perceive sensory stimuli, such as touch, pain, and changes in temperature, it can be determined whether a specific nerve root has been affected by injury or disease. Conclude the neurological portion of the examination by testing the patient's patellar (L2–L4) and calcaneal (L5–S1) tendon reflexes.[8,9,16]

Musculoskeletal Imaging

Because of the role these body regions play in supporting body weight and posture, they possess significant bony strength. This makes fractures to these bones, particularly the pelvis and femur, extremely significant. Indeed, these injuries are often accompanie by serious neurovascular complications. Consequently, be sure to consider this when deciding on which imaging techniques to order.

Order an anteroposterior (AP) radiograph of the pelvis after trauma to either the hip or the pelvis, because doing so provides an x-ray image of both hip joints and the pelvis. Also obtain a lateral plain-film image for suspected injury to the hip. If these views reveal a defect, consider ordering a unilateral AP view, because this projection

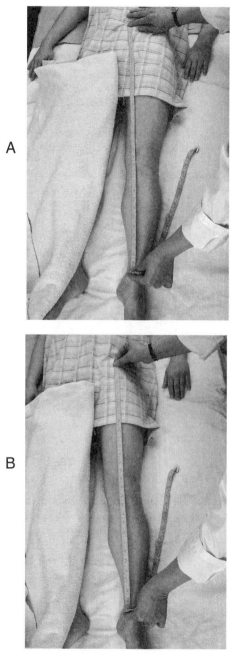

FIGURE 10.18 Testing for leg length discrepancy (LLD). (A) Testing for an apparent LLD. (B) Testing for a true LLD.
From Dillon: *Nursing Health Assessment: A Critical Thinking, Case Studies Approach.* 2003.
Philadelphia: F.A. Davis Company, Measuring Leg Length, A and B, pg 617, with permission.

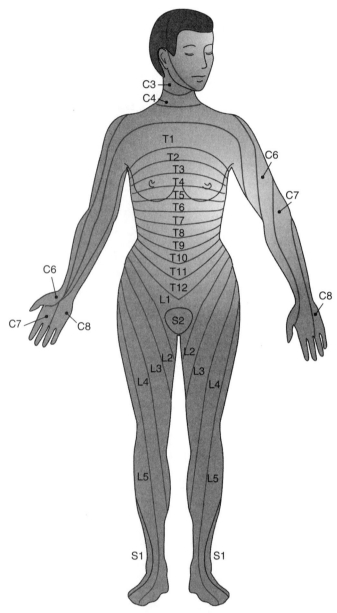

FIGURE 10.19 Dermatome pattern of the body.
From Dillon: *Nursing Health Assessment: A Critical Thinking, Case Studies Approach.* 2003. Philadelphia: F.A. Davis Company, Fig. 10-4B, pg 247, with permission.

better shows the integrity of the acetabulum, femoral head and neck, proximal femur, and greater trochanter. Because traumatic hip injuries often involve the pelvis, it is important to obtain an oblique view of the pelvis in these situations. Also, use these projections to assess unexplained hip and pelvic pain, degenerative disease, and osseous changes due to metabolic disease, nutritional deficiencies, or congenital disorders. Because certain conditions may not be initially evident on x-ray, consider ordering magnetic resonance imaging (MRI) in cases in which diseases related to hip degeneration, such as avascular necrosis of the femoral head, are suspected. Additionally, MRI is also sensitive for detecting the development of femoral stress fractures in their early stages.[2,17,18]

For bony pathologies of the lumbar spine, order AP, lateral, and oblique x-ray views of this region. The AP and lateral projections provide a three-dimensional view of the area, whereas the oblique views are excellent for evaluating the health of the facet joints. Although intervertebral disks cannot be seen well on x-rays, standard radiographs are useful for examining the space these disks occupy. Conversely, an MRI is helpful when visualizing the disks themselves. Use a bone scan or computed tomography when the presence of subtle bony abnormalities, such as a stress fracture or the beginning stages of **spondylolysis** (discussed later in this chapter), are suspected. In some cases, verifying the presence of a bone abnormality requires comparing the results of more than one imaging technique. This may also be true when trying to determine whether a defect is new or old.[17]

Conditions of the Hip, Pelvis, and Sacrum

Recall that the hip and pelvis form the structural junction between the trunk and the lower extremity, meaning that injury to these areas has the potential of affecting the lower extremities and/or the lumbar spine. Keep this in mind as specific hip and SI conditions are reviewed, because the evaluation of these regions must be performed as merely one part of a more comprehensive evaluation. Also, because traumatic injury to the hip joint usually causes the patient major disability, these conditions are more likely to be seen in the emergency care setting. Thus, this review of hip conditions is limited to those typically encountered in the primary care setting.

Contusion to the Iliac Crest (Hip Pointer)

The iliac crest is a common site of injury because this bony prominence has little soft tissue protection. When it becomes contused, the patient is said to have a **hip pointer**, a common misnomer because it is the pelvis, not the hip, that has been injured. Nevertheless, injury to this area results in extreme pain, swelling, bruising, and dysfunction, because many muscles attach here (Fig. 10.20). In fact, it is not uncommon that the amount of pain and dysfunction the patient experiences with this injury is disproportionate to the severity.[5,8,19]

History and Physical Examination

A patient with a hip pointer relates that he or she sustained blunt-force trauma to the iliac crest. The acute response to this mechanism of injury (MOI) is localized swelling, redness, and intense discomfort. Pain increases when the patient takes a deep breath, coughs, or sneezes. The region is tender when palpated, and spasm is present, owing

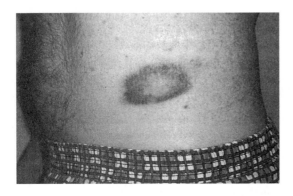

FIGURE 10.20 A "hip pointer" (contusion to the iliac crest).

to injury of the muscles that attach to the iliac crest. Any attempt to move the trunk through its full ROM causes the person extreme pain, particularly when the patient attempts to laterally flex to the side opposite of the injury. Be sure to rule out injury to the abdominal organs as described in Chapter 14.[2,18,19]

The name *hip pointer* is misleading, because this injury actually occurs at the iliac crest of the pelvis.

Management
Treat patients with this condition by reducing inflammation and pain and by decreasing the tensile strain from the muscles which attach to the iliac crest. Do this by prescribing cryotherapy treatments and advising the patient to avoid excessive movement of the trunk. Order x-rays to rule out an underlying fracture. Refer all confirmed cases of fracture to an orthopedist, and all suspected cases of intra-abdominal injury to an internist. Instruct all other patients to avoid vigorous activity until pain subsides and full motion of the trunk returns. Upon return to activity, advise all athletes participating in a collision or contact sport to wear protective padding over the site of injury.[18]

Iliotibial Band Friction Syndrome
Iliotibial band friction syndrome occurs as the ITB passes over the lateral condyle of the femur on its way to its attachment site on the tibia. This condition is commonly seen in people who participate in sports or activities that require repeated knee flexion and extension movements, such as running. Often, malalignments of the hip, knee, ankle, or foot contribute to iliotibial band friction syndrome, because these abnormalities can cause the ITB to become short and tight, a primary risk factor for the development of this condition.[20]

History and Physical Examination
Patients with iliotibial band friction syndrome report a sharp or burning pain over the lateral femoral condyle, sometimes extending distally into the lateral calf. They state this pain is present during and/or after activity. In the early stages of injury, the area

may appear normal because the initial signs commonly associated with musculoskeletal pathology, such as redness and swelling, are usually absent. However, the lateral femoral condyle is almost always painful when palpated, as is the ITB's tibial insertion site. Active knee flexion and extension also cause pain, because these actions cause the ITB to pass over the lateral femoral condyle. **Noble's compression test** is an excellent special test to use to confirm the presence of pain with knee motion.[20,21] To perform this test (Fig. 10.21):

• Instruct the patient to lie supine.
• Stand to the lateral side of the affected lower extremity.
• Apply pressure with your thumb to the ITB just superior to the affected lateral femoral condyle.
• Passively flex and extend the patient's knee with your opposite hand.
• A positive test occurs when the patient reports pain beneath your thumb.

Another exceptional test to use on patients suspected of having iliotibial band friction syndrome is **Ober's test**, which determines whether the ITB has been shortened enough to place it at risk of becoming injured.[2,9,18] To perform this test (Fig. 10.22):

• Instruct the patient to lie on the unaffected side.
• Stand behind the patient, and support the affected extremity by grasping the leg above the ankle.
• With the patient's knee flexed, abduct and extend the patient's affected hip.
• Allow the extremity to passively adduct toward the table.
• Ober's test is positive if the leg is unable to adduct past parallel.

Management
Instruct patients with iliotibial band friction syndrome to modify activity and to use ice massage to control pain and inflammation. To improve ITB flexibility, tell the patient to perform the Ober's test at home, because this maneuver can also be used as a rehabilitative tool. After the ITB has been stretched, prescribe hip abduction strengthening exercises, as shown and described in PTH 10.1, because strengthening this muscle group allows the ITB to maintain its new, lengthened position. Once symptoms subside, gradually return the patient to full activity, being sure to avoid all situations that irritate the ITB.[5,6,18,22]

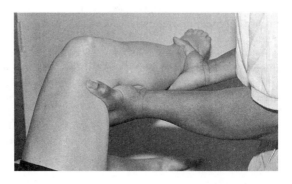

FIGURE 10.21 Noble's compression test for iliotibial band friction syndrome.
From Starkey and Ryan: *Evaluation of Orthopedic and Athletic Injuries,* 2nd ed. 2002. Philadelphia: F.A. Davis Company, Box 6-21A, pg 236, with permission.

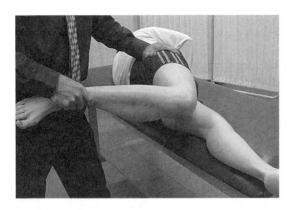

FIGURE 10.22 Ober's test for iliotibial band tightness.

Snapping Hip Syndrome and Greater Trochanter Bursitis

Although technical and complicated, snapping hip syndrome refers to a condition where the patient reports "snapping" in the hip, with or without discomfort. This syndrome arises from friction buildup as the proximal portion of the ITB, the tendon of the gluteus maximus muscle, or both pass over the femur's greater trochanter. This MOI also causes the trochanteric bursa to be irritated. The typical etiology of these conditions includes the following steps[5,18,23,24]:

- the ITB continually rubs over the greater trochanter;
- the greater trochanteric bursa becomes inflamed; and
- snapping hip syndrome develops.

Underlying causes for this rubbing-type mechanism include structural malalignment of the hips and pelvis and imbalances in strength and/or flexibility of the muscles in the area. Women are more susceptible to development of these conditions because of the female's naturally larger Q angle (discussed in Chapter 9). These conditions are also more prevalent in people who participate in activities such as running that require the body to perform the repetitive motions of hip flexion and extension for extended periods.[25,26]

History and Physical Examination

Patients with either of these conditions feel, and may hear, a snapping occurring in the area of the hip when they walk or run. Indeed, a telltale sign of snapping hip syndrome is the audible "snap" patients report that they hear during hip movement. This is usually associated with pain over the greater trochanter, often referring into the buttock. Pain typically increases with hip flexion and extension activities, such as running, climbing stairs, or rising from a seated position. The patient's discomfort increases when he or she actively flexes and extends the hip as you palpate the greater trochanter. In some instances, the soft tissues can be felt as they move over this structure, though this sign cannot be reproduced in all patients. People with either of these conditions usually have an LLD, a positive Ober's test, and/or a positive Trendelenburg sign.[5,6,22]

A telltale sign of snapping hip syndrome is the audible "snap" the patient reports hearing during normal hip motion.

Management

As with iliotibial band friction syndrome, initially treat people with either of these conditions by modifying the patient's activity level and by telling the patient to stretch the ITB using Ober's maneuver. Have the patient strengthen the hip abductors by prescribing the exercises shown and described in PTH 10.1. If necessary, correct LLD as described earlier in this chapter and treat the area with cryotherapy. Rarely do either of these conditions require further intervention, particularly if treatment is started when symptoms first appear.[5,6,18,26]

Adductor Strain (Groin Strain)

As with most muscle strains, an adductor, or groin, strain results from an overstretching of the muscle, often occurring in conjunction with an eccentric muscle contraction. This injury can be quite debilitating, causing disability ranging from pain while walking or standing to difficulty when playing sports. Keep in mind that conditions such as a sports hernia, discussed in Chapter 14, and a **slipped capital femoral epiphysis**, discussed later in this chapter, present with similar signs and symptoms as a groin strain. Thus, always consider the possible presence of these conditions when formulating a differential diagnosis after injury to the hip adductors and their respective attachment on the pubis.[27,28]

Pain in the groin region can be a sign of a groin strain, a sports hernia, or a slipped capital femoral epiphysis.

History and Physical Examination

The patient with a groin strain reports discomfort over the inner thigh just distal to where the adductors attach to the pubis. Often, the MOI is forced abduction with concurrent contraction of the adductor muscle group. Inspection of the groin area reveals swelling, bruising, and/or a visual defect, the extent of which is directly related to the severity of the injury. The area is point tender near the muscle group's pubic attachment, with a palpable defect almost always present in a second or third degree strain. In these instances, the strength of the patient's adductors and the ability of the person to fully abduct the hip are also diminished. Be sure to consider the possible presence of a pubic avulsion fracture in patients who are in extreme pain. Also, realize that any localized hardening of these injured tissues indicates that myositis ossificans may have developed (discussed in Chapter 9), necessitating quick referral for follow-up care.[18,27]

Management

Initially treat a patient with a groin strain as you would any acute injury, with rest and the application of cold to the injured area. Ice massaging the region while stretching the adductors is a particularly effective way to initially manage this injury. If walking is extremely painful, fit the patient for crutches, as outlined in PTH 6.1. Instruct the patient to support the area by wearing neoprene shorts (Fig. 14.7 on page 463), because this provides support and decreases discomfort. If you suspect that the muscle group has avulsed from its pubic origin or has developed myositis ossificans, send the patient for radiograph evaluation. If x-rays confirm either of these conditions, immediately refer the patient for orthopedic consultation. For all others, prescribe adductor stretching and strengthening exercises, shown in PTH 10.1. Instruct the patient to perform these exercises within pain limits. As the injury progresses, add general lower extremity stretching and strengthening exercises shown in PTH 10.1. Only return the person to vigorous activity when he or she has achieved full pain-free strength and ROM.[6,26,28]

Sacroiliac Joint Dysfunction

Sacroiliac joint dysfunction occurs as a result of both acute and chronic mechanisms. Acute injuries typically result from a person directly falling on the pelvis or from blunt-force trauma. Overuse cases of SIJ dysfunction occur in patients who participate in activities that place extreme stresses on the pelvis, such as rowing. Structural deviations of the body, such as LLD, muscle strength imbalance, and hypoflexibility and hyperflexibility of the trunk and hip muscles, also contribute to instances of chronic SIJ dysfunction. Additionally, conditions of the lumbar disk (discussed later in this chapter) and pathologies of the hip, such as degenerative joint disease, may refer pain into this area. Thus, a thorough examination of these body parts should always occur when a patient presents with SIJ pain. Unfortunately, the fact that other conditions can be masked by SIJ pain often makes SIJ dysfunction a diagnosis of exclusion.[1,3,6]

Lumbar spine and hip pathologies often refer pain to the SI region. Therefore, it is critical to complete a thorough evaluation of all of these areas when a patient presents with SIJ pain.

History and Physical Examination

Regardless of cause, patients with SIJ dysfunction typically report pain and discomfort in the low back and buttock region near the area of the PSIS. This pain may also refer to the hip, thigh, and groin and down the posterior thigh. Patients may also report a history of ankle, foot, or knee injury that immediately preceded the development of SIJ pain. Pain usually increases with repetitive, overload activity and/or with prolonged periods of sitting with the low back and pelvis unsupported. A distinguishing feature of SIJ dysfunction is a lack of pain above the L5 level, a key point when trying to differentiate between SIJ pain and pain produced by lumbar spine injury (discussed later in this chapter). In addition, the type, location, and quality of pain described by those with SIJ dysfunction differ greatly among patients. For example, some describe pain as being sharp and intermittent, whereas others report a constant, dull ache. Furthermore, the person's pain may be concentrated in a single area, or it can be more diffuse.[3,6,29,30]

(P E A R L)

Though pain caused by SIJ dysfunction may also refer to the hip, thigh, and groin and down the posterior thigh, it typically does not refer above the level of L5.

When observed with the patient in the standing position, the SIJs of a patient with this condition usually maintain some degree of pelvic tilt. Disruptions to the way the patient walks, such as decreases in stride length and the presence of a noticeable limp, are also present. These lead to the development of a Trendelenburg gait, a sign seen in many people with SIJ dysfunction. When palpated, these patients almost always have pain over the area of the PSIS on the involved side. Because the sacrum articulates with the lumbar spine, most people experience some level of discomfort when ROM of the lumbar spine is tested. Tightness of the hamstrings and iliopsoas complex, leading to a positive Thomas test, is usually present. The beginning stage of the double straight leg test also causes the patient pain. It is also typical for people with SIJ dysfunction to have an LLD. When SIJ dysfunction occurs in isolation from a lumbar spine condition, results of the patient's neurological evaluation are normal.[1,3,6,29]

Unfortunately, clinical special tests that consistently and accurately identify SIJ pain and dysfunction do not exist. Nevertheless, conclude the assessment by performing the **SIJ compression** and **distraction tests**; **Gaenslen's test**; and the **FABERE** (*f*lexion, *ab*duction, *e*xternal *r*otation, and *e*xtension of the hip) **test**, otherwise known as *Patrick's* test, because SIJ dysfunction typically produces pain with any or all of these tests.[1,3,6,9,29–32] Recognize, however, that a negative finding for any of these does not exclude a finding of SIJ dysfunction.

To perform the SIJ compression test (Fig. 10.23):

• Instruct the patient to lie supine.
• Standing beside the patient, cross your hands, placing your right hand on the patient's right ASIS and your left hand on the patient's left ASIS.
• Compress the patient's SIJ by applying outward pressure to the ASISs.

To perform the SIJ distraction test (Fig. 10.24):

• Ask the patient to assume a side-lying position.
• Standing behind the patient, place both hands on the anterior portion of the person's ilium.
• Distract the patient's SI joint by pressing downward on the ilium.

To perform the FABERE test (Fig. 10.25):

• Instruct the patient to lie supine, with one ankle crossed over the opposite thigh, creating a figure-four position.
• Standing next to the patient on the side of the flexed knee, position one hand over the opposite ASIS and one hand on the flexed knee.
• While stabilizing the ASIS, gently apply downward pressure on the flexed knee. This externally rotates the hip and places pressure on the SI joint.
• Though pain occurring in the SI region indicates SI pathology, pain elicited from the groin area indicates hip pathology.

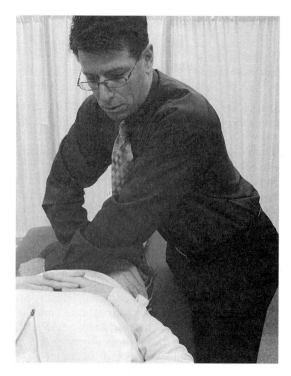

FIGURE 10.23 Sacroiliac joint compression test for sacroiliac joint dysfunction.

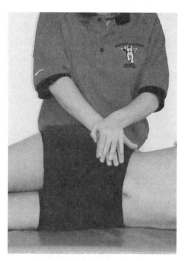

FIGURE 10.24 Sacroiliac joint distraction test for sacroiliac joint dysfunction.
From Starkey and Ryan: *Evaluation of Orthopedic and Athletic Injuries*, 2nd ed. 2002. Philadelphia: F.A. Davis Company, Box 10-18B, pg 362, with permission.

To perform Gaenslen's test (Fig. 10.26):

• Ask the patient to lie supine, close to the edge of the table.
• Standing beside the patient, use one hand to stabilize his or her shoulder
• Instruct the patient to hang the lower extremity closest to you over the side of the table.

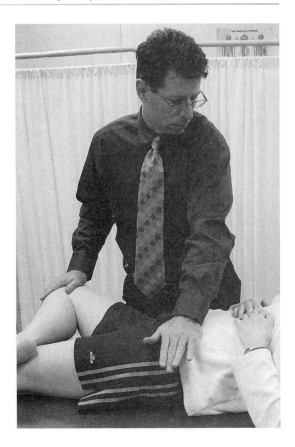

FIGURE 10.25 FABERE test for sacroiliac joint dysfunction.

- Simultaneously, ask the person to use his or her hands to hug the knee of the extremity opposite to the patient's chest.
- Move the hip of the hanging extremity into hyperextension by gently applying downward pressure to the patient's thigh.

Management

Though obtaining x-rays of the SIJ for patients with SIJ pain is certainly advocated by some, imaging techniques used to evaluate this joint provide minimal feedback because they cannot distinguish asymptomatic from symptomatic people. Thus, use the cause and severity of the patient's pain as a guide when managing this condition. Initially, modify the patient's activity and employ therapeutic techniques, such as the application of cryotherapy, to control patient discomfort. Implement a general strengthening and stretching exercise routine, as outlined in PTHs 10.1, 3.1, and 3.2, for the entire pelvic and low back regions. If needed, correct for LLD and poor posture. Slowly return the person to physical activity as pain and discomfort allow. However, stress to patients the importance of continuing a pelvic and low back strengthening and stretching regimen even after pain has disappeared. Refer to an orthopedist patients who do not improve with conservative measures.[1,6,29,30]

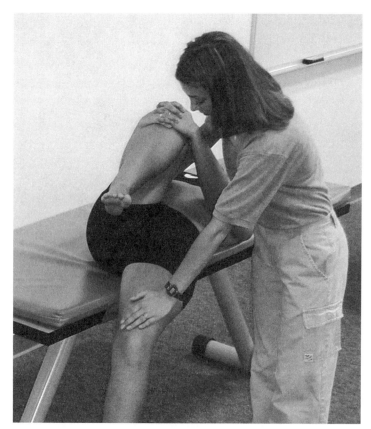

FIGURE 10.26 Gaenslen's test for sacroiliac joint dysfunction.
From Starkey and Ryan: *Evaluation of Orthopedic and Athletic Injuries*, 2nd ed. 2002.
Philadelphia: F.A. Davis Company, Box 10-20, pg 364, with permission.

Conditions of the Lumbar Spine

In general, patients identified as having low back problems are those who experience pain between the lower ribs and the proximal thighs. Recall, however, that this area also includes the SIJs and that pain that occurs below the level of L5 is most likely due to pathology of these joints versus pathology of the lumbar region. This means that, in some instances, lumbar spine and SIJ pathology often occur together. Keep this in mind as the conditions of the lumbar spine are discussed.

General Low Back Pain

General low back pain is a very common complaint in the United States. In any given year, approximately 50% of adults in this country report experiencing at least one episode of moderate to severe pain in this region. Indeed, this is one of the most common reasons patients visit their primary health care provider. It is also the leading cause of disability in those younger than 45 years.[8,33]

History and Physical Examination

In most instances, patients with general low back problems report an idiopathic onset of pain, and 70% of these people report pain that is nonspecific in nature. Most present with decreased lumbar spine motion that may or may not be associated with spasm of the erector spinae muscle group. These patients also have trouble standing, sitting, or lying in any one position for an extended period. Typically, the double straight leg test causes pain after 70° of hip flexion is achieved, though this test may be positive throughout the entire range if the SIJ is also injured. Ultimately, a diagnosis of general low back pain is made as long as the patient does not present with any of the "red flag" indicators listed in Box 10.2. Typically, a patient's low back pain can be attributed to a more serious cause if any of these indicators are present. In these situations, further investigation as to the cause of the patient's pain is warranted.[33,34]

Management

In the absence of "red flag" indicators, treat patients with general low back pain conservatively with the interventions outlined in Box 10.3. Fortunately, most patients recover in 4 to 6 weeks, though at times the person's pain may persist for up to 3 months. Indeed, 90% of these patients improve within a month.[8,33–35]

Intervertebral Disk Herniation

Of the "red flag" indicators, neurological deficits of the lower extremity associated with low back pain are commonly seen in the physically active population. These deficits are usually associated with some form of injury to the lumbosacral nerve roots and/or nerves in the region. Pinpointing the exact cause of nerve root or nerve involvement can be extremely challenging for even the most seasoned health care provider. Indeed, this leads many practitioners to assign a nonspecific diagnosis, such as **radiculopathy** or **sciatica**, to patients with low back pain. Though many things can irritate a nerve root or cause sciatica, a **herniated intervertebral lumbar disk**, otherwise referred to as a *herniated disk*, is one of the most common.[33,35,36]

BOX 10.2
RED FLAGS FOR POTENTIAL SERIOUS CONDITIONS FOR PATIENTS REPORTING WITH LOW BACK PAIN

Acute trauma	Recent bacterial infection
Age (over 50 or under 20)	Intravenous drug use
Fever	Immune suppression
Chills	Lower extremity neurological deficit
Unexplained weight loss	• weakness
Unexplained pain	• paresthesia
• when supine	• radiating pain
• at night	Chronic use of corticosteroids
Bladder dysfunction	

Adapted from U.S. Department of Health and Human Services. Acute low back problems in adults: assessment and treatment. *J Am Acad Nurse Pract* 1995;7(6):287; Harvard Medical School. Low back pain: causes, symptoms, and diagnosis. *Harv Mens Health Watch* 2006;11(4):1; Kinkade S. Evaluation and treatment of acute low back pain. *Am Fam Physician* 2007;75:1181.

BOX 10.3

INITIAL TREATMENT PARAMETERS FOR PATIENTS WITH GENERALIZED LOW BACK PAIN

Advise the patient to avoid prolonged bed rest.

Modify the patient's activity, but instruct the patient to stay as active as the pain allows.

Use acetaminophen to manage pain.

Avoid prescribing muscle relaxants and oral steroids, because neither has been shown to be effective and both have significant side effects.

Refrain from ordering x-rays, MRIs, or other imaging techniques, because these provide little, if any, feedback in the early stages of low back pain.

Adapted from U.S. Department of Health and Human Services. Acute low back problems in adults: assessment and treatment. *J Am Acad Nurse Pract* 1995;7(6):287; Harvard Medical School. Low back pain: causes, symptoms, and diagnosis. *Harv Mens Health Watch* 2006;11(4):1; Kinkade S. Evaluation and treatment of acute low back pain. *Am Fam Physician* 2007;75:1181.

Radiculopathy and *sciatica* are terms often used to describe any neurological condition of the low back that causes pain to radiate to the lower extremities.

A herniated disk occurs when the nucleus pulposus portion of the disk protrudes through the annulus fibrosis (Fig. 10.27). Commonly called a *slipped disk*, most herniations occur posterolaterally, meaning that they protrude directly into the intervertebral space. Recall that it is within this space that the nerve roots exit the spinal cord. More than 90% of lumbar disk herniations occur at the levels of L4/L5 and L5/S1, and most occur in people between the ages of 20 and 50 years.[8,33,34,37]

PEARL

Most disks herniate posterolateral into the intervertebral space, increasing the chance that they will impinge on a nerve root.

History and Physical Examination

All patients with an acute herniation of a lumbar disk report general back pain, and 95% of them also present with sciatica. Indeed, the presence of pain that follows the path of the sciatic nerve is a telltale sign of a disk herniation. This makes it extremely difficult to clinically diagnose a disk herniation in those who do not present with sciatica. When sciatica is present, patients typically relate feeling a sharp or burning sensation in the buttocks that travels down the posterolateral aspect of the thigh, continuing distal to the knee. The most commonly affected areas are the dorsal and lateral aspects of the foot, because these are the body regions supplied by the nerve roots arising from L4/L5 and L5/S1. In some instances, the pain patients experience in the leg is so severe that it often overshadows the pain they experience in the back. This pain may or may not be associated with paresthesia and/or muscle weakness in the affected areas. If the motor aspect of the L4/L5 nerve root is affected, MMT reveals weakness when the patient dorsiflexes the ankle and extends the great toe (Fig. 10.27), whereas ankle plantar flexion and toe flexion are weak in patients with pathology at the L5/S1 nerve root level.

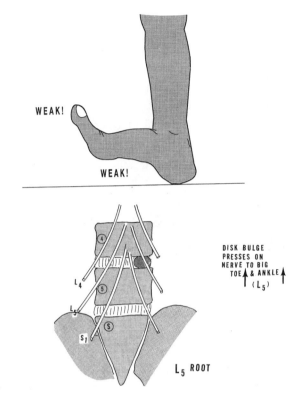

FIGURE 10.27 A herniated L4/L5 lumbar disk. From Cailliet: *Soft Tissue Pain and Disability*, 3rd ed. 1996. Philadelphia: F.A. Davis Company, Fig. 12-47, pg 423, with permission.

The patient's calcaneal reflex may be diminished if the L5/S1 nerve root is involved. Confirm the presence of a pressure on these nerve roots by performing the **straight leg test.**[8,33,34,37,38] To perform this test (Fig. 10.28):

- Instruct the patient to lie supine.
- Passively raise the involved lower extremity, with the knee extended to between 30° and 70° of hip flexion, because this is when tension on the nerve roots begins to occur.
- Reproduction of sciatic pain distal to the knee with this maneuver is positive for a herniated disk.

Next, perform the straight leg test on the contralateral side. Known as the **cross straight leg test**, pain on the involved side with this test is also indicative of a herniated disk.[8,32,37,38]

Management

Order an MRI for those with a suspected herniated disk, because this is the most sensitive test to detect this condition. After the presence of a herniated disk has been confirmed, deciding on how to properly manage this condition can be difficult because controversy surrounding operative, versus conservative, treatment protocols exist. Most experts believe, however, that as long as motor involvement is not affected, the prognosis for patients with a lumbar disk herniation is favorable when the condition is treated conservatively.[36,38]

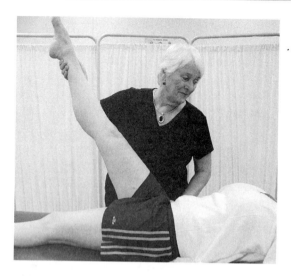

FIGURE 10.28 Straight leg test for lumbar disk herniation.

(PEARL)

As long as motor involvement is not affected, treat patients with a herniated lumbar disk conservatively.

Initially advise these patients to participate in low-level aerobic activities, such as walking, because herniations of this type respond well to low-intensity exercise activities. Instruct the patient to perform lumbar extension exercises as outlined in PTH 10.1. These exercises relieve nerve root tension and decrease the compressive forces the disk places on the affected nerve root(s). If the conservative approach is successful, most people experience a decrease in symptoms in 4 to 6 weeks. Refer for immediate neurological consultation those patients who do not respond to conservative treatment and those who experience progressive neurological deficits, bilateral sciatica, or weakness of any muscles of the lower extremity. Surgical intervention includes a partial discectomy and, if needed, partial laminectomy.[8,33,38]

Spondylolysis and Spondylolisthesis

Spondylolysis is a defect that occurs in the pars interarticularis of a vertebra (Fig. 10.29). Though this condition can happen anywhere along the lumbar spine, the fourth and fifth lumbar vertebrae are most affected. Spondylolysis can be either unilateral or bilateral and results from repetitive hyperextension loading of the lumbar spine, ultimately leading to a stress fracture–type injury. If left undetected, spondylolysis can develop into **spondylolisthesis** (Fig. 10.29). This condition can also result from degeneration due to overuse. Commonly seen in children and adolescents, spondylolysis and spondylolisthesis occur more in young athletes than in the general population. Because they must constantly hyperextend the lumbar spine during activity, offensive linemen in football, female gymnasts, and dancers are particularly vulnerable to development of either of these conditions.[39,40]

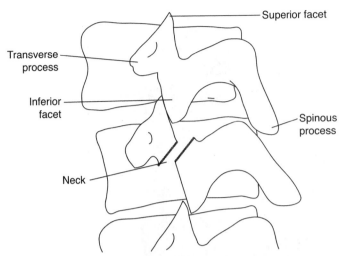

FIGURE 10.29 Spondylolysis and spondylolisthesis. In spondylolysis, the "neck," or pars interarticularis, of the "scotty dog" is fractured, with no slippage of the pars interarticularis. In spondylolisthesis, a forward slippage of the pars interarticularis occurs, leading to a "decapitation" of the neck of the scotty dog (shown in figure).
Adapted from Starkey and Ryan: *Evaluation of Orthopedic and Athletic Injuries,* 2nd ed. 2002. Philadelphia: F.A. Davis Company, Fig. 10-28, pg 359, with permission.

History and Physical Examination

Patients with spondylolysis or spondylolisthesis initially report low back pain that increases when the lumbar spine is hyperextended. Though this pain initially subsides when activity is ended, it eventually occurs with ADLs and at rest. The patient's pain may radiate to one or both lower extremities following the path of the sciatic nerve. Indeed, the presence of sciatica indicates that the patient may have either of these conditions.[35,39]

Patients with spondylolysis or spondylolisthesis present with marked hyperlordosis. These patients also maintain limited lumbar spine ROM in all directions, and tight hamstrings prevent them from being able to touch their toes. A palpable **step-off deformity**, where the spinous process of the affected vertebrae cannot be palpated because of its forward slippage, is clearly evident in cases of spondylolisthesis. Confirm the presence of either of these conditions by performing the stork test.[39,41] To perform this test (Fig. 10.30):

- Stand behind the patient.
- Tell the patient to place his or her hands on the hips.
- Instruct the patient to lift one leg by flexing the knee and hip.
- Have the patient arch his or her back into hyperextension. Make sure the patient does not fall.
- Repeat the test with the patient standing on the opposite leg.
- Pain in the lumbar spine area is indicative of spondylolysis or spondylolisthesis.

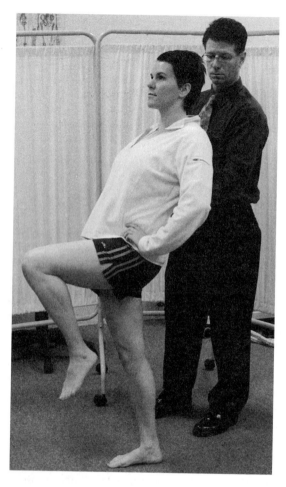

FIGURE 10.30 The stork test for spondylolysis and spondylolisthesis.

Management

Obtain AP, lateral, and bilateral oblique radiographic views for patients with lumbar pain caused by hyperextension activities, particularly in instances in which the pain has lasted for more than 3 weeks. When spondylolysis is present, the appearance on the oblique view reveals the classic "neck of the scotty dog" fracture (Fig. 10.29). That is, the pars interarticularis, the portion of the vertebra that makes up the neck of a scotty dog whose body shape is formed by the bony landmarks in the region, is fractured. If spondylolisthesis is present, the scotty dog appears decapitated, owing to the forward slippage of one vertebra on another.[41]

Refer all patients with suspected and confirmed cases of either spondylolysis or spondylolisthesis to an orthopedist. Treatment consists of relative rest, analgesics, and, if the condition is bad enough, bracing for up to a year. The patient's long-term prognosis is favorable if spondylolysis is detected early and treated properly. Those with spondylolisthesis have a greater chance of having prolonged disability. The ability of the patient to be physically active is usually self-limiting. That is, many with these conditions participate regularly in sports within pain limits.[39]

Lifespan Considerations

Evaluating disorders of the hip, pelvis, and sacral and lumbar spines is not always a straightforward process. Specific pathologies can masquerade as other injuries, making proper diagnosis and timely management critical. This section reviews those conditions that should always be considered when assessing injury to these regions. Note that most of these involve the hip, and because this joint plays an important role in weight-bearing, these conditions can be very debilitating. Also, though some of these conditions are more prevalent in certain populations, such as adolescents or the elderly, realize they all occur across the life span. In general, it is common for many of the patients presenting with one of these hip conditions to have an LLD, and the hip scoring test is almost always positive. Obtain x-rays, and refer all patients suspected of having any of these conditions to an orthopedist.

Hip Degeneration (Osteoarthritis)

Osteoarthritis of the hip, the most common hip disorder seen within the general population, affects both men and women equally as they age. Indeed, those over the age of 50 are most likely to have this condition. Other factors that contribute to its development include repetitive stresses placed on the hip, obesity, and a history of previous hip injury. When it occurs in the younger population, it most often results from acute trauma. Regardless of cause, over time the arthritic hip becomes irregular in shape, and its surrounding musculature becomes weak and inflexible.[6,42]

PEARL

Because of the weight-bearing role it plays, osteoarthritis in the hip
can be very debilitating.

Consider a diagnosis of hip osteoarthritis for those older than 50 years who report an insidious onset of hip pain with activity and for younger people who report persistent hip discomfort after a traumatic event. Conservative treatment includes modifying the patient's activity by advising him or her to avoid those things that increase pain and by prescribing oral anti-inflammatory medication. These steps usually keep the patient's symptoms under control. For those who desire to maintain or increase fitness levels, suggest that they participate in low-impact activities, such as aquatic exercise, cycling, and walking, because these do not place undue stress on the hip. Use PTHs 3.1 and 3.2 as a guide to instruct proper warm-up and strengthening techniques. Provide nutrition and weight control information, as described in Chapters 3 and 4, to patients who are overweight or obese.[42,43]

Avascular Necrosis

By definition, avascular necrosis is death of bone tissue due to decreased or total loss of blood supply. Especially common in the hip, its occurrence is linked to many different things, including anabolic steroid use, corticosteroid use, vascular disruption, and alcoholism. Some people are congenitally predisposed to development of some forms of hip necrosis, as in the case of Legg-Calvé-Perthes disease (discussed later in this chapter), whereas in others necrotic hip develops as the result of repetitive trauma. Still others experience an idiopathic onset of this condition. In general, the incidence of hip necrosis typically occurs in males between the ages of 30 and 70 years and often in conjunction with osteoarthritis.[6,44,45]

Initially, people with a necrotic hip may be asymptomatic. However, as the disease progresses, the person experiences unexpected hip or groin pain that occurs during weight-bearing and subsides with rest. Eventually, the person's gait pattern changes and the patient reports constant pain, ultimately diminishing the function of the joint. It is at this time that patients usually seek medical attention. A decision between conservative and surgical management depends on the underlying cause of the necrosis, the stage of the disease, the age of the individual, and the reported symptoms. Detecting this debilitating disease early increases the chance that the patient will experience a positive outcome.[6,44]

PEARL

When treating a patient with a necrotic hip, early detection is the key
to increasing the likelihood that the patient will experience
a positive outcome.

Legg-Calvé-Perthes Disease

Congenital avascular necrosis of the femoral neck, otherwise known as *Legg-Calvé-Perthes disease*, most typically occurs in males between the ages of 2 and 12 years. Idiopathic in nature, it results when the head of the patient's femur, in an attempt carry through with the normal process of replacing dead tissue with normal, healthy bone cells, is unable to do so. It is believed that the area's naturally poor blood supply contributes to its development. Nevertheless, the degenerative changes associated with its development may have implications well into the patient's adult years.[7]

People with Legg-Calvé-Perthes disease report an insidious onset of a limp, which may or may not be painful. Indeed, in most instances, the child's parent or guardian seeks medical advice only after noticing that the child walks or runs with a limp. If present, pain is nonspecific and mild, refers to the knee, and increases with physical activity. In some cases, the presence of pain is associated with stiffness and decreased hip strength, ultimately limiting the child's mobility. Telltale signs of Legg-Calvé-Perthes disease include decreased active abduction and internal rotation of the hip. Because there are four phases associated with its degeneration/regeneration process, treatment of this condition is patient specific, depending on the stage of disease and the severity of the patient's pain and disability. Though management choices include both conservative and surgical options, the process of bone regeneration can last many years.[7,5,46]

Slipped Capital Femoral Epiphysis

The slipped capital femoral epiphysis is one of the most common hip pathologies in the adolescent population. This condition occurs when the growth plate slips posteriorly in relation to the femoral head (remember that the epiphysis is the area of growth near the end of the bone). Though a slipped capital femoral epiphysis can occur acutely, most of the time its cause is insidious. Overweight African American males between the ages of 10 and 15 years are most at risk for development of this condition. It almost always presents itself during an adolescent growth spurt. In most instances, chronic inflammation and nutritional deficiencies contribute to its development. Early diagnosis of this condition helps prevent the development of short-term complications such as avascular necrosis of the femoral head and longer-term problems such as osteoarthritis.[7,47]

PEARL

A slipped capital femoral epiphysis often occurs insidiously in overweight individuals during an adolescent growth spurt.

The patient with a slipped capital femoral epiphysis reports an insidious onset of chronic medial thigh or knee pain with or without associated hip pain. Because hip pain may not occur with this condition, it is common for the primary care provider to misdiagnose the problem. Patients may or may not tolerate weight-bearing and typically walk with the affected leg in an externally rotated position as compared with the uninvolved side. Passive internal rotation of the hip causes discomfort, and the hip externally rotates during passive flexion. Additionally, the affected hip abductors are weak, making the Trendelenburg sign positive. Symptoms usually manifest and increase in severity over the course of months, meaning the condition progressively worsens. Treatment depends on the severity of the condition and ranges from conservative to surgical intervention.[7,47]

Apophyseal Avulsion Fractures

Recall that apophyseal avulsion fractures commonly occur at sites where soft tissues, such as muscles, attach to bone. In the pelvis, the bony areas typically affected, and the muscles attached to these sites, include the AIIS (rectus femoris), ischial tuberosity (hamstrings), ASIS (sartorius), and pubis (hip adductors). In these regions, this injury usually results from a sudden, eccentric type force applied to the lower extremity. It also results less frequently from incidences of repetitive overuse or microtrauma. However, these cases are less obvious to identify because symptoms are often similar to those of a muscle strain or tendonitis. Those aged 14 to 17 years who are physically active are at greatest risk of incurring this type injury.[5–7]

Patients with an apophyseal avulsion fracture usually report a sharp pain in the area of the avulsion, leading to a functional loss of the affected muscles. The most common clinical signs that an avulsion has occurred include swelling and point tenderness over the affected area and increased pain with passive stretching of the involved muscle(s). Most heal well through conservative management by modifying activity until the injury mends.[5,7,48]

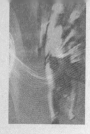

CASE STUDY
Conditions Involving the Hip, Pelvis, and Sacral and Lumbar Spines

SCENARIO

A 14-year-old male cross-country runner reports to your office after approximately 3 weeks of anterior hip pain. Since the beginning of the cross-country season, he reports a gradual onset of pain during, and more recently after, running. He admits that he had not trained during the off-season, and since practice started 4 weeks ago, his training volume and intensity have been higher than what he was accustomed to. Until the past week, the athlete has been able to continue his training regimen through regular stretching and cryotherapy. About 5 days ago, however, he reports feeling a more vigorous pain in the area after a speed workout. He now walks with a slight limp and is unable to continue to run.

PERTINENT HISTORY

Medications: None.

Family History: No pertinent history noted.

PERSONAL HEALTH HISTORY

Tobacco Use: Denies smoking cigarettes or using oral tobacco products.

Recreational Drugs: Denies drug use.

Alcohol Intake: Denies alcohol use.

Caffeinated Beverages: Reports drinking various caffeinated beverages (cola, coffee, etc.) before practice.

Exercise: In addition to running cross-country, the patient participates in physical education class during school.

Past Medical History: No pertinent past medical history.

PERTINENT PHYSICAL EXAMINATION*

Mild swelling over the ASIS, but no bruising or obvious deformity noted. Point tender over the ASIS, with diffuse tenderness into the groin. Decreased active and passive hip extension, abduction, and external rotation ROM on the involved side, along with acute pain at the ASIS with seated hip flexion and external rotation strength tests. Positive Thomas test on involved side. Decreased apparent leg length on the involved side. No neurological motor or sensory deficit.

*Focused examination limited to key points for this case.

RED FLAGS FOR THE PRIMARY HEALTH CARE PROFESSIONAL TO CONSIDER

- Adolescent age of the patient may lead you to consider injury to the growth plate (apophysitis or apophyseal avulsion fracture).
- Insidious onset may indicate a chronic condition.
- Marked increase in training volume and intensity will also lead to chronic overuse injuries.
- Decreased ROM, decreased strength, and pain over the ASIS indicated injury to the attachment of the sartorius tendon or the apophysis.

RECOMMENDED PLAN

- Refer for radiographic analysis and orthopedic evaluation to rule out apophyseal avulsion fracture.
- Do not allow the athlete to return to athletics until the results of the radiographic analysis and strength and ROM are normal.
- Prescribe acetaminophen to assist in decreasing pain.
- Continue with cryotherapy, but discontinue stretching until the results of the radiographic analysis are obtained.

REFERENCES

1. Brolinson PG, Kozar AJ. Sacroiliac joint dysfunction in athletes. *Curr Sports Med Rep* 2003;2:47.
2. Safran MR. Evaluation of the hip: history, physical examination, and imaging. *Oper Tech Sports Med* 2005;13:2.
3. Chen YC, Fredericson M, Smuck M. Sacroiliac joint pain syndrome in active patients. *Phys Sportsmed* 2002;30(11):30.
4. Shindle MK, Ranawat AS, Kelly BT. Diagnosis and management of traumatic and atraumatic hip instability in the athletic patient. *Clin Sports Med* 2006;25:309.
5. Weiss JM, Ramachandran M. Hip and pelvic injuries in the young athlete. *Oper Tech Sports Med* 2006:14:212.
6. Prather H. Pelvis and sacral dysfunction in sports and exercise. *Phys Med Rehabil Clin N Am* 2000;11:805.
7. Kocher MS, Tucker R. Pediatric athlete hip disorders. *Clin Sports Med* 2006;25:241.
8. U.S. Department of Health and Human Services. Acute low back problems in adults: assessment and treatment. *J Am Acad Nurse Pract* 1995;7(6):287.
9. Braly BA, Beall DP, Martin HD. Clinical examination of the athletic hip. *Clin Sports Med* 2006;25:199.
10. Pearsall MAW. Assessing acute hip injury. *Phys Sportsmed* 1995;23(6):36.
11. Van Dillen LR, McDonnell MK, Fleming DA, et al. Effect of knee and hip position on hip extension range of motion in individuals with and without low back pain. *J Orthop Sports Phys Ther* 2000;30:307.
12. Schache AG, Blanch PD, Murphy AT. Relation of anterior pelvic tilt during running to clinical and kinematic measures of hip extension. *Br J Sports Med* 2000;34:279.
13. Harvey, D. Assessment of the flexibility of the elite athlete using the modified Thomas test. *Br J Sports Med* 1998;32:68.
14. Harris I, Hatfield A, Walton J. Assessing leg length discrepancy after femoral fracture: clinical examination or computed tomography? *ANZ J Surg* 2005;75:319.
15. Timgren J, Soinila S. Reversible pelvic asymmetry: an overlooked syndrome manifesting as scoliosis, apparent leg-length difference, and neurologic symptoms. *J Manipulative Physiol Ther* 2006;29:561.
16. Lyle MA, Manes S, McGuinness M, et al. Relationship of physical examination findings and self-reported symptom severity and physical function in patients with degenerative lumbar conditions. *Phys Ther* 2005:85:120.
17. McKinnis LN. *Fundamentals of Musculoskeletal Imaging*, 2nd ed. Philadelphia, PA: FA Davis Co., 2005.
18. Adkins SB, Figler RA. Hip pain in athletes. *Am Fam Physician* 2000;61:2109.
19. Blazina ME. The "hip-pointer," a term to describe a specific kind of athletic injury. *Calif Med* 1967;106:450.
20. Fairclough J, Hayashi K, Toumi H, et al. The functional anatomy of the iliotibial band during flexion and extension of the knee: implications for understanding iliotibial band syndrome. *J Anat* 2006;208:309.
21. Ekman EF, Pope T, Martin DF, et al. Magnetic resonance imaging of iliotibial band syndrome. *Am J Sports Med* 1994;22:851.
22. Noble CA. The treatment of iliotibial band friction syndrome. *Br J Sports Med* 1979;13:51.
23. Winston P, Awan R, Cassidy JD, et al. Clinical examination and ultrasound of self reported snapping hip syndrome in elite ballet dancers. *Am J Sports Med* 2007;35:118.
24. Allen WC, Cope R. Coxa saltans: the snapping hip revisited. *J Am Acad Orthop Surg* 1995;3:303.
25. Beals RK. Painful snapping hip in young adults. *West J Med* 1993;159:481.
26. Paluska SA. An overview of hip injuries in running. *Sports Med* 2005;35:991.
27. LeBlanc KE, LeBlanc KA. Groin pain in athletes. *Hernia* 2003;7:68.
28. Morelli V, Smith V. Groin injuries in athletes. *Am Fam Physician* 2001;64:1405.
29. Zelle BA, Gruen GS, Brown S, et al. Sacroiliac joint dysfunction. *Clin J Pain* 2005;21;446.
30. Cohen, SP. Sacroiliac joint pain: a comprehensive review of anatomy, diagnosis, and treatment. *Anesth Analg* 2005;101:1440.
31. Potter NA, Rothstein JM. Intertester reliability for selected clinical test of the sacroiliac joint. *Phys Ther* 1985:1671.

32. Kenna C, Murtagh J. Patrick or fabere test to test hip and sacroiliac joint disorders. *Aust Fam Physician* 1989;18:375.
33. Kinkade S. Evaluation and treatment of acute low back pain. *Am Fam Physician* 2007;75:1181.
34. Harvard Medical School. Low back pain: causes, symptoms, and diagnosis. *Harv Mens Health Watch* 2006;11(4):1.
35. Markova T, Dhillon BS, Martin SI. Treatment of acute sciatica. *Am Fam Physician* 2007;75:100.
36. Rhee JM, Schaufele M, Abdu W. Radiculopathy and the herniated lumbar disc. *J Bone Joint Surg Am* 2006;88:2070.
37. Deyo RA, Rainville J, Kent DL. What can the history and physical examination tell us about low back pain. *JAMA* 1992;268:760.
38. Lively MW, Bailes JE. Acute lumbar disk injuries in active patients: making optimal management decisions. *Phys Sportsmed* 2005;33(4):21.
39. Cassas KJ, Cassettari-Wayhs A. Childhood and adolescent sports-related overuse injuries. *Am Fam Physician* 2006;73:1014.
40. Congeni J, McCulloch J, Swanson K. Lumbar spondylolysis: a study of natural progression in athletes. *Am J Sports Med* 1997;25:248.
41. Solomaon R, Brown T, Gerbino PG, et al. The young dancer. *Clin Sports Med* 2000;19:717.
42. Manek NJ, Lane NE. Osteoarthritis: current concepts in diagnosis and management. *Am Fam Physician* 2000;61:1795.
43. Zimmy NJ. Clinical Reasoning in the evaluation and management of undiagnosed chronic hip pain in a young adult. *Phys Ther* 1998;78:62.
44. Aldridge JM III, Urbaniak JR. Avascular necrosis of the femoral head: etiology, pathophysiology, classification, and current treatment guidelines. *Am J Orthop* 2004;33:327.
45. Boettcher EG, Bonfiglio M, Hamilton HH, et al. Non-traumatic necrosis of the femoral head. *J Bone Joint Surg Am* 2007; 52A:312.
46. Stulberg SD, Cooperman DR, Wallensten R. The natural history of Legg-Calvé-Perthes disease. *J Bone Joint Surg Am* 1981;63:1095.
47. Johnson BC, Klabunde LA. The elusive slipped capital femoral epiphysis. *J Athl Train* 1995;30:124.
48. Rossi F, Dragoni S. Acute avulsion fractures of the pelvis in adolescent competitive athletes: prevalence, location and sports distribution of 203 cases collected. *Skeletal Radiol* 2001;30:127.

SUGGESTED READINGS

Hahne AJ, Ford JJ. Functional restoration for a chronic lumbar disk extrusion with associated radiculopathy. *Phys Ther* 2006;86:1168.
Moeller JL, Rifat SF. Spondylolysis in active athletes. *Phys Sportsmed* 2001;29(12):27.
Sponseller PD. Evaluating the child with back pain. *Am Fam Physician* 1996;54:1933.

WEB LINKS

http://www.nlm.nih.gov/medlineplus/hipinjuriesanddisorders.html. Accessed 8/4/08.
   Comprehensive Web site related to hip disorders. Outlines specific disorders, diagnosis, symptoms, rehabilitation, and recovery. Provides links to research and professional organizations.

http://www.spineuniverse.com/displayarticle.php/article1394.html. Accessed 8/4/08.
   Diagrams of lumbar spine, nerves, and blood supply. Provides links to low back pain, sciatica, and lumbar radiculopathy. Outlines protocols used to treat lumbar conditions.

http://orthoinfo.aaos.org/menus/spine.cfm. Accessed 8/4/08.
   Web site that provides an overview of common orthopedic conditions of the spine, including spondylolysis, spondylolisthesis, sciatica, and herniated disk.

Conditions Involving the Cervical Spine, Shoulder Complex, and Arm

● **Brian J. Toy, PhD, ATC**

The cervical spine, shoulder, and arm are highly interrelated structures, with injury to one affecting the others. Because these body parts work in unison, they are discussed here collectively, as evaluating one of these body parts necessitates that all three be assessed simultaneously.

Anatomy of the Cervical Spine, Shoulder Complex, and Arm

The anatomy of these regions is extremely complex. Pertinent anatomic tissues of the cervical region include bones, muscles, nerves, and the intervertebral disks, while bones, ligaments, capsules, muscles, tendons, and bursae are important structures of the shoulder complex and arm.

Bones and Joints

As previously discussed in Chapter 10 and shown in Figure 10.3 on page 270, the cervical spine consists of seven vertebrae that form a concave curve. These small vertebrae, in addition to protecting the spinal cord as it runs in the vertebral canal, help move and keep the head erect. The third through seventh cervical vertebrae consist of the same bony landmarks as most vertebrae (Fig. 10.4 on page 271) and maintain the same articulations (Fig. 10.3 on page 270) as the lumbar spine (see Chapter 10 to review this information). In contrast, the first cervical vertebrae, also referred to as the *atlas*, and the second cervical vertebrae, otherwise known as the *axis*, maintain many different bony landmarks. This arrangement allows these bones to articulate with one another at the atlantoaxial joint. The atlas also has processes that articulate with the skull's occipital bone, forming the atlanto-occipital joint.

Bones that compose the shoulder complex and arm include the humerus, scapula, clavicle, and sternum (Fig. 11.1). The humerus is the largest long bone of the upper extremity. Its proximal portion is composed of the humeral head and greater and lesser tubercles, both located anterolaterally. Between these tubercles is the longitudinal aligned bicipital groove, or *intertubercular sulcus*, which houses the long head of the biceps brachii tendon, simply known as the *long head of the biceps* (LHB), discussed in more detail later in this chapter. Adjacent to the humerus is the triangle-shaped scapula. While the axillary and vertebral borders of this bone form an inferior angle, its vertebral and superior borders form a superior angle. The shallow glenoid fossa, which articulates with the humeral head to form the glenohumeral joint (GHJ) (Fig. 11.2), is formed as the scapula's axillary and superior boarders meet. This fossa is lined by the glenoid labrum, a fibrocartilage that improves joint stability by increasing the fossa's depth. Medial to the glenoid fossa, and protruding anteriorly from the scapula's superior border, is the coracoid process.

PEARL

The GHJ is formed between the articulation of the humeral head and the glenoid fossa of the scapula.

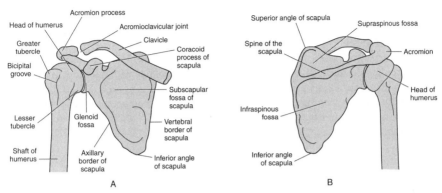

FIGURE II.I Bony anatomy of the shoulder complex. (A) Anterior view. (B) Posterior view. Adapted from McKinnis: *Fundamentals of Musculoskeletal Imaging*, 2nd ed. 2005. Philadelphia: F.A. Davis Company, Fig. 12-1, pg 412, with permission.

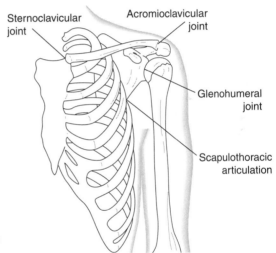

FIGURE II.2 The shoulder complex. From Lippert: *Clinical Kinesiology and Anatomy*, 4th ed. 2006. Philadelphia: F.A. Davis Company, Fig. 8-1, pg 94, with permission.

When viewed from the front, the majority of the scapula's anterior surface is composed of the subscapular fossa. It is this fossa and the subscapularis muscle located within it that articulate with the rib cage to form the scapulothoracic articulation (STA) (Fig. 11.2), commonly referred to as the *shoulder girdle*. Posteriorly, the spine of the scapula traverses laterally from the vertebral border and divides the scapula into supraspinous and infraspinous fossae. The spine ends as the anteriorly curved acromion process.

The clavicle is a long bone whose shaft is divided into proximal, middle, and distal thirds. Proximally, it articulates with the sternum to form the sternoclavicular joint (SCJ) (Fig. 11.2). As it traverses distally, it bends at the junction of the proximal and middle thirds, giving the bone an *S*-shaped appearance. Distally, the clavicle articulates with the acromion to form the acromioclavicular joint (ACJ) (Fig. 11.2). The clavicle is the only bony attachment the upper extremity has with the axial skeleton.

Though most people consider the GHJ to be the "shoulder joint" because it is this structure that performs the motions commonly associated with shoulder movement, the shoulder complex is a multifaceted structure composed of the GHJ, ACJ, SCJ, and STA. Though the soft tissues associated with these structures, such as ligaments, capsules, muscles, and tendons, help stabilize and protect the region from injury, in general the GHJ sacrifices strength for motion. This not only makes the GHJ the most freely moveable joint in the body, it also predisposes the entire shoulder complex to both overuse and acute injury.

PEARL

The GHJ, the most freely moveable joint in the body, sacrifices strength for motion, which predisposes the entire shoulder complex to both overuse and acute injury.

Motions

Like the lumbar spine, the cervical region acts like ball-and-socket joint because of the motions it produces (Fig. 11.3). Rotation is primarily produced by at the atlantoaxial joint, whereas the majority of flexion and extension occurs at the atlanto-occipital joint. The remaining amount of flexion, extension, and rotation and all of lateral flexion derive from a combination of the small amounts of movement occurring between each intervertebral joint (IVJ) and facet joint (FJ) of C3–C7. Average ranges of motion (ROMs) for each cervical movement are listed in Box 11.1.

Although three joints and one articulation compose the shoulder complex, only STA and GHJ motions can be seen and measured. However, the small motions performed by the SCJ and ACJ allow the STA and GHJ to work properly. Motions of the STA include scapular elevation; depression; abduction, or *protraction*; adduction, or

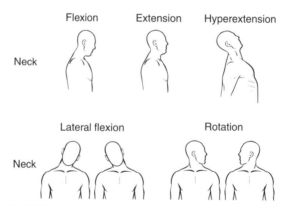

FIGURE 11.3 Motions of the cervical spine.
Adapted from Lippert: *Clinical Kinesiology and Anatomy*, 4th ed. 2006. Philadelphia: F.A. Davis Company, Fig. 14-2, pg 184, with permission.

BOX 11.1
ACTIVE RANGES OF MOTION OF THE CERVICAL SPINE

60° Flexion
75° Hyperextension
45° Lateral flexion (R and L)
80° Rotation (R and L)

as *retraction*; and upward and downward rotation (Fig. 11.4). The scapula can also "tilt," meaning the bone's superior border moves anteriorly and the inferior angle moves posteriorly. In general, scapular elevation, depression, protraction, and retraction can occur in isolation of GHJ motion, whereas the other STA motions only occur in combination with GHJ motion.

Classified as a ball-and-socket joint, motions of the GHJ are shown in Figure 11.5. Remember that, by definition, the action of extension brings the GHJ to anatomical position from a flexed position, with movement beyond this position classified as hyperextension. Also, recognize that internal and external GHJ rotation occurs in many planes. For example, these motions occur with the GHJ abducted, as shown in Figure 11.5; they can occur with the GHJ fully extended; and they can occur when the

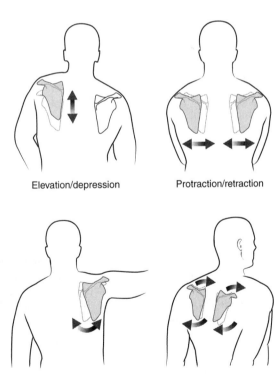

Elevation/depression

Protraction/retraction

Upward rotation/
downward rotation

Scapular tilt

FIGURE 11.4 Motions of the scapulothoracic articulation. From Lippert: *Clinical Kinesiology and Anatomy,* 4th ed. 2006. Philadelphia: F.A. Davis Company, Fig. 8-9, pg 97, with permission.

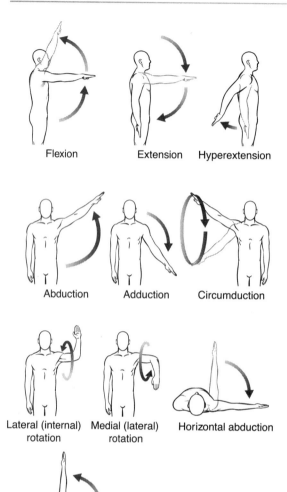

Flexion   Extension   Hyperextension

Abduction   Adduction   Circumduction

Lateral (internal)   Medial (lateral)   Horizontal abduction
rotation   rotation

Horizontal adduction

FIGURE 11.5 Motions of the glenohumeral joint. Adapted from Lippert: *Clinical Kinesiology and Anatomy*, 4th ed. 2006. Philadelphia: F.A. Davis Company, Fig. 9-2, pg 108, with permission.

GHJ is flexed. It cannot be emphasized enough that for the GHJ to experience full ROM in all planes, the STA must work properly. This is most true when the GHJ fully flexes or abducts, because as much as one-third of the total range allowed by these motions is attributed to the STA. Average ranges-of-motion (ROM) for each GHJ movement are listed in Box 11.2.

PEARL

For the GHJ to experience full **ROM** in all planes, the **STA** must work properly.

BOX 11.2
ACTIVE RANGES OF MOTION OF THE GLENOHUMERAL JOINT

180° Flexion
40° Hyperextension
180° Abduction
55° Internal rotation
45° External rotation
45° Horizontal abduction
90° Horizontal adduction

Ligaments, Bursae, Nerves, and Intervertebral Disk

As mentioned in Chapter 10, the spinal column maintains 31 pairs of spinal nerves, and these nerve roots exit the spinal column through individual intervertebral foramen (Fig. 10.3 on page 270). The nerve roots that form the sciatic nerve provide the majority of the lower extremity with its neurological function, whereas most of the entire upper extremity is supplied by the brachial plexus, formed by the C5–T1 nerve roots (Fig. 10.5 on page 271). Like the lumbar vertebrae, the bodies of the third through seventh cervical vertebrae are each separated by an intervertebral disk (Fig. 10.3 on page 270). See Chapter 10 to review this information.

Ligaments in the shoulder complex primarily support the ACJ, SCJ, and GHJ (Figs. 11.6 and 11.7). The ACJ is supported by the acromioclavicular ligament (ACL) and conoid and trapezoid portions of the coracoclavicular ligament (CCL). While the ACL supports the ACJ's capsule and holds the clavicle next to the acromion, the CCL attaches the coracoid to the clavicle and prevents superior displacement of the clavicle at the ACJ. The SCJ is supported by three ligaments: sternoclavicular (SCL), costoclavicular (CoCL), and interclavicular (ICL). Attaching the sternum to the clavicle, the SCL provides primary support for the SCJ's capsule and limits anterior and posterior motions of the clavicle's sternal end. The CoCL, which attaches the costal cartilage of the first rib and the rib itself to the clavicle, prevents superior displacement of the clavicle at the SCJ. The ICL connects the sternal portions of the right and left clavicles and limits inferior displacement of the clavicle's sternal end. The GHJ is supported anteriorly by glenohumeral ligaments (GHLs). These ligaments are thickened portions of the joint's capsule and attach the glenoid labrum to the humerus. These ligaments provide the GHJ with most of its anterior and inferior stability, though they do support the joint in all planes. Also attached directly to the joint's capsule, the coracohumeral ligament (CHL) reinforces the superior aspect of the GHJ as it travels from the coracoid to the humerus. This ligament combines with the GHLs to secure the LHB within the bicipital groove.

Though not directly responsible for GHJ stability, the coracoacromial ligament (CAL), which runs from the coracoid to the acromion, protects the humeral head from moving superiorly into the subacromial space, an area that houses the tendon of the supraspinatus muscle, the LHB, and the subacromial bursa. This bursa acts as a cushion between the tendon of the supraspinatus and the **coracoacromial arch** when the humerus is elevated (Fig. 11.8).

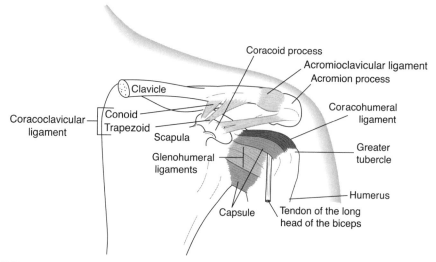

FIGURE 11.6 Ligaments of the glenohumeral and acromioclavicular joints.
Adapted from Lippert: *Clinical Kinesiology and Anatomy*, 4th ed. 2006. Philadelphia: F.A. Davis Company,
Fig. 9-5, pg 110 with permission.

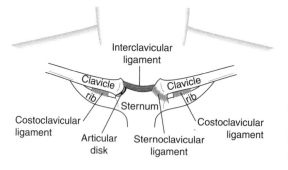

FIGURE 11.7 Ligaments of the sternoclavicular joint.
From Lippert: *Clinical Kinesiology and Anatomy*, 4th ed. 2006. Philadelphia: F.A. Davis Company, Fig. 8-6, pg 96 with permission.

(PEARL)

The subacromial space houses the tendon of the supraspinatus muscle, the long head of the biceps brachii tendon, and the subacromial bursa.

Muscles and Tendons

Posteriorly, the muscles that extend the neck are termed the *cervical erector spinae* (Fig. 10.12 on page 277). They are also responsible for keeping the head erect when standing and sitting. Anterior and lateral neck muscles are responsible for rotating and flexing the cervical spine.

Muscles of the shoulder complex include those that move the GHJ and those that act on the STA (Figs. 11.9, 11.10, and 11.11). The major muscles acting on the GHJ are divided into two groups: superficial and deep. Superficial muscles are those that

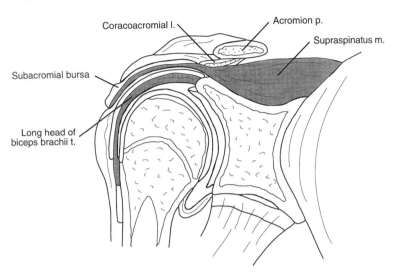

Coracoacromial l.

Acromion p.

Supraspinatus m.

Subacromial bursa

Long head of
biceps brachii t.

FIGURE 11.8 The coracoacromial arch and the structures of the subacromial space.
From Starkey and Ryan: *Evaluation of Orthopedic and Athletic Injuries,* 2nd ed. 2002. Philadelphia:
F.A. Davis Company, Fig. 13-35, pg 470, with permission.

can be easily palpated and include the pectoralis major, deltoid, latissimus dorsi, and teres major. The pectoralis major, or *chest muscle*, encompasses most of the anterior chest wall and forms the anterior axillary fold. Composed of anterior, middle, and posterior portions, the triangle-shaped deltoid, or shoulder muscle, gives the GHJ its rounded appearance. The latissimus dorsi and teres major form the posterior axillary fold. Deep muscles include the supraspinatus, infraspinatus, teres minor, and subscapularis. The supraspinatus, infraspinatus, and subscapularis each arise from their corresponding fossa on the scapula, whereas the teres minor originates just below the infraspinatus. From anterior to posterior, the supraspinatus, infraspinatus, and teres minor insert on the greater tubercle, while the subscapularis inserts on the lesser tubercle. Otherwise known as the *SITS* (supraspinatus, infraspinatus, teres minor, and subscapularis) muscles in recognition of where they attach on the humerus, this **rotator cuff** muscle group functions to hold the head of the humerus in the glenoid fossa, providing the GHJ with much of its stability. Stabilizing the humeral head in this fashion also helps prevent the head from migrating superiorly into the subacromial space. Remember that the tendon of the supraspinatus is the only rotator cuff muscle tendon to pass through this space. Table 11.1 lists the primary actions the major muscles of the shoulder have on the GHJ.

PEARL

The primary function of the rotator cuff muscle group is to hold the
head of the humerus in the glenoid fossa.

Though usually thought of as the muscles that flex and extend the elbow, the biceps brachii, located on the anterior portion of the arm, and the triceps brachii,

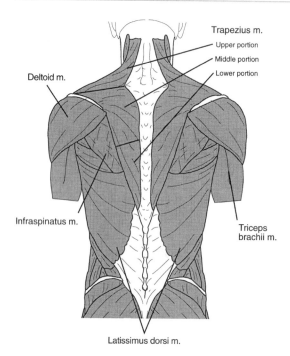

FIGURE 11.9 Posterior muscles acting on the shoulder complex. From Starkey and Ryan: *Evaluation of Orthopedic and Athletic Injuries*, 2nd ed. 2002. Philadelphia: F.A. Davis Company, Fig. 13–13, pg 432, with permission.

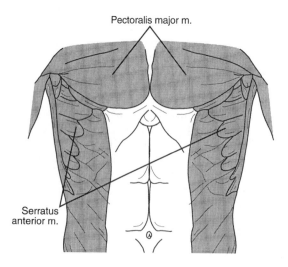

FIGURE 11.10 Pectoralis and serratus anterior muscles. From Starkey and Ryan: *Evaluation of Orthopedic and Athletic Injuries*, 2nd ed. 2002. Philadelphia: F.A. Davis Company, Fig. 13-16, pg 433, with permission.

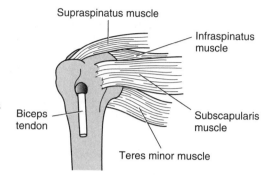

FIGURE 11.11 Rotator cuff muscles with a view of the long head of the biceps tendon.
From McKinnis: *Fundamentals of Musculoskeletal Imaging*, 2nd ed. 2005. Philadelphia: F.A. Davis Company, Fig. 12-2A, pg 412, with permission.

TABLE 11.1 Primary actions of the major muscles that move the glenohumeral joint

MUSCLE	PRIMARY ACTIONS
Pectoralis major	Flexion, horizontal adduction
Deltoid	
• Anterior third	Flexion, horizontal adduction
• Middle third	Abduction
• Posterior third	Extension, horizontal abduction
Latissimus dorsi	Extension, adduction, internal rotation
Teres major	Extension, adduction, internal rotation
Supraspinatus	Abduction
Infraspinatus	External rotation
Teres minor	External rotation
Subscapularis	Internal rotation
Biceps brachii	Flexion
Triceps brachii	Extension

located on the arm's posterior portion, flex and extend the shoulder, respectively. Remember that the LHB is held in the bicipital groove by the CHL and GHLs. Proximally, this tendon attaches to the glenoid rim and the superior portion of the glenoid labrum, exposing it to injury when the labrum is traumatized.

The primary movers of the STA include the trapezius, pectoralis minor, rhomboid major and minor, levator scapulae, and serratus anterior. Only the trapezius and serratus anterior can be easily palpated, because the levator scapulae and rhomboid muscles lie deep to the trapezius and the pectoralis minor lies deep to the pectoralis major. These muscles serve the shoulder complex in a variety of ways. First, they produce the movements of scapula elevation, depression, protraction, and retraction with or without GHJ motion (Table 11.2). Second, by moving the STA, they facilitate GHJ motion. For example, for the GHJ to reach full abduction, the scapula must rotate upward. Finally, during certain motions, these muscles stabilize the scapula by holding it to the chest wall, allowing certain GHJ motions to occur unimpeded.

Examination of the Cervical Spine, Shoulder Complex, and Arm

It should be apparent that understanding how the cervical spine and shoulder complex work is complicated, making evaluation of these areas extremely challenging.

TABLE 11.2 Primary actions of the major muscles that move the scapulothoracic articulation

MUSCLE	PRIMARY ACTIONS
Trapezius	
• Upper portion	Elevation
• Middle portion	Retraction
• Lower portion	Depression
Rhomboid major	Retraction, elevation
Rhomboid minor	Retraction, elevation
Levator scapulae	Elevation, downward rotation
Serratus anterior	Protraction, upward rotation
Pectoralis minor	Protraction, anterior tilt

Systematically approaching this process by combining the information presented here with what is offered in Chapter 7 ensures that all essential aspects of the evaluation are covered.

History

As with any musculoskeletal assessment, a comprehensive examination begins with a thorough review of how the injury occurred. Indeed, a thorough history reveals the cause of shoulder pain in most patients and also provides the basis for establishing a diagnosis of cervical injury. Promptly assess the patient's chief concerns, which usually include pain, instability, stiffness, locking, catching, and swelling for shoulder pathology and pain, numbness, and weakness for cervical spine injury. Though not a usual sign, the patient may also have deformity, which is mostly associated with injury of the ACJ, clavicle, and SCJ.[1–3]

After the patient's chief concerns are determined, ask whether the injury occurred as the result of a macrotrauma event or from overuse. In the case of shoulder injury, if the patient describes an acute mechanism of injury (MOI), he or she usually states, "I hurt my shoulder." In these instances, ask the patient to reproduce the MOI using the uninjured extremity for demonstration purposes. Most frequently, the patient places his or her upper extremity in front of, to the side of, or behind the body and states, "I got hurt when I placed my arm out to break my fall" or "I fell on my outstretched arm," as shown in Figure 11.12. This exposes the entire upper extremity to injury, because the force produced by this MOI is transmitted from the hand to the wrist, forearm, elbow, and arm, ultimately reaching the shoulder complex. Another common response to the question "How did you injure your shoulder?" is "My arm got pushed back while it was in the air." That is, with the person's GHJ abducted, the joint was forced into extreme external rotation. This MOI places intense pressure on the soft tissues supporting the anterior aspect of the GHJ and is the primary reason this joint becomes unstable after acute injury. "I fell [or got hit] on the tip [or top] of my shoulder" is a third common way a patient describes how he or she acutely injured this region. This mechanism places the ACJ at risk and usually occurs when a patient performs a forward roll in response to falling from a great height, such as what happens when a person falls from a horse.[1,2,4]

PEARL

Falling on the "outstretched arm" is the most common way to acutely injure the shoulder complex.

Though patients presenting with an acute cervical spine condition often reveal injury mechanisms similar to those that cause a traumatic shoulder injury, people with an acute cervical injury also report neck involvement at the time of injury. Thus, when a patient presents with neck or shoulder pain, always ask what position the head and neck were in at the time of injury. Common cervical spine injury mechanisms include compression, which forces the vertebrae to collapse on one another, such as what happens when a football player makes helmet-to-helmet contact with another player and forced neck rotation combined with lateral flexion.[3]

If a patient presents with a case of shoulder pathology due to overuse, he or she usually states "My shoulder hurts" without being able to identify a traumatic episode

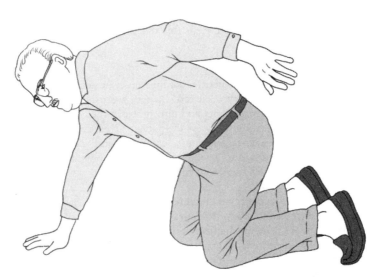

FIGURE 11.12 When a person falls on the "outstretched arm," the force entering the body is transmitted through the upper extremity as follows: (1) hyperextended wrist, (2) forearm, (3) extended elbow, (4) arm, (5) glenohumeral joint, (6) acromioclavicular joint, (6) clavicle, and (7) sternoclavicular joint.
From Levangie and Norkin: *Joint Structure and Function: A Comprehensive Analysis*, 4th ed. 2005. Philadelphia: F.A. Davis Company, Fig. 7-10, pg 239, with permission.

responsible for the pain. Other symptoms include weakness, stiffness, locking, and catching. In these instances, inquire what activities the patient was doing the days and weeks immediately preceding the onset of symptoms. Usually, patients report performing repetitive activities with the upper extremity above the head. For example, a baseball pitcher may report that he has been doing a lot of throwing in preparation for the upcoming season, whereas the tennis player may report that she has been practicing her serves. This MOI, known as performing overhead activities above the 90° plane, is the most common way overuse injury occurs in the soft tissues of the shoulder complex.[1,2,4]

(P E A R L)

Performing activities above the 90° plane is the most common way overuse injury occurs in the soft tissues of the shoulder complex.

Patients with a chronic neck condition usually present with an insidious onset of neck and arm pain that can be either diffuse or concentrated. If a nerve root is involved, this pain often radiates beyond the level of the elbow, a rare occurrence if the patient's pain originates from the shoulder. Indeed, determining whether pain radiates beyond the level of the elbow is a key way to differentiate between shoulder and cervical pathology. Chronic neck pain in older patients is usually related to a previous neck injury or a long history of generalized neck pain.[1,3]

⟮PEARL⟯

The pain associated with a shoulder injury rarely radiates beyond the level of the elbow, whereas radiating pain into the forearm, wrist, and hand is indicative of cervical spine pathology.

Physical Examination

Begin the physical examination with observation and palpation, followed by ROM and strength testing. Complete the examination by applying stress and special tests designed to evaluate the neck and shoulder complex and by performing a neurological assessment of the upper extremity.

Observation

While completing the history portion of the examination, observe the patient's head and neck posture, because people with cervical spine pathology typically hold the neck stiffly and laterally flex the neck away from the side of injury. In contrast, patients with an acutely injured shoulder usually support the involved extremity in the sling position, as shown in Figure 6.1 on page 129. Ask the patient to remove his or her shirt, because patients with functional deficits and patients with pain during shoulder movement have trouble disrobing. With the patient standing, obtain posterior, lateral, and anterior views of the neck and shoulder complex. Assess for deformity, muscle atrophy, and asymmetry between the involved and uninvolved sides. Note that the dominant shoulder naturally rides lower than the nondominant, a fact that is extenuated when the shoulder is viewed posteriorly and when the patient grasps a heavy object with the dominant hand. Bilaterally compare the status of the patient's ACJs, clavicles, and SCJs. Because these bony landmarks are very superficial, abnormalities are easily identified by noted deformity of the injured structure. Check the area of the deltoid muscle for the normally rounded appearance associated with an intact GHJ. A flattened looking deltoid is indicative of GHJ pathology.[1,3]

Next, compare the positions of the patient's right and left scapulae. The spine of each scapula should be level with the third thoracic vertebrae, and all borders and angles should ride flat against the posterior chest wall. Determine whether **Sprengel's deformity** is present, because this is the most common congenital abnormality affecting the shoulder complex. Though this condition may not affect scapula function, if it does, the usual clinical manifestation is decreased motion of the affected shoulder. Check for the presence of postural **kyphosis**, otherwise known as *roundback*, which typically becomes noticeable during adolescence. Assess for **scapula winging** by asking the patient to perform a "push-up" maneuver against a wall. Mild cases of this deformity are commonly associated with many shoulder disorders, including GHJ instability. In these instances, the serratus anterior muscle, which is responsible for keeping the vertebral border against the body, becomes fatigued and/or is weakened, causing a muscle strength imbalance in the region. In more severe cases, scapula winging is caused by pathology to the long thoracic nerve that innervates this muscle.[1]

Palpation

In preparation to palpate these regions, instruct the patient to stand with his or her hands at the sides of the body. Standing behind the patient, begin by palpating the spinous processes of the cervical vertebrae. Start with C7, otherwise known as the *vertebral prominens*, or the most prominent vertebrae. To find C7, instruct the patient to flex the neck slightly, because doing so highlights this bony landmark. Working superiorly, palpate the spinous process of each vertebrae, realizing that the spinous processes of C4 and C3 are extremely difficult to palpate because of their small size and that C2 and C1 are not palpable because they do not have spinous processes. Next, palpate the cervical erector spinae, which typically are tender and/or in spasm in response to cervical pathology. Complete this part of the cervical examination by palpating the anterior muscles of the neck, though doing so usually does not reveal abnormal findings.[3]

Next, systematically palpate the shoulder complex by touching, in order, the SCJ, clavicle, and ACJ, because doing so simultaneously checks bone, joint, and ligament integrity. Injury to these structures produces a palpable deformity. Palpate the borders, angles, and scapula spine. Though the bony landmarks of the scapular are not injured often, identifying them allows for soft tissues in the area to be better identified. Doing this also prepares for the evaluation of scapula motion during the ROM portion of the examination.[1]

Once bone palpation is completed, instruct the patient to place his or her hands on the hips. With the patient in this position, palpate the pectoralis major, deltoid, latissimus dorsi, teres major, and axilla. Pain or deformity in these regions indicates pathology to the underlying GHJ. Extend the patient's GHJ and feel just distal to the anterolateral corner of the acromion for the insertion of the supraspinatus, the muscle most responsible for causing rotator cuff pain. With the humerus in the anatomical position, palpate the LHB as it passes through the bicipital groove.[1]

Range-of-Motion and Strength Testing

Check the active ROM of the patient's cervical spine, GHJ, and STA by having the patient perform the motions illustrated in Figures 11.3, 11.4, and 11.5. Assess for the presence of a **painful arc**, which is frequently associated with overuse shoulder pathologies. Perform **Apley's scratch tests** (Fig. 11.13), because these tests allow for the gross evaluation of a variety of shoulder motions. Follow active testing with passive testing of all cervical and GHJ motions.[1,3–5]

PEARL

Perform the Apley's scratch tests to evaluate active motion of
the shoulder complex.

Once the patient's ROM is established, test the strength of the cervical spine by resisting the motions shown in Figure 11.3. To manual muscle test (MMT) these motions, apply resistance on the patient's forehead to test flexion, on the occiput to test extension, on the side of the head to test lateral flexion (being sure not to irritate the patient's ears), and on the side of the forehead to test rotation. MMT the GHJ by resisting the motions shown in Figure 11.5. Apply resistance above the level of the elbow when testing the motions of flexion, extension, abduction, adduction, and horizontal abduction and adduction. For internal and external rotation, apply resistance at the wrist. While pushing down on the right and left upper trapezius, instruct the patient to perform a shoulder shrug. This tests the strength of the scapula elevators and is the only MMT needed for motions of the STA.

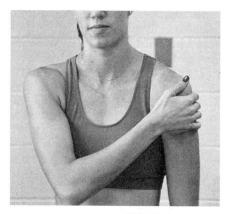
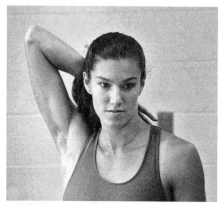
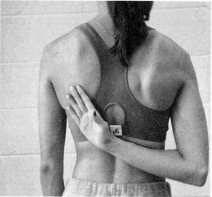

FIGURE 11.13 Apley's scratch tests are used to simultaneously assess multiple motions of the shoulder complex.
From Starkey and Ryan: *Evaluation of Orthopedic and Athletic Injuries*, 2nd ed. 2002. Philadelphia: F.A. Davis Company, Box 13-3, pg 447, with permission.

Stress and Special Testing

Stress and special tests of the shoulder complex evaluate the health of the GHJ, ACJ, STA, and structures located in the subacromial space, whereas tests of the cervical spine evaluate nerve root integrity. The most accurate and commonly used stress and special tests used to evaluate injury in these regions are presented in conjunction with the specific musculoskeletal conditions covered in this chapter.

Neurological Examination

Assessing injury to these regions dictates that a complete neurological examination of the upper extremity be completed, especially when pathology of the cervical spine is suspected. This neurological evaluation includes assessing the patient's motor and sensory functions, as well as performing reflex testing.

As with the lower extremity, determining the health of the patient's motor nerves occurs via strength testing. However, to ensure that all motor function is intact, test the strength of the entire upper extremity, because doing so assesses the health of the whole brachial plexus. Thus, in addition to strength testing the cervical spine and shoulder, use the information provided in Chapter 12 to MMT the rest of the upper extremity's major muscle groups. Evaluate for sensory deprivation by testing the patient's dermatomes, following the patterns shown in Figure 10.19 on page 286, because doing so determines whether a specific nerve root has been affected by injury or disease. Conclude the neurological examination by testing the patient's biceps brachii (C5–C6), brachioradialis (C5–C6), and triceps (C7–C8) reflexes.[3]

Musculoskeletal Imaging

Plain-film radiography remains the first diagnostic test ordered for patients presenting with cervical spine injury. Thus, order anteroposterior (AP), lateral, and oblique x-ray views for patients suspected of having cervical spine pathology. Include an open-mouth view, which evaluates the integrity of the atlantoaxial joint, for patients who have undergone a traumatic event. However, be aware that the use of plain-film radiographs are limited in what they can detect and be aware that by the age of 60, most people have some form of cervical degenerative change that can be identified through x-rays. This makes the use of x-rays less effective when trying to identify the exact cause of a person's chronic neck pain in this population. Use magnetic resonance imaging (MRI), if needed, to detect pathology of the cervical spine, because this technique has become the imaging technique of choice to evaluate this region.[3,6]

Though standards are scarce with regard to when to radiograph the shoulder, be sure to order x-rays in all cases of acute trauma, when ROM is diminished and when severe pain exists. Though obtaining x-rays during the initial management of overuse shoulder injury is usually not necessary, obtain plain-film radiographs if shoulder pain resulting from a chronic injury has not improved after a few weeks of conservative treatment. Common shoulder complex projections are listed in Box 11.3. Recognize that it is not necessary to obtain all of these views for every shoulder injury. Indeed, determining the views needed for a specific condition depends on the differential diagnosis. However, be sure to include AP views with the GHJ in internal and external rotation in all radiographic studies. Consider ordering a trauma series, consisting of AP, axillary, and scapular "Y" views, after acute shoulder injury, because these are the best views to use to rule out fractures and dislocations.[2,5,7–9]

BOX 11.3
COMMON PLAIN–FILM RADIOGRAPH VIEWS OF THE SHOULDER COMPLEX

AP–GHJ in internal rotation★	40° cephalic tilt (serendipity)–clavicle;
AP–GHJ in external rotation★	SCJ
Axillary★	Supraspinatus outlet
Scapular "Y" (anterior oblique)★	

★Trauma series view.

AP = anteroposterior; GHJ = glenohumeral joint; SCJ = sternoclavicular joint.

◖ P E A R L ◗

Include AP x-rays with the GHJ in internal and external rotation in all radiographic studies of the shoulder.

Whereas plain-film radiography identifies bone and joint abnormalities, MRI is the gold standard for diagnosing soft tissue injury of the shoulder. Thus, order MRI studies when the clinical evaluation indicates soft tissue injury, such as a tear to the rotator cuff. Also, obtain an MRI to help identify areas of pathology in instances where radiographs are normal after trauma but significant clinical symptoms, such as severe pain, weakness, and decreased motion, persist after a course of conservative management.[5,8,10]

Conditions of the Cervical Spine

Though many specific conditions of the cervical spine exist, most fall under the category of **cervical radiculopathy**. In sports, injury to the brachial plexus is a common occurrence among athletes who participate in collision and contact activities.

Cervical Radiculopathy

Cervical radiculopathy can be caused by many things, including a herniated intervertebral disk (Fig. 11.14). Indeed, in younger people, an acute disk herniation and impingement of a nerve root as it exits the foramen are the primary causes of this condition. Student athletes who participate in sports such as football and wrestling are at an increased risk of experiencing a cervical nerve root injury, owing to the compressive and rotational forces these activities place on the intervertebral foramen. In older patients, cervical radiculopathy commonly results from narrowing of the intervertebral foramen due to **osteophyte** formation. In many instances, a combination of factors causes this condition, as when a herniated disk occurs in conjunction with degenerative changes. Regardless, the sixth and seventh nerve roots are most commonly affected, causing symptoms to appear throughout the upper extremity. This fact causes cervical radiculopathy to be misdiagnosed as an injury to the rotator cuff, subacromial bursitis, bicipital tendonitis (all discussed later in this chapter), and lateral epicondylitis (discussed in Chapter 12).[3,11]

History and Physical Examination

Patients with cervical radiculopathy report an insidious onset of neck and arm discomfort, which ranges from a dull ache to a severe, burning pain. This pain typically radiates down the upper extremity corresponding with the involved nerve root. Tingling and numbness also occur along the involved nerve root dermatome. These symptoms are relieved when the patient abducts the shoulder on the involved side and places the hand behind his or her head, because this decreases symptoms by taking pressure off the irritated nerve root. When palpated, the area of the cervical erector spinae muscle group on the side of the involved nerve root is tender. These muscles may also be in spasm. Tenderness and spasm may also occur in the muscles where symptoms are referred. For example, the posterior compartment of the forearm (discussed in Chapter 12) may be painful, and the muscles within the compartment may spasm, if the C6 nerve root is

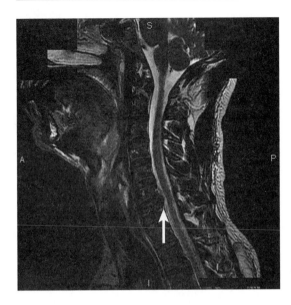

FIGURE 11.14 Herniated C6/C7 intervertebral disk placing pressure on nerve root C7.

affected. Laterally flexing the neck to the same side of the injury increases pain in patients with an impinged nerve root, whereas laterally flexing the neck to the opposite side of the injury causes pain in patients with an intervertebral disk herniation. Muscles supplied by the affected nerve root may become weak, but recognize that a loss of strength almost always occurs secondary to sensory loss. Reflexes may be affected if the nerve root supplying the reflex is involved.[3,11]

Use **Spurling's test**, otherwise known as the *foramen compression test*, to clinically determine the presence of cervical radiculopathy. To perform this test[4]

- Instruct the patient to sit, neck extended and rotated toward the involved side.
- After positioning yourself posterior to the patient, apply downward pressure on the patient's head.
- Reproduction of pain confirms cervical nerve root pathology.

Management

Prescribe the use of a cervical collar, and immediately refer patients for neurological consultation if they report experiencing progressive neurological deficits or if the physical examination reveals bilateral symptoms, because these could be signs of spinal cord injury. Do the same for people who have upper extremity weakness, because these patients may require surgical intervention. Though a cervical collar does not aid healing, in many instances using it increases patient comfort. For all other patients, prescribe a cervical collar and order an MRI, because the best way to confirm the presence of a radiculopathy is to determine the cause of the patient's symptoms. After pathology has been confirmed, refer patients for neurological consultation. Initial treatment consists of reducing pain and inflammation with therapeutic modalities and pharmacological agents and instructing patients to avoid body positions that increase symptoms.[3,11]

Brachial Plexus Injury

Injury to the brachial plexus, otherwise known as a *burner* or *stinger*, has a high rate of occurrence in collision and contact sports. Indeed, this is the most frequent cervical spine–related injury in football. The resulting neuropraxia occurs when either a compressive or tension force is applied to the plexus. A compressive force impinges on the roots of the plexus as they exit the spinal cord, whereas a tension force stretches the nerves beyond what the plexus can handle. A tension injury is experienced when blunt-force trauma occurs on the side of the head, causing the neck to laterally flex and rotate to the side opposite of where the damage occurs. For example, a blow delivered to the left side of a person's head forces the neck to laterally flex and rotate to the right, stretching and exposing the left brachial plexus to injury. College and professional athletes are most likely to sustain a brachial plexus injury by impinging a nerve root, whereas high school athletes usually sustain a stretch-type injury. The upper portions of the brachial plexus, namely C5 and C6, are at greatest risk from this injury mechanism.[3,12,13]

History and Physical Examination

Patients with a traumatized brachial plexus report feeling a shock-like sensation consisting of pain, tingling, burning, and numbness that radiated from the neck to the shoulder, arm, forearm, and hand at the time of injury. They always relate that these symptoms occurred unilaterally and usually state that they resolved within minutes, though in rare instances a patient may report that symptoms persisted longer. When the condition is caused by a compression mechanism, the patient may report lingering neck pain, whereas this is not the case if the condition is caused by a tension injury. Regardless, the patient's cervical ROM is usually normal, as is neck and shoulder strength. Occasionally, weakness is present, but unless severe, this usually does not alter the prognosis. Because the C5 and C6 nerve roots are injured most often, when weakness does occur, the deltoid, biceps brachii, supraspinatus, and infraspinatus are most commonly affected. In some instances, a patient may present with chronic burner syndrome, a condition characterized by significant weakness of the deltoid. Chronic burner syndrome is caused by nerve root compression at the intervertebral foramen secondary to disk disease, and 70% of patients with this syndrome have a positive Spurling's test.[12–14]

Management

When the injury is not associated with neck pain or limitation of neck movement and if all motor and sensory symptoms resolve within seconds to minutes from the time of injury, it is safe to clear for competition patients who have a brachial plexus injury. If sensory complications or weakness persist more than a few minutes, order an MRI of the cervical spine to rule out a herniated disk or other compressive pathology. Disqualify from competition, and refer for neurological consultation, patients who have symptoms for 24 hours or more, multiple episodes, or persistent neck pain.[12,13]

Conditions of the Glenohumeral Joint

Though a variety of injuries occur at the GHJ in response to playing sports, the most common condition seen is joint instability. By and large, GHJ instability is caused by traumatic and atraumatic events, with many acute instabilities ultimately becoming chronic.

Acute Dislocation of the Glenohumeral Joint

An acute GHJ dislocation, referred to simply as a *shoulder dislocation*, occurs when the head of the humerus dislodges from the glenoid fossa. This condition happens quite often in sports because the GHJ is the most frequently dislocated major joint in the body.[15]

Because the humeral head moves in many different directions, the type of acute GHJ dislocation a person experiences is classified according to the direction the humeral moves and the position it assumes. For example, in an anterior, or *subcoracoid*, dislocation, the head of the humerus moves forward and becomes lodged under the coracoid process. In an inferior, or *subglenoid*, dislocation, the humeral head migrates below the glenoid fossa. The head of the humerus becomes positioned under the spine of the scapula in a posterior, or *subspinous*, dislocation. The anterior shoulder dislocation occurs by far most often, accounting for up to 90% of all acute GHJ dislocations. However, in certain instances, inferior instability accompanies an anterior GHJ dislocation.[4,16–18]

PEARL

The GHJ most commonly dislocates anteriorly, causing the head of the humerus to lodge under the coracoid process.

An anterior shoulder dislocation most commonly occurs when a force is applied to the upper extremity with the GHJ abducted and externally rotated. This mechanism forces the humeral head anteriorly, placing great stress on the joint's capsule and GHLs. When the force applied is greater than what the capsule and ligaments can handle, the head of the humerus dislodges from the glenoid fossa. Though not as common, other MOIs include a direct blow to the shoulder and a fall on the outstretched arm. Anterior GHJ instability is particularly common in active adolescents and young adult males younger than 25 years.[1,2,4,15,17–19]

PEARL

Anterior shoulder dislocations occur from forced GHJ abduction and external rotation and are particularly common in active adolescents and young adult males younger than 25 years.

Be aware that certain complications accompany the traumatic anterior GHJ dislocation. In some cases, this injury disrupts the anterior, inferior margin of the joint's labrum, commonly referred to as a *Bankart lesion*. Occasionally, the LHB tears away from its attachment on the labrum, producing an injury to the anterior and posterior portions of the superior labrum, otherwise known as a *SLAP* (superior labrum from anterior to posterior) *lesion*. A posterolateral humeral head impression fracture, also known as a *Hill-Sachs lesion*, forms when the posterior humeral head, as it dislodges from the glenoid fossa, abuts the anterior edge of the glenoid. It is also common for the brachial plexus to become injured in an anterior dislocation. These conditions must be considered as part of the differential diagnosis of an acute anterior GHJ dislocation.[15,18,19]

In most cases, a person with an acute anterior GHJ dislocation that has not been reduced is usually transported immediately to an emergency medical facility for treatment. There may be instances, however, when a patient reports to the primary care setting with a nonreduced dislocation. In addition, instead of completely dislocating, the joint may subluxate. These patients usually report symptoms that are similar to but less intense than symptoms of people with a GHJ dislocation.[18]

History and Physical Examination

Regardless of whether the humeral head is still dislodged, the patient with a GHJ dislocation supports the injured extremity in either a position of comfort or a position of necessity. For example, the patient whose joint is still dislocated may hold the extremity in abduction and external rotation because the humeral head may be "stuck" in this position. In contrast, the patient who has experienced a spontaneous reduction may, in an attempt to protect the joint from further injury, present by supporting the upper extremity with the shoulder adducted and internally rotated, as if the upper extremity were in a sling (Fig. 6.1 on page 129). In addition, the shoulder of the patient whose GHJ has reduced appears close to normal, whereas the shoulder of someone with an active dislocation looks square or flat, and the acromion process appears prominent. In these instances, the humeral head is not in position to provide the rounded contour of the deltoid typically seen in the healthy shoulder. The humeral head can also be felt in the axilla of patients with an active dislocation, because of its being lodged under the coracoid process, in an anterior dislocation, or, less frequently, under the glenoid fossa, in an inferior dislocation. In these instances, the patient's distal circulation and sensation may be compromised by the humeral head because it places pressure on the nerves and vessels in the region. If the history, observation, and palpation portions of the evaluation lead to a diagnosis of an active GHJ dislocation, do not perform GHJ ROM, strength, or special and stress tests. Rather, treat these patients as described in the management portion of this section.[1,2,15,18]

PEARL

When evaluating a patient with an acute anterior GHJ dislocation, carefully examine for distal circulation and sensation, because the head of the humerus may place pressure on the nerves and vessels in the region.

Though the joint may appear to be normal, patients who have experienced an acute GHJ dislocation that has reduced present with shoulder stiffness and apprehension. This is typically accompanied by decreases in both active and passive shoulder movement, though the patient's shoulder strength may or may not be affected. Ultimately, the results of the **GHJ apprehension test** and **GHJ relocation test** are used to document a case of anterior GHJ instability, whereas the presence of a **sulcus sign** confirms inferior instability.[4,18,19]

In preparation for performing the GHJ apprehension and relocation tests, place the patient supine, with the GHJ abducted and externally rotated and the upper extremity situated off the edge of the table. Position yourself either lateral to the extremity or adjacent to the patient's head. To perform the GHJ apprehension test (Fig. 11.15)[1,2,4,15,18,19]:

- Place one hand on the patient's wrist and the other hand on the posterior aspect of the proximal humerus.
- Apply a gentle anterior translation force by pushing back on the patient's wrist and pushing forward on the patient's humerus.
- Monitor the patient's response, because a positive test is indicated by discomfort and the apprehension the person feels as the joint reaches impending instability. The patient may actively internally rotate the shoulder in an effort to avoid having the GHJ dislocate.

With the patient in the same position used for the apprehension test, perform the relocation test by applying posterior pressure to the anterior aspect of the proximal humerus while pushing back gently on the patient's wrist. Push back to relocate the joint if the humeral head migrates anteriorly. This constitutes a positive sign for anterior GHJ instability. Because this test attempts to relocate, versus dislocate, the GHJ, most patients respond to the relocation test much better than to the apprehension test.[1,4,15,19]

To determine whether a sulcus sign exists (Fig. 11.16)[1,2]:

- Position yourself laterally to the standing patient.
- Grasp the distal end of the patient's forearm with one hand.
- Place your other hand over the ACJ.
- Apply a distraction force to the humerus by pulling down on the forearm.
- As the humerus is distracting, look for the formation of a sulcus, or divot, just inferior to the acromion.

After confirming that the patient has experienced a GHJ dislocation, determine whether the glenoid labrum has been injured by performing the **clunk test** and **biceps tension test**, or *SLAP test*. To perform the clunk test, instruct the patient to lie supine. With the patient completely relaxed, passively circumduct and compress the humeral head into the glenoid fossa. Pain, catching, or a clunk-like sensation is indicative of a labral tear. Next, instruct the patient to stand with the forearm supinated, elbow extended, and shoulder abducted to 90°. Attempt to push the forearm downward,

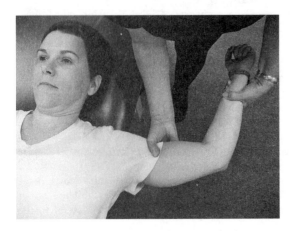

FIGURE 11.15 The apprehension test for anterior glenohumeral joint instability. Perform the relocation test with the patient in the same position by applying pressure to the anterior aspect of the proximal humerus as you gently push back on the patient's wrist.

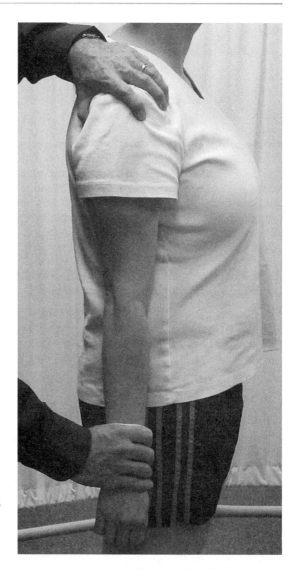

FIGURE 11.16 The sulcus sign for inferior glenohumeral joint instability. When this test is used to determine whether the acromioclavicular joint has been sprained, it is called the *acromioclavicular distraction test.*

instructing the patient to resist this action. Pain or weakness with this test indicates the presence of a SLAP lesion, particularly when these occur in the posterior aspect of the GHJ.[1,2,19,20]

Management

Obtain plain-film radiographs on all patients with suspected GHJ instability. If the humeral head is still dislodged, x-rays confirm the diagnosis. Use the shoulder trauma series to determine the direction of the nonreduced dislocation and to rule out bony pathology. The axillary view of this trauma series also evaluates for the presence of a posterior dislocation.[2,8,9,15,18,19]

Prompt reduction is the treatment of choice for patients with a dislocated GHJ. In cases of an anterior dislocation, reduction is easiest, and is best performed, immediately after injury. Doing so prevents additional soft tissue injury, decreases the chance that the surrounding musculature will spasm, relieves pain, and decreases the chance of neurovascular injury. However, be aware that patients with a first time anterior GHJ dislocation who do not respond to reduction efforts may require general anesthesia for the joint to be successfully relocated. In contrast, patients with dislocations that happen after an initial occurrence are easier to relocate. Indeed, after instances of multiple dislocations, many patients are able to spontaneously relocate a dislocated GHJ.[2,18]

If your scope of practice allows and if you have been properly trained, attempt to reduce the anteriorly dislocated GHJ. Though many reduction methods exist, **Stimson's maneuver** is an easy-to-use, effective, and fairly safe-to-administer method to relocate a GHJ. To execute Stimson's maneuver[15]

• Place the patient prone, with the involved extremity dangling over the side of a table.
• Fasten a 10- to 15-pound weight to the wrist and hand on the involved side. Avoid having the patient grasp the weight with the hand, because doing so causes the muscles to contract, impeding the desired outcome of maintaining full relaxation so the joint can relocate.
• Reduction typically occurs within 20 minutes.

Repeat the neurovascular examination once the reduction is completed and order postreduction x-rays to ensure that the reduction was successful. If reduction is not obtained, immobilize the joint in a position of comfort and immediately refer the patient to an orthopedist or to an emergency department. If postreduction plain-film radiographs, or x-rays of the patient who reports with a recently reduced joint, reveal additional pathology, such as a SLAP or Hill-Sachs lesion, refer the patient to an orthopedist. In these cases, surgical intervention is indicated. Also immobilize, and refer to an orthopedist or emergency department, patients with inferior or posterior GHJ dislocations.[1,15,18]

After a successful reduction, and for people who report with a recently reduced joint, conservative treatment is the initial recommended course of action. Thus, for these patients, immobilize the injured shoulder for 3 to 6 weeks by placing the upper extremity in a sling, as shown in Figure 6.1 on page 129. Keep the immobilization period as short as possible so that adhesive capsulitis (discussed later in this chapter) does not develop. This is particularly important for older patients because adhesive capsulitis is highly prevalent in this population. Though the use of conservative measures is the preferred course of treatment for most patients with GHJ instability, the risk of recurrent instability developing with conservative treatment is directly proportional to the activity level the person pursues and is inversely proportional to age. That is, the recurrence rate is greater for young, active people and decreases as a person ages and becomes less active. Indeed, up to 80% of young, active patients experience episodes of recurrent dislocations.[3,15,18]

The ultimate goal of conservative treatment for a patient with a dislocated GHJ is to slowly increase the joint's ROM and to strengthen the muscles that surround and support the joint, namely, the rotator cuff, deltoid, and pectoral muscles. Do this by initiating ROM exercises, as presented in Patient Teaching Handout (PTH) 11.1, as soon as pain and discomfort allow. Start isometric strengthening exercises, as described in PTH 11.1, at 3 to 4 weeks after injury. Once the patient regains full ROM, pursue more advanced strengthening exercises, shown in PTH 11.1. Avoid placing the patient in the at-risk position of GHJ abduction and external rotation for the first 6 weeks of the rehabilitation process.[15,18]

PEARL

During the rehabilitation process, the patient should avoid exercise activities that place the GHJ in the at-risk position of abduction and external rotation.

Recurrent Glenohumeral Joint Instability

Recurrent or chronic GHJ instability results from either a history of an initial GHJ dislocation followed by other instances of dislocation and/or subluxation, or from atraumatic causes occurring without a history of previous acute episodes of dislocation. In these latter instances, the patient is usually involved in an activity requiring strenuous repetitive overhead shoulder motions, which, over time, stretch out the joint's capsule. For example, swimmers and gymnasts often develop chronic GHJ instability because of the stresses these activities place on the shoulder. Remember that in the adolescent and young adult populations, an acutely dislocated, or subluxed, GHJ has a high risk of recurring, resulting in recurrent anterior GHJ instability. Also, recurrent episodes of anterior dislocation are associated with Bankart and SLAP lesions, tears of the rotator cuff (particularly in older patients), the development of impingement syndrome, and brachial plexus trauma in the form of a stinger injury. Rotator cuff tears and impingement syndrome are discussed later in this chapter.[1,18,19]

PEARL

Recurrent GHJ instability commonly occurs in people who participate in activities requiring strenuous repetitive overhead shoulder motions, such as gymnastics and swimming, which, over time, stretch out the joint's capsule.

History and Physical Examination

Regardless of what caused the condition, a person with recurrent GHJ instability usually reports frequent episodes of subluxation associated with spontaneous reduction and short-lived disability. These patients also relate a sensation of constant "looseness" of the shoulder, particularly when they carry heavy objects. **Dead arm syndrome**, caused by the humeral head pressing against the underlying neurovascular structures each time the joint subluxates, is another common complaint of patients with this condition. Both muscle atrophy and signs of asymmetry are absent, because these patients usually maintain normal GHJ ROM and strength. As with people who have had an acute dislocation that has spontaneously reduced, the apprehension and relocation tests are usually positive when performed on patients with chronic GHJ instability. If inferior instability is present, the sulcus sign may also be positive.[18,19]

Management

Refer all patients with recurrent GHJ instability to an orthopedist, because surgical intervention may be necessary, particularly if the patient desires to continue participating in the activity that produced the instability. Though many different open and arthroscopic surgical techniques are used to repair GHJ laxity, all come with limitations and require that the patient be dedicated to a fairly lengthy rehabilitation process. Indeed, in some instances, chronic GHJ instability results in a permanent discontinuation of the offending activity.

Conditions of the Acromioclavicular and Sternoclavicular Joints

Though some overuse conditions of the ACJ and SCJ do exist, injury to these joints almost always results from an acute MOI, resulting in sprains.

Acromioclavicular Joint Sprain

The ACJ is one of the most commonly injured structures of the shoulder complex. An ACJ sprain, regularly referred to as a *shoulder separation*, usually occurs when the patient receives a direct blow to the joint (Figs. 11.17 and 11.18). In sports, this happens when a player falls to the ground from a great height and, instead of placing his or her hand out to break the fall, absorbs the blow by landing on the shoulder, sometimes in an attempt to perform a forward roll. This also happens when a person bends from the waist and "lowers" the shoulder to make contact with someone, or something, during competition. For example, a defensive player in football frequently lowers the shoulder when attempting to tackle an offensive player who is carrying the ball. An ice hockey or lacrosse player sometimes inadvertently lowers the shoulder just before impacting an immovable object, such as a goalpost (it is for this reason that shoulder pads are a mandatory piece of protective equipment in the collision sports of football, ice hockey, and lacrosse). In these instances, the resulting force moves the acromion inferiorly and the clavicle superiorly, traumatizing the ACJ. Indeed, it is the amount of force delivered to the joint that determines the resulting amount of instability, deformity, and pain.[2,21]

PEARL

The primary reason why the use of shoulder pads is mandatory in the sports of football, ice hockey, and lacrosse is to protect the ACJ from injury.

History and Physical Examination

Regardless of injury severity, the patient with an ACJ sprain usually reports an MOI similar to what has just been described. The person's chief concern is ACJ pain, which, the person states, has affected the amount that he or she can move the shoulder. Because this joint is superficial, a **step deformity** is easily seen (Fig. 11.18). In addition, pushing

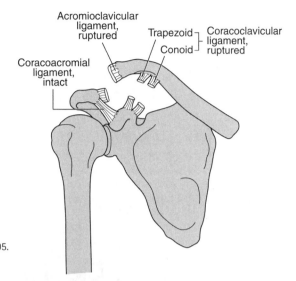

FIGURE 11.17 A third degree acromioclavicular joint sprain. Note that both the acromioclavicular and the coracoclavicular ligaments have been totally ruptured.
From McKinnis: *Fundamentals of Musculoskeletal Imaging,* 2nd ed. 2005. Philadelphia: F.A. Davis Company, Fig. 12–47, pg 436, with permission.

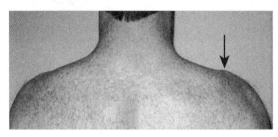

FIGURE 11.18 A sprain of the right acromioclavicular joint. Note the presence of a step deformity, caused by the distal end of the clavicle riding higher than the acromion process.

down on the distal end of the clavicle causes it to move up and down, otherwise known as the *piano key sign*. Being able to displace the clavicle in this fashion indicates that both the ACL and the CCL have been injured. ACJ pathology also causes the patient pain when he or she abducts the GHJ past 120°, particularly if the injury is in the subacute or chronic stages. The **crossover test**, in which the patient reaches across the chest and touches the contralateral acromion process, compresses the ACJ and causes pain to patients with a sprain to this joint.[1,4,5,21]

Perform the **distraction test** and **shear test**, otherwise known as the *compression test*, to verify ACJ pathology. To perform these tests, position yourself laterally to the standing patient. To execute the shear test (Fig. 11.19):

- Place one hand in front of and the other hand behind the GHJ. Interlock your fingers over the top the ACJ, effectively cupping the shoulder complex.
- Squeeze your hands together, because this compresses the ACJ.
- Monitor the patient's response, because this test is positive if the patient experiences increased pain.

To perform the distraction test, complete the sulcus sign maneuver, explained previously and shown in Figure 11.16. When using this test to determine the integrity of

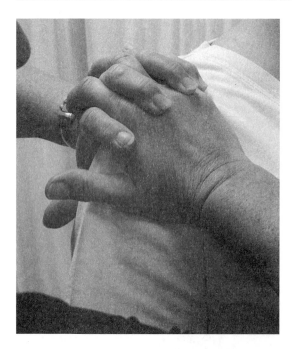

FIGURE 11.19 The acromioclavicular joint shear test is used to assess the integrity of the acromioclavicular joint.

the ACJ, watch and feel for a step deformity as the humerus and scapula of the injured ACJ move downward in relation to the clavicle.

Once the presence of an ACJ sprain is documented, its severity is graded by the amount of pain, instability, and deformity present. This is determined by the degree of ACL and CCL injury (Table 11.3). Though grading an ACJ sprain allows for the severity of injury to be determined, doing so has little bearing on the influence the injury may have on future shoulder function. Indeed, once an ACJ sprain heals, athletic performance is not affected greatly, regardless of injury severity.[2]

Management

When the clinical evaluation leads to a diagnosis of an ACJ sprain, order shoulder trauma series x-rays. The axillary view of this series determines whether there has been any AP displacement of the clavicle and can rule out any other associated shoulder pathology. Once this condition is verified, treat patients with a first or second degree sprain conservatively with sling immobilization, as shown in Figure 6.1 on page 129, until pain subsides. In these instances, initiate ROM and strengthening exercises, as shown in PTH 11.1, as soon as pain allows. Usually, these can be started within the first few weeks after injury. Refer patients with a third degree sprain to an orthopedist. Initially, this condition is almost always treated conservatively, because the outcome of conservative intervention is the same as that of surgical intervention. However, surgical intervention may be considered if conservative treatment fails.[21]

Sternoclavicular Joint Sprain

Sprains to the SCJ usually occur from a fall on the outstretched arm (Fig. 11.12). Because this is the same mechanism that injures the clavicle (discussed later in this

TABLE 11.3 Grading acromioclavicular joint sprains

GRADE	STRUCTURES INJURED	CLINICAL SIGNS
I	<50% ACL torn CCL intact	No visual deformity; mild pain on palpation; no instability noted; GHJ ROM not affected
II	>50% ACL torn <50% CCL torn	Mild step deformity present; moderate pain on palpation; mild to moderate pain associated with special tests; pain with GHJ motion, particularly above 120° abduction
III	>50% ACL torn >50% CCL torn	Severe step deformity; severe pain on palpation and with all special tests; gapping present with AC distraction test; unable to move the GHJ throughout its full ROM

ACL = acromioclavicular ligament; CCL = coracoclavicular ligament; GHJ = glenohumeral joint; ROM = range of motion.

chapter), be aware that clavicular fractures are much more common than SCJ sprains. This is because the force produced by such a fall usually concentrates at the mid clavicle, rarely reaching the SCJ. Though SCJ sprains are fairly uncommon, when they do happen their diagnosis is frequently delayed, because these sprains typically occur in combination with other upper extremity injuries, making it easy for the examiner to overlook this condition.[1,22]

PEARL

Though rarely injured in sports, an SCJ sprain is often overlooked because it usually occurs in combination with other upper extremity injuries.

When the SCJ is injured, the proximal end of the clavicle moves either anteriorly or posteriorly, with anterior dislocations being most common. Regardless, a sprain to the SCJ indicates that the SCL, CoCL, and ICL have been injured. Though rare, posterior dislocations are more dangerous than anterior because of the proximity of the clavicle's proximal end to the underlying trachea and blood vessels. These injuries typically occur in younger people whose clavicular medial epiphyseal plate is still open. Indeed, an SCJ sprain in this population often occurs in conjunction with a fracture through this growth plate. Thus, when evaluating injury to this region, take extra care to rule out posterior SCJ dislocation and proximal clavicular fracture in adolescents and young adults.[1,22–24]

PEARL

When evaluating injury to the SCJ in adolescents and young adults, rule out the presence of a posterior dislocation and/or a proximal clavicular fracture, because these conditions could place pressure on the underlying trachea and blood vessels.

History and Physical Examination

A history that includes a fall on the outstretched arm with point tenderness over the SCJ indicates that the person has injured this joint. Patients with a mild SCJ sprain usually do not need to support the upper extremity in any specific fashion, because there is no displacement of the clavicle in relation to the sternum in these instances. In contrast, people with a second or third degree anterior sprain present by holding the shoulder in the sling position, as shown in Figure 6.1 on page 129, with the neck rotated and flexed toward the involved side. In these cases, deformity in the form of a prominent proximal clavicle on the involved side is usually quite apparent. Regardless of injury severity, the SCJ is usually painful when touched, a symptom that is increased when the GHJ is moved while the joint is palpated. Also, note that the patient with a second or third degree sprain is unable to horizontally adduct the GHJ. Differentiating between a moderate and a severe sprain can be accomplished by noting the amount of mobility present in the proximal end of the patient's clavicle. Though this portion of the bone maintains increased mobility in both conditions, the clavicle of a person with a second degree injury moves without dislocation, whereas the clavicle of a person with a third degree sprain is easily dislocated from its attachment to the sternum.[22]

When evaluating the patient with a traumatized SCJ, a posterior dislocation may not be as apparent as an anterior injury. Indeed, the patient with this injury presents with decreased prominence of the clavicle's proximal end, which, when compared with an anterior deformity, is harder to identify clinically. In these instances, look for a depression deformity of the skin overlying the joint, and recognize its injury symptoms. These include a tingling feeling in the throat, shortness of breath, choking, and difficulty swallowing, all caused by the clavicle placing pressure on the underlying trachea. Though these symptoms may not be present during the initial evaluation, they may appear over time. Thus, instruct all patients who experience trauma to this region to seek medical attention immediately if any of these symptoms develop, because a posterior dislocation can have life-threatening consequences.[23,24]

PEARL

Instruct all patients who experience a tingling feeling in the throat, shortness of breath, choking, and difficulty swallowing after trauma to the SCJ to immediately seek medical attention, because a posterior dislocation of this joint can have life-threatening consequences.

Management

Radiographic evaluation is mandatory to confirm an SCJ sprain. Thus, verify this injury by obtaining a shoulder trauma series and cephalic tilt x-ray views. The cephalic tilt view shows the clavicle projecting above or below the horizontal plane, depending on the type of dislocation. If a definitive diagnosis cannot be made through plain-film radiography, confirm the diagnosis through CT scanning, particularly if a posterior dislocation is suspected.[22,23,25]

Treat patients with first degree anterior SCJ sprains conservatively with sling immobilization, as shown in Figure 6.1 on page 129. Within the first 2 weeks after injury, add ROM and strengthening exercises, as shown in PTH 11.1, as pain allows. Refer all patients with suspected second and third degree anterior sprains and all patients with suspected posterior dislocations to an orthopedist. Anterior instabilities can usually be treated with closed reduction followed by the wearing of a figure-eight bandage splint for 3 to 6 weeks, whereas the posterior dislocation requires either closed reduction under anesthesia or an open repair.[22-24]

Conditions of the Clavicle

Injuries to the clavicle resulting from sports participation include fractures caused by acute trauma and overuse conditions, most notably **osteolysis**.

Clavicular Fracture

The clavicle is the most commonly fractured bone of the shoulder complex, with roughly 75% of all cases involving people younger than 13 years. It is usually fractured from a fall on the outstretched arm (Fig. 11.12) or from a direct blow. The middle third is at greatest risk for injury due to the bone's *S* shape at this location. However, fracture to the distal end can be troubling because of the incidence of nonunion and delayed union at this site. And, as previously discussed, a fractures of a young person's proximal clavicle often affects the growth plate in this region.[2,9,21,22,24]

History and Physical Examination

The patient with a fractured clavicle usually relates hearing and feeling the clavicle break on impact. They report immediate pain and disability after the incident, making use of the shoulder complex nearly impossible. In most instances, the person presents by supporting the involved extremity in a sling position, as shown in Figure 6.1 on page 129, with the head tilted toward the injured shoulder and the chin rotated toward the uninjured side. The injured area is swollen and deformed, signs that are easily seen because of the superficial nature of the clavicle. Crepitus and point tenderness are present when the fracture site is palpated. Though distal circulation and sensation are usually unaffected, in certain instances a fractured clavicle may cause sensory, motor, and circulatory deficits due to the underlying neurovascular structures being injured.[2,9,21,22,24]

Management

Initially immobilize a suspected fracture by placing the upper extremity of the affected person in a sling, as shown in Figure 6.1 on page 129. Immediately refer patients experiencing neurovascular complications to an orthopedist or neurosurgeon. For all others, obtain trauma series and cephalic tilt x-ray views to verify the clinical diagnosis. Although a fracture in an adult most often results in a complete break to the bone, x-rays of an adolescent usually reveal the presence of a greenstick fracture. Refer these patients, and people with fractures of the clavicle's proximal or distal ends, to an orthopedist. Treatment of proximal and distal end fractures is controversial, with some clinicians advocating a conservative approach and others believing in surgical intervention.[2,21]

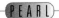

PEARL

X-ray films of an adolescent's fractured clavicle usually reveal the presence of a greenstick fracture.

Once confirmed, treat a fracture of the middle third of the clavicle with a figure-eight bandage splint, and, if needed, place the upper extremity in a sling as shown in Figure 6.1 on page 129. Use clinical signs, such as decreased pain and increased shoulder motion, along with follow-up x-rays, to verify healing and to determine when it is safe to remove the splint and/or sling. This usually can occur after 4 to 8 weeks of immobilization. Start ROM and isometric strengthening exercises, as presented in PTH 11.1, as soon as pain allows, which is usually by the end of the second week after injury. Most clavicular fractures have a favorable prognosis and heal uneventfully with conservative treatment, making surgical intervention necessary only in severe cases.[2,9]

Osteolysis of the Distal Clavicle

Osteolysis of the distal clavicle either develops secondary to acute ACJ injury or results from overuse. When caused by macrotrauma, it usually occurs as a consequence of blunt-force trauma to the ACJ. Repetitive incidences of microtrauma to the shoulder complex are the underlying cause of atraumatic cases. This frequently occurs in patients participating in weight-lifting activities, making overuse the primary cause of osteolysis of the distal clavicle in sports. Be aware that lifting weights may be a secondary activity for patients with this condition, as in the case of a football player lifting weights in preparation for an upcoming season, making all who participate in heavy resistive training activities at risk for development of osteolysis.[21,26,27]

Patients involved in heavy resistance training exercise, such as weight lifters and football players, are at great risk of developing osteolysis of the distal clavicle.

History and Physical Examination

Be sure to obtain a complete history of past episodes of acute shoulder trauma for all patients reporting with distal clavicular pain, because the injury that initiated the development of osteolysis may have occurred years before the patient sought medical care. In contrast, people without this history usually report an insidious onset of symptoms that include a constant, dull ache over the ACJ, which may radiate to the anterior deltoid or trapezius; pain when performing push-ups, dips, and bench-press exercises; and reduced overall strength of the involved extremity. However, most patients primarily report diffuse pain occurring when they abduct the shoulder above 90°. Patients may also state that symptoms decrease when the shoulder is rested, only to have them return almost immediately when the offending activity is resumed. When observed, the patient's shoulder appears perfectly normal but is point tender to touch. The patient is also unable to horizontally adduct the GHJ without pain. These signs are also present in an ACJ sprain, so be aware that it is easy to confuse a sprain of the ACJ with osteolysis in this region.[21,26,27]

Management

Obtain AP plain-film radiographic views of the ACJ and clavicle for patients with suspected osteolysis of the distal clavicle. If the injury is in the early stages, x-rays may appear normal. In these instances, reschedule the patient for follow-up views in

2 to 4 weeks. However, if the condition has been present for months or years, a loss of subchondral bone at the distal end of the clavicle and a widening of the ACJ are clearly evident. Once this condition is diagnosed, treat it conservatively by advising the patient to discontinue the offending activity. Though doing so allows the body to repair the damage in 4 to 6 months, the space between the acromion and the clavicle remains widened permanently. Even after this period of healing, any return to the offending activity causes the condition to reoccur. Refer patients who do not get better with conservative treatment, and people who insist on continuing to participate in the offending activity, to an orthopedist, because one of the treatment options is resection of the distal clavicle. Patients who have this surgery do quite well and can usually return to full, unrestricted activity.[21,26,27]

Conditions of the Rotator Cuff and Subacromial Structures

The rotator cuff muscle group is by far the most common shoulder structure injured with **subacromial impingement syndrome**, referred to simply as *impingement syndrome*, the leading cause of rotator cuff injury. It comes as no surprise, then, that this condition, along with tears of the rotator cuff, are the most common shoulder disorders encountered in the primary care setting. They are also extremely disabling, making their treatment frustrating for both the primary health care provider and patient. Because they are so closely related, for this discussion the History and Physical Examination and Management sections for these conditions have been combined.[5,28,29]

PEARL

Subacromial impingement syndrome and tears to the rotator cuff are the most common shoulder disorders encountered in the primary care setting.

Subacromial Impingement Syndrome

Remember that the supraspinatus tendon and the LHB, as well as the subacromial bursa, are all located under the coracoacromial arch in the subacromial space (Fig. 11.8). The potential for injuring these structures increases when the size of this space becomes too small to accommodate them, a situation that naturally occurs when the GHJ is elevated above the 90° plane. That is, when a person raises his or her hand above the head, the size of this space decreases. This is because for the GHJ to achieve overhead motion, the humeral head must elevate, causing it to migrate superiorly. Though other causes of impingement syndrome, such as acute trauma to the region, also occur, the migration of the humeral head into the subacromial space from performing repetitive, overhead activities remains the leading cause of impingement syndrome.[2,5,10,29,30]

PEARL

The migration of the humeral head into the subacromial space from performing repetitive, overhead activities is the primary cause of impingement syndrome.

Though the head of the humerus naturally moves superiorly during overhead activities, most of the time the rotator cuff muscles are able to stabilize the head by placing a downward force on the humerus. This prevents the humeral head from impinging the structures in the subacromial space against the coracoacromial arch. However, weakness of the rotator cuff caused by a lack of strength in the muscle group, fatigue, or chronic GHJ instability, as previously described, results in a loss of humeral head depression. This results in humeral invasion into the subacromial space, ultimately impinging on the supraspinatus tendon.[10,29]

Because the adolescent and young adult populations maintain fairly high rates of chronic GHJ instability, impingement syndrome occurs more in people younger than 30 years than in older people. Also, it is the supraspinatus tendon, followed by the LHB, that are at most risk for injury, because irritation to the subacromial bursa in the form of bursitis usually occurs secondary to supraspinatus impingement.[30]

Rotator Cuff Tears

Though a tear of the rotator cuff muscle group can occur from a singular macrotrauma event, much like what happens when other muscle groups in the body are injured, this injury usually results from the patient participating in repetitive overhead activities. In addition to causing impingement syndrome, over time these activities degenerate the supraspinatus tendon. Initially, this degeneration causes microtearing of the tendon and, if not diagnosed and treated, microtears develop into macrotears. Indeed, a tear of the supraspinatus tendon is almost always precipitated by the patient having impingement syndrome for years. Supraspinatus tendon degeneration also occurs because the tendon is naturally **hypovascular** at its insertion on the greater tubercle of the humerus. Otherwise referred to as the tendon's *critical zone*, repetitively impinging this area decreases its ability to supply enough blood needed to keep the tissue healthy. This combination of factors makes the supraspinatus the most often torn of the rotator cuff muscle group.[30–34]

PEARL

The supraspinatus is the most often torn of the rotator cuff muscle group.

Because it takes years for supraspinatus tendon degeneration to occur, tears of the rotator cuff typically occur in people older than 40 years. In addition, as a person ages, the risk of having a more severe injury also increases. A patient closer to the age of 40 years usually experiences a partial-thickness, or *singular*, tear to the supraspinatus tendon, whereas older people are more likely to have a full-thickness, or *complete*, tear of the tendon. It is also common for older patients not to realize they have injured the rotator cuff. Indeed, one-third of all asymptomatic patients and half of all people older than 60 years have asymptomatic tears of the rotator cuff.[2,30-34]

PEARL

Impingement syndrome occurs more in those younger than 30 years, whereas people older than 40 years are more likely to experience a tear to the rotator cuff muscle group.

History and Physical Examination

Based on previous discussions, it should be obvious that the history portion of the assessment should determine the extent to which the patient is participating in overhead activities and the patient's age. Thus, opening questions should concentrate on these points. Once this information has been gathered, question the patient regarding the pain he or she is experiencing, because pain, accompanied by weakness and limited shoulder motion, is a hallmark sign of rotator cuff involvement. These patients usually report nonspecific tenderness around the shoulder, which is characteristically troublesome at night. This is particularly true if the person has a rotator cuff tear versus impingement syndrome. The patient may relate that pain radiates down the involved upper extremity, but recall that in these cases radiating pain rarely goes below the elbow.[1,4,10,29]

PEARL

Pain, weakness, and limited **ROM** are hallmark signs of rotator cuff injury.

When observed, the person with rotator cuff pathology may have noticeable atrophy of the deltoid, because this muscle is often affected by tears and impingement of the supraspinatus. These patients are also tender over the anterolateral part of the shoulder. People with impingement syndrome also experience pain within the painful arc, because it is in this range that the supraspinatus tendon compresses against the coracoacromial arch. In severe cases of impingement syndrome and in moderate to severe cases of a rotator cuff tear, the person is unable to abduct the GHJ fully, with the amount of abduction lost directly related to the severity of injury (i.e., the more abduction is lost, the more serious the injury is). In some but not all cases of a torn rotator cuff, the patient experiences limited passive GHJ motion. Those with impingement of the subacromial bursa without a rotator cuff tear often demonstrate weakness of the rotator cuff secondary to pain, particularly when the upper extremity moves through the painful arc.[1,5,29,32]

Pain produced by **Neer's impingement test** and/or the **Hawkins-Kennedy test** confirms the presence of impingement syndrome. To perform these tests, position yourself either lateral or posterior to the standing patient. Administer Neer's test by passively flexing the shoulder with the elbow extended and the GHJ in internal rotation (Fig. 11.20). As maximum flexion is approached, monitor the patient's response, because pain is indicative of impinging the supraspinatus tendon and/or LHB.[31]

To perform the Hawkins-Kennedy test (Fig. 11.21)[4,5]

- Instruct the patient to flex both the shoulder and the elbow to 90°.
- While supporting the upper extremity, passively internally rotate the GHJ.
- As maximum internal rotation is approached, monitor the patient's response. Pain occurs when the supraspinatus tendon becomes impinged between the greater tubercle and the coracoacromial arch.

Use the **drop arm test, empty can test,** and **full can test** to determine whether the patient has a torn rotator cuff. Positive signs for the empty and full can tests, though more sensitive for a supraspinatus tear, may also indicate the presence of impingement syndrome. For all of these tests, position yourself directly in front of the standing or seated patient. To perform the drop arm test (Fig. 11.22)[4,5,30]

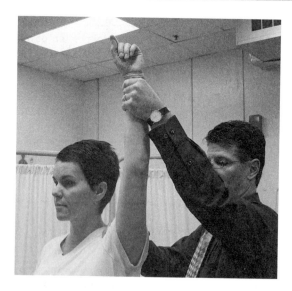

FIGURE 11.20 Neer's impingement test is used to determine whether subacromial impingement syndrome exists.

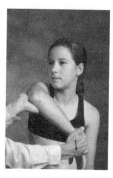

FIGURE 11.21 Hawkins-Kennedy impingement test is used to determine whether subacromial impingement syndrome exists.
From Gulick: *Ortho Notes, Clinical Examination Pocket Guide.* Philadelphia: F.A. Davis Company, pg 52, with permission.

• Instruct the patient to fully abduct the GHJ.
• With the patient in this position, tell the patient to slowly lower the raised upper extremity.
• Though the patient may be able to control the extremity's descent for the first 90°, a positive test occurs if the person "drops" the upper extremity to the side during the last 90° of motion, because a torn rotator cuff prohibits the upper extremity from controlling the extremity's descent throughout the range.

In preparation to administer the empty and full can tests, instruct the patient to abduct the GHJ to 90°. With the patient in this position, move the affected shoulder into 30° horizontal adduction. To perform the empty can test, tell the patient to point the thumb to the floor, mimicking the motion one would perform to empty a can of soda. Instruct the patient to resist your attempts to push down on the forearm (Fig. 11.23). To perform the full can test, tell the patient to point the thumb up, mimicking the motion one would perform to hold a full can of soda. As with the empty can test, instruct the patient to resist your attempts to push down on the

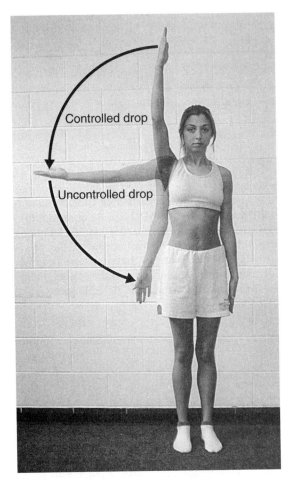

Controlled drop

Uncontrolled drop

FIGURE 11.22 The drop arm test determines whether the rotator cuff has been torn.
From Starkey and Ryan: *Evaluation of Orthopedic and Athletic Injuries*, 2nd ed. 2002. Philadelphia: F.A. Davis Company, Box 13-4, pg 449, with permission.

forearm. Positive full and empty can signs occur if these tests elicit pain or if the patient cannot fully resist the pressure you apply, and these positive signs are indicative of supraspinatus pathology.[4,5]

Management

As previously stated, obtaining x-rays during the initial management of overuse shoulder injury is usually not necessary. Thus, treat patients with rotator cuff and impingement injuries conservatively, because this remains the gold standard for managing these conditions. Initiate ROM and strengthening exercises as shown in PTH 11.1. Limit overhead activities until the patient has full ROM without pain. If improvements are not noted after 6 to 12 weeks, obtain AP, axillary, and supraspinatus outlet x-ray views. The AP view reveals superior migration of the humeral head, whereas the supraspinatus outlet view identifies narrowing of the subacromial space. Use the axillary radiograph to document evidence of GHJ instability commonly associated with impingement syndrome and rotator cuff injury.[2,8,30,31,35]

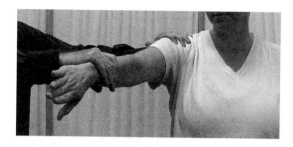

FIGURE 11.23 The empty can test. To perform the full can test, apply resistance to the patient's upper extremity with the thumb pointed up. These tests evaluate the integrity of the supraspinatus muscle tendon and determine the presence of subacromial impingement syndrome.

If plain-film radiographs reveal pathology or are inconclusive, obtain an MRI, because this is the preferred imaging technique for evaluating rotator cuff and impingement syndrome pathology. In addition to being able to diagnose partial- and full-thickness tears, an MRI can demonstrate the extent of cuff retraction and can evaluate the integrity of other soft tissues, including the subacromial bursa and LHB. Refer the patient to an orthopedist if the MRI or plain-film radiographs reveal pathology. If the results of these tests are negative, continue conservative treatment for another few months. If 6 months of nonoperative treatment fails, refer the patient for orthopedic evaluation and possible surgical intervention.[5,8,10,29,30,36]

PEARL

MRI is the preferred imaging technique for evaluating rotator cuff pathology.

Conditions of the Long Head of the Biceps Brachii Tendon

Pathological conditions of the LHB include injury to the tendon's attachment on the glenoid labrum (SLAP lesion), impingement within the subacromial space, rupture, tendonitis, and cases of subluxation and dislocation from the bicipital groove. Because SLAP lesions and impingement syndrome have already been discussed, this section concentrates on LHB rupture, tendonitis, subluxation, and dislocation.

Tendonitis, Subluxation, and Dislocation

As discussed in Chapter 1, most cases of tendonitis that occur throughout the body are actually tendinosis conditions. Though this holds true in most instances in which the LHB becomes irritated, the term *tendonitis* is used throughout this discussion, because this is what is traditionally used in the clinical setting. Furthermore, because LHB tendonitis is closely associated with tendon subluxation and, to some extent, tendon dislocation, these conditions are presented together.

Because the LHB is held within the bicipital groove by the CHL and the superior GHL, pathology involving these structures, including GHJ instability, can injure the LHB. In addition, because the LHB is located in the subacromial space, the same mechanisms that traumatize the supraspinatus also injure this tendon. Consequently, this means that most cases of LHB tendonitis, and all instances of subluxation and dislocation, are associated with impingement syndrome and/or supraspinatus tears. Furthermore, when the LHB dislocates, it does so medially, causing the tendon to invade the substance of the subscapularis near its attachment on the lesser tubercle of the humerus. This action tears the subscapularis, making injury to this muscle, along with supraspinatus pathology, present in all cases of LHB dislocation.[31,37,38]

PEARL

Most cases of LHB tendonitis, and all instances of subluxation and dislocation, are associated with impingement syndrome and tears of the supraspinatus and subscapularis.

Whereas all instances of LHB instability are associated with rotator cuff injury, only cases of secondary tendonitis are related to rotator cuff pathology. As its name implies, this condition occurs secondary to another condition, the most common being impingement syndrome. It results from the LHB wearing away as it rubs against the coracoacromial arch and is usually seen in the latter stages of impingement syndrome. Secondary tendonitis also occurs when the LHB becomes irritated as it rubs over the lesser tubercle of the humerus in cases of subluxation and dislocation. In contrast, primary tendonitis of the LHB occurs in isolation of rotator cuff pathology, only affecting the portion of the tendon located in the bicipital groove. It accounts for a small fraction of all LHB tendonitis cases, and when it does arise, it is usually seen in younger people, because primary tendonitis rarely occurs in older patients.[31,38,39]

History and Physical Examination

As might be expected, it can be difficult to distinguish LHB pathology from rotator cuff involvement, because the patient's history and reported symptoms caused by these conditions are very similar. For example, as with most cases of impingement syndrome, people with LHB pathology usually cannot recall definitive traumatic episodes that caused the onset of pain. Patients also report general shoulder pain that increases when they perform overhead activities, worsens at night, and radiates down the arm— all common symptoms of a rotator cuff tear and/or impingement syndrome.[38]

To differentiate among these conditions, ask the patient to pinpoint the painful area. If LHB pathology is present, the patient usually identifies the anterior portion of the shoulder as being the most painful. This can be confirmed by palpating the LHB in the bicipital groove. A subluxating LHB can be documented by feeling and listening for a snap as the patient actively moves the GHJ through its ROM. Pain occurring in the bicipital groove as the patient flexes the shoulder against resistance with the elbow extended, known as *Speed's test*, indicates the presence of tendonitis. **Yergason's test** is used to check for both tendonitis and subluxation. To perform this test (Fig. 11.24)[1,19,29,31,38,39]

- Instruct the patient to pronate the forearm and flex the elbow to 90°, keeping the upper extremity firmly positioned at the side of the body.
- Standing next to the patient, hold the person's wrist and elbow.
- Resist the patient as you tell him or her to supinate the forearm, flex the elbow, and externally rotate the GHJ.
- Pain in the bicipital groove is positive for tendonitis; a dislodging of the tendon from the bicipital groove is indicative of a subluxation.

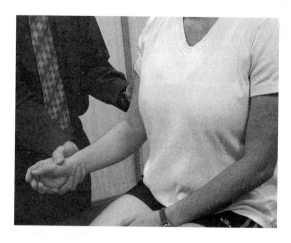

FIGURE 11.24 Yergason's test assesses for long head of the biceps brachii tendonitis and subluxation.

Because the prevalence of LHB tendonitis, subluxation, and dislocation are closely associated with impingement syndrome and rotator cuff tears, be sure to evaluate for these conditions when assessing the LHB. Also, administer the **lift-off test**, shown in Figure 11.25, to check the strength of the subscapularis muscle, because weakness with this test is indicative of LHB pathology.[5,38]

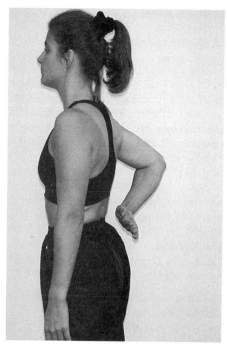

FIGURE 11.25 The lift-off test. An inability to lift the hand off the spine indicates subscapularis weakness, which is indicative of long head of the biceps brachii tendon pathology.
From Starkey and Ryan: *Evaluation of Orthopedic and Athletic Injuries*, 2nd ed. 2002. Philadelphia: F.A. Davis Company, Box 13-7, pg 455, with permission.

Management

Manage secondary LHB tendonitis by focusing on treating the associated rotator cuff pathology. Thus, initially use the conservative treatment protocol outlined for rotator cuff tears and impingement syndrome for this condition. Refer people who do not respond to conservative treatment to an orthopedist. In contrast, immediately refer to an orthopedist all patients with suspected LHB subluxation or dislocation. These conditions are treated either conservatively or surgically, depending on the severity of the condition and physician preference. Both conservative and operative treatments for LHB instability concentrate on treating the underlying rotator cuff pathology.[38]

Biceps Rupture

Traumatic rupture of a healthy LHB is an uncommon event. Thus, an LHB tear is typically a consequence of impingement syndrome, rotator cuff tear, or secondary tendonitis. However, when rotator cuff irritation occurs in conjunction with secondary tendonitis of the LHB, the supraspinatus tendon is much more apt to rupture than is the biceps tendon. When the LHB does rupture, the tear usually occurs around the site of the bicipital groove, sparing from injury its attachment at the glenoid labrum.[31,38]

A rupture of the LHB is usually the consequence of impingement syndrome, rotator cuff tear, or secondary tendonitis pathology.

History and Physical Examination

While obtaining a patient history, be sure to ask the person whether they had been experiencing discomfort before the injury, because an LHB rupture is usually preceded by a prolonged period of anterior shoulder pain. At the time of injury, the patient reports hearing an audible "pop" or "snap," which made this pain disappear. Extensive bruising traveling the length of the anterior portion of the person's arm and forearm is common after this injury. Though affected patients are able to flex the elbow and supinate the forearm, motions that are performed by the biceps brachii, they do so with decreased strength. Manual muscle testing for these actions, as discussed in Chapter 12, confirms these strength deficits. Note that when the biceps brachii contracts, a bunching of the injured muscle and tendon occurs in the distal portion of the anterior arm. Otherwise known as the *Popeye sign*, this refers to the bulge created by the bunching. Use **Ludington's test** to confirm an LHB rupture. To perform this test (Fig. 11.26)[1,38]

- Instruct the patient to place his or her interlocked fingers on top of the head.
- Standing behind the patient, bilaterally palpate the bicipital grooves.
- Tell the patient to contact the biceps by pushing his or her hands down against the top of the head.
- A positive sign is elicited if you cannot feel the long head of the biceps tendon in its groove or if no contraction is felt on the involved side.

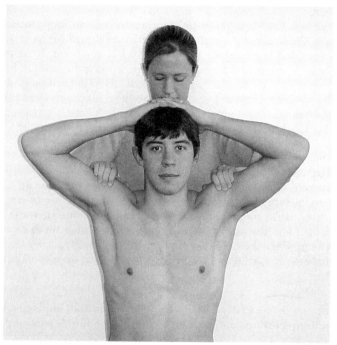

FIGURE 11.26 Ludington's test assesses the integrity of the long head of the biceps brachii tendon.
From Starkey and Ryan: *Evaluation of Orthopedic and Athletic Injuries,* 2nd ed. 2004. Philadelphia: F.A. Davis Company, Box 13-22, pg 479, with permission.

Management
Immediately place the upper extremity of the patient with an LHB rupture in sling, as shown in Figure 6.1 on page 129, and refer the patient to an orthopedist. A decision on conservative versus surgical treatment is based on a number of factors, including the patient's age and future planned activity level. Surgical intervention is indicated for patients who desire to return to physical activity, whereas those who need only to perform activities of daily living usually do fine with conservative measures. Regardless, all patients are also treated for whatever underlying rotator cuff pathology exists.[1,31,38]

Lifespan Considerations

Though not necessarily caused by sports participation, adhesive capsulitis, otherwise known as *frozen shoulder syndrome* (FSS), deserves special mention because of the effects it has on the shoulder complex and entire upper extremity.

Adhesive Capsulitis
Identified by painful restriction of active and passive GHJ motion, FSS develops because of prolonged immobilization of the shoulder complex, either by having

the upper extremity in a sling for an extended period or from not using the shoulder because of some underlying pathology. It is most commonly seen in patients aged 40 to 70 years and affects women more than men. Additionally, people with diabetes mellitus, hyperthyroidism, ischemic heart disease, and cervical spondylolysis maintain an increased risk of developing this condition.[2,35]

FSS is most commonly seen in patients aged 40 to 70 years and affects women more than men.

When FSS develops from being immobilized in a sling, the reason for the immobilization may or may not be an injured shoulder. For example, the upper extremity may be immobilized for GHJ instability, or it may be in a sling as part of a treatment plan for elbow pathology. In either case, it is extremely important to prevent this condition from occurring. Do this by initiating shoulder ROM exercises as outlined in PTH 11.1 as soon as possible after any injury that necessitates immobilization of the shoulder.[35]

Prevent FSS by initiating shoulder ROM exercises as soon as possible after any injury that necessitates immobilization of the shoulder.

When FSS results from underlying pathology, patients limit the amount they use the shoulder because of pain. Doing this leads to increased discomfort when patients attempt to move the GHJ. Subsequently, this discomfort causes patients to further limit the amount they use the shoulder. The result of repeating the vicious cycle of not using the shoulder because of pain results is an almost total loss of shoulder function.[2]

The primary concerns from patients with FSS are shoulder stiffness and a loss of motion. Other concerns include pain, localized discomfort near the deltoid's insertion on the humerus, and an inability to sleep on the affected side. Before settling on a diagnosis of FSS, determine how long the patient has experienced these symptoms. Make the diagnosis if painful loss of shoulder motion, with or without underlying pathology, has either plateaued or worsened over a period of 1 month. Though all motions of the GHJ can be affected, the most common include[1,4,35]

- active abduction,
- assisted internal rotation,
- passive flexion,
- external and internal rotation with the GHJ at 90° abduction, and
- external rotation with the GHJ.

Once a diagnosis of FSS is made, determine whether the patient's limited shoulder motion is related to cervical spine pathology. Thus, perform cervical ROM and strength tests, and check the patient's upper extremity neurological status, as described previously in this chapter. If any neurological abnormalities are detected, refer the patient to an orthopedist or neurosurgeon.[35]

Once cervical spine injury has been ruled out, obtain AP, axillary, and supraspinatus outlet plain-film radiographs of the shoulder for patients with FSS. Though x-rays cannot detect the presence of this syndrome, use them to check for the presence of other shoulder pathology. If x-rays are negative, proceed with restoring the patient's shoulder function by reducing the person's pain and by increasing motion. Instruct the patient to perform ROM exercises as outlined in PTH 11.1. Even though FSS is one of the most difficult dysfunctions of the shoulder to treat, in most cases shoulder function returns to its preinjury state.[2,35]

In instances in which FSS has been present for more than 2 months and in cases where the patient is in severe pain, consider initiating a tapered course of oral corticosteroid treatment, such as prednisone, in lieu of other anti-inflammatory agents. If this treatment option is pursued, use it for only a few weeks, making sure the patient is free of conditions that are contraindicated for oral corticosteroid use, such as diabetes mellitus. If 3 months of conservative treatment does not produce the desired results, refer the patient to an orthopedist for possible surgical intervention.[2,35]

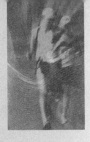

CASE STUDY
Conditions Involving the Cervical Spine, Shoulder Complex, and Arm

SCENARIO
A 47-year-old man comes to your practice reporting ongoing left shoulder pain. He cannot pinpoint an exact date of injury, only stating a gradual onset of pain and discomfort over the past few years. Though he maintains an office job that does not require a great deal of strenuous activity, he does participate in a year-round tennis league requiring him to play once a week. He also partakes in an occasional weekend tournament. When he was younger, he was an active baseball player, playing until he graduated from college at age 22. He then participated in competitive softball in his 20s, only to discontinue playing in his early 30s, in part because of a diagnosed case of shoulder impingement syndrome, a condition he had experienced on and off since college. At age 40, he began playing tennis to lose weight, lower his total cholesterol count, and get into better physical shape. Though he reports experiencing discomfort and pain for quite some time, these symptoms have only recently affected his ability to play tennis.

PERTINENT HISTORY
Medications: Currently taking sporadic doses of aspirin when his shoulder pain increases. No other medications except for a daily multivitamin.

Family History: Father died of prostate cancer at age 67. No other significant family history.

PERSONAL HEALTH HISTORY
Tobacco Use: Denies smoking cigarettes or oral tobacco use.

Recreational Drugs: Denies use.

Alcohol Intake: 1 to 2 drinks per day, sometime more on weekends, particularly when he participates in a tennis tournament.

Caffeinated Beverages: 2 to 3 morning cups of coffee per day.

Exercise: Tennis once per week and an occasional weekend tournament requiring anywhere from two to six matches of play.

Past Medical History: Physical examination at age 40 revealed borderline high total cholesterol, which is currently within normal limits. Childhood mumps and chickenpox, though he cannot remember the ages at which these occurred.

PERTINENT PHYSICAL EXAMINATION*
The patient carries the left upper extremity normally, and the involved shoulder appears symmetrical with the uninvolved. His rotator cuff is point tender at its insertion site on the greater tubercle of the humerus. Though he maintains full ROM pain increases during the terminal ends of GHJ abduction and flexion. Strength is normal except for GHJ abduction, which is considerably weaker than on the contralateral side. The drop arm and empty and full can tests are positive, as are the Neer's and Hawkins-Kennedy tests.

*Focused examination limited to key points for this case.

(case study continues on page 358)

CASE STUDY
Conditions Involving the Cervical Spine, Shoulder Complex, and Arm (continued)

RED FLAGS FOR THE PRIMARY HEALTH CARE PROFESSIONAL TO CONSIDER

- A person older than 40 years with a history of impingement syndrome maintains a higher risk of developing a tear to the rotator cuff.
- A positive drop arm test is indicative of a supraspinatus tear.
- Positive drop arm and empty and full can tests indicate a supraspinatus tear or impingement of this muscle's tendon.
- Positive Neer's and Hawkins-Kennedy tests indicate the presence of impingement syndrome.

RECOMMENDED PLAN

- Refer to an orthopedist for evaluation because a definitive diagnosis between a supraspinatus tear and impingement syndrome must be made. Both conditions may be present.
- Change the course of oral anti-inflammatory treatment to ibuprofen 800 mg tid.
- Provide the patient with a written home management care plan that he can use while waiting to see the orthopedist. Include in this plan shoulder ROM and strengthening exercises, avoiding the risk-increasing activities of terminal GHJ flexion and abduction.

REFERENCES

1. Clarnette RG, Miniaci A. Clinical exam of the shoulder. *Med Sci Sports Exerc* 1998;30(4 suppl):S1.
2. Glockner SM. Shoulder pain: a diagnostic dilemma. *Am Fam Physician* 1995;51:1677.
3. Malanga GA. The diagnosis and treatment of cervical radiculopathy. *Med Sci Sports Exerc* 1997;29(7 suppl):S236.
4. Woodward TW, Best TM. The painful shoulder, part I: clinical evaluation. *Am Fam Physician* 2000;61:3079.
5. Stevenson JH, Trojian T. Evaluation of shoulder pain. *J Fam Pract* 2002;51:605.
6. Gore DR, Sepic SB, Gardner GM. Roentgenographic findings of the cervical spine in asymptomatic people. *Spine* 1986;11:521.
7. American College of Radiology Practice Guidelines for the Performance of Radiography of the Extremities, 2003 (Res. 11). Effective 10/1/03. Retrieved from: http://www.acr.org. Accessed 8/28/08.
8. American College of Radiology Appropriate Radiographic Criteria for Acute Shoulder Trauma. Retrieved from: http://www.acr.org. Accessed 8/28/08.
9. McKinnis LN. *Fundamentals of Musculoskeletal Imaging*, 2nd ed. Philadelphia, PA: FA Davis Co., 2005.
10. Ertl JP, Kovacs G, Brugr RS. Magnetic resonance imaging of the shoulder in the primary care setting. *Med Sci Sports Exerc* 1998;30(4 suppl):S7.
11. Radhakrishnan K, Litchy WJ, O'Fallon WM. Epidemiology of cervical radiculopathy: a population-based study from Rochester, Minnesota, 1976 through 1990. *Brain* 1994;117:325.
12. Cantu RC. Stingers, transient quadriplegia, and cervical spinal stenosis: return to play criteria. *Med Sci Sports Exerc* 1997;29(7 suppl):S223.
13. Page S, Guy JA. Neurapraxia, "stingers," and spinal stenosis in athletes. *South Med J* 2004;97:766.
14. Levitz CL, Reilly PT, Torg JS. The pathomechanism of chronic recurrent cervical nerve root neurapraxia: the chronic burner syndrome. *Am J Sports Med* 1997;25:73.
15. Park MC, Blaine TA, Levine WN. Shoulder dislocation in young athletes: current concepts in management. *Phys Sportsmed* 2002;30(12):41.
16. Cofield RH, Irving JF. Evaluation and classification of shoulder instability: with special reference to examination under anesthesia. *Clin Orthop Relat Res* 1987;223:32.
17. Ceroni D, Sadri H, Leuenberger A. Radiographic evaluation of anterior shoulder dislocation of the shoulder. *Acta Radiol* 2001;41:658.
18. Warme WJ, Arciero RA, Taylor DC. Anterior shoulder instability in sport: current management recommendations. *Sports Med* 1999;28(3):209.
19. Line L, Murret L. Labral tears: diagnosis, treatment and rehabilitation. *Athl Ther Today* 1999;4(4):18.
20. Field LD, Savoie FH. Arthroscopic suture repair of superior labral detachment lesions of the shoulder. *Am J Sports Med* 1993;21:783
21. Turnbull JR. Acromioclavicular joint disorders. *Med Sci Sports Exerc* 1998; 30(4 suppl):S26.
22. Wroble RR. Sternoclavicular injuries: managing damage to an overlooked joint. *Phys Sportsmed* 1995;23(9):19.
23. Williams C. Posterior sternoclavicular joint dislocation. *Phys Sportsmed* 1999;27(2):105.
24. Prime HT, Boig SG, Hooper JC. Retrosternal dislocation of the clavicle: a case report. *Am J Sports Med* 1991;19:92.
25. Heare MM, Heare TC, Gillespy T. Diagnostic imaging of pelvic and chest wall trauma. *Radiol Clin North Am* 1989;27:873.
26. Stephens M, Wolin PM, Tarbet JA, et al. Osteolysis of the distal clavicle: readily detected and treated shoulder pain. *Phys Sportsmed* 2000;28(12):35.
27. Scavenius M, Iversen BF. Nontraumatic clavicular osteolysis in weight lifters. *Am J Sports Med* 1992;20:463.
28. Van der Windt DA, Koes BW, De Jong BA, et al. Shoulder disorders in general practice: incidence, patient characteristics and management. *Ann Rheum Dis* 1995;54:959.
29. Rodgers JA, Crosby LA. Rotator cuff disorders. *Am Fam Physician* 1996;54:127.

30. Trojian T, Stevenson JH, Agrawal N. What can we expect from nonoperative treatment options for shoulder pain? *J Fam Pract* 2005;54(3):216.
31. Neer CS. Impingement lesions. *Clin Orthop* 1983;173:70.
32. Norwood LA, Barrack R, Jacobson KE. Clinical presentation of complete tears of the rotator cuff. *J Bone Joint Surg Am* 1989;71:449.
33. Lohr JF, Uhthoff HK. The microvascular pattern of the supraspinatus tendon. *Clin Orthop* 1990;254:35.
34. Sher JS, Urbie JW, Posada A, et al. Abnormal findings on magnetic resonance images of asymptomatic shoulders. *J Bone Joint Surg Am* 1995;77-A:10.
35. Pearsall AW, Speer KP. Frozen shoulder syndrome: diagnostic and treatment strategies in the primary care setting. *Med Sci Sports Exerc* 1998;30(4 suppl):S33.
36. Mantone JK, Burkhead WZ, Noonan J. Nonoperative treatment of rotator cuff tears. *Orthop Clin North Am* 2000;31:295.
37. Walch G, Nové-Josserand L, Boileau P, et al. Subluxations and dislocations of the tendon of the long head of the biceps. *J Shoulder Elbow Surg* 1998;7:100.
38. Patton WC, McCluskey GM. Biceps tendonitis and subluxation. *Clin Sports Med* 2001;20:505.
39. Post D, Benca P. Primary tendonitis of the long head of the biceps. *Clin Orthop* 1989;246:117.

SUGGESTED READINGS

Quillen DM, Wuchner M, Hatch RL. Acute shoulder injuries. *Am Fam Physician* 2004;70:1947.

Whiteside JW. Management of head and neck injuries by the sideline physician. *Am Fam Physician* 2006;74:1357.

Woodward TW, Best TM. The painful shoulder, part II: acute and chronic disorders. *Am Fam Physician* 2000;61:3291.

WEB LINKS

http://www.emedicine.com/sports/topic115.htm. Accessed 8/28/08.

Web site devoted to the rotator cuff. Provides an in-depth look at rotator cuff injury, including functional anatomy, sports biomechanics, and imaging studies related to the rotator cuff.

http://www.nlm.nih.gov/medlineplus/shoulderinjuriesanddisorders.html. Accessed 8/28/08.

All-inclusive government Web site dedicated to shoulder injuries and disorders. Useful for both patients and practitioners.

http://www.hughston.com/hha/pdf/vol13no1.pdf. Accessed 8/28/08.

Health alert publication reporting on shoulder injuries in children and adolescents. Excellent resource for providers working with these populations.

12

Conditions Involving the Elbow, Forearm, Wrist, and Hand

● **Brian J. Toy, PhD, ATC**

The elbow and forearm compose the area of the upper extremity between the arm and the wrist, whereas the wrist and hand compose the areas distal to the forearm. These body parts are complex structures. This is particularly true when talking about the wrist and hand, which ultimately present a challenge to any health care provider attempting to evaluate musculoskeletal injury to them.

Anatomy of the Elbow, Forearm, Wrist, and Hand

Pertinent anatomical structures of the elbow, forearm, wrist, and hand include bones, ligaments, muscles, tendons, bursae, and nerves. Remember that all directional terms used relate to the body in its anatomical position. Though true when discussing anatomy throughout the body, this fact is particularly relevant here because pronating (palm down) and supinating (palm up) the forearm vastly changes the position of these structures.

Bones and Joints (Figs. 12.1 and 12.2)

Bones that encompass the elbow and forearm include the humerus, radius, and ulna. Those of the wrist and hand include the carpals, metacarpals, and phalangeals.

Remember that the humerus is the largest long bone of the upper extremity. Its bony prominences in this area include the capitulum, trochlea, and lateral and medial epicondyles. The olecranon fossa, a posteriorly situated depression, is located at the distal end of the humerus, whereas the cubital tunnel is situated just lateral to the medial epicondyle. It is through this tunnel that the ulnar nerve passes as it traverses from the arm to the forearm. The elbow joint is formed when the distal portions of the humerus articulate with the proximal portions of the radius and ulna. Specifically, the head of the radius articulates with the capitulum, the trochlea notch of the ulna articulates with the trochlea, and the olecranon process of the ulna fits into the olecranon fossa. The radius is smaller proximally and larger distally, whereas the ulna's proximal segment is larger than its distal portion. The radius and ulna also articulate with one another to form the proximal radioulnar joint (PRUJ) and distal radioulnar joint (DRUJ). The shafts of these bones are attached by an interosseous membrane that runs the length of the forearm from the PRUJ to the DRUJ. Finally, the radius and ulna each maintain a styloid process at their terminus.

Composed of eight irregularly shaped bones, the carpal region is divided into two rows of four bones each. Together, these are commonly referred to as the *wrist bones*. From lateral to medial, the proximal row consists of the scaphoid, lunate, triquetrum, and pisiform. It is primarily the scaphoid and lunate that articulate with the distal radius to form the wrist joint, otherwise known as the *radiocarpal joint* (RCJ). This is the joint that produces the motions most commonly associated with the wrist (discussed later in this chapter). Note that because the ulna does not project as far distal as the radius, it is not involved in the bony makeup of the wrist joint. Also, be aware that for many years, the scaphoid was referred to as the *navicular*, though currently most health providers use the term *scaphoid* to identify this bone.

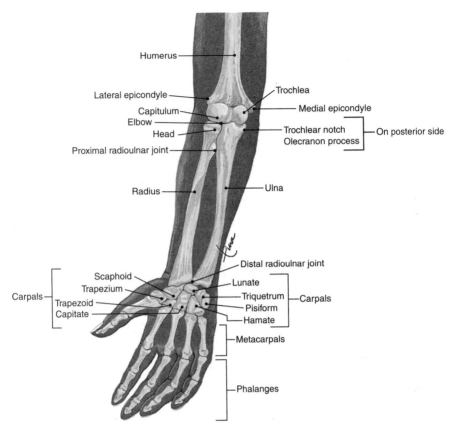

FIGURE 12.1 Bones and joints of the elbow, forearm, wrist, and hand.
Adapted from Scanlon: *Essentials of Anatomy and Physiology*, 5th ed. 2007. Philadelphia: F.A. Davis Company, Fig. 6-12, pg 124, with permission.

The distal row of carpal bones includes the trapezium, trapezoid, capitate, and hamate. The hamate maintains a "hook" that arises from its ventral aspect. This structure forms the roof of Guyon's canal, a passage that allows the arteries, veins, and, most importantly, the ulnar nerve, to pass from the wrist to the hand. Though by and large the bones of the proximal row articulate with at least one bone of the distal row, it is the scaphoid that provides the primary link between the two rows of carpals. As a group, the articulations that occur between adjoining carpal bones are referred to as the intercarpal (IC) joints. The small amount of motion produced by each of these gliding joints allows the RCJ to function properly. Of note is the scapholunate joint (SLJ), because this is the IC joint most commonly involved in instances of carpal instability.

Lying distal to the carpals, the five metacarpals, or *hand bones*, are numbered one through five going lateral to medial. They function to connect the carpals to the phalanges. Composed of 14 long bones, the phalangeal region is composed of five digits

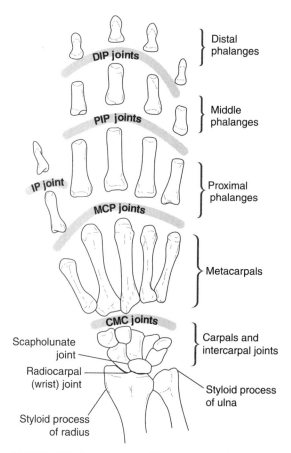

FIGURE 12.2 Bones and joints of the wrist and hand. CMC = carpometacarpal; DIP = distal interphalangeal; IP = interphalangeal; MCP = metacarpophalangeal; PIP = proximal interphalangeal. Adapted from Lippert: *Clinical Kinesiology and Anatomy*, 4th ed. 2006. Philadelphia: F.A. Davis Company, Fig. 12-1, pg 144, with permission.

that are divided into four fingers and a thumb. Whereas each finger maintains a proximal, middle, and distal phalanx, the thumb has only a proximal and distal phalanx. When observed medial to lateral, the fingers are designated as follows: little, ring, middle, and index.

With so many bones composing it, the hand maintains an abundance of articulations. These include the carpometacarpal (CMC) joints, which are formed by the distal row of carpal bones articulating with the metacarpals. Though the second through fifth CMC joints do not move much, the first CMC joint is extremely mobile. Distally, the metacarpophalangeal (MCP) joints are formed when each metacarpal articulates with its corresponding proximal phalange. In layperson's terms, these joints are referred to as the *knuckles*. The proximal interphalangeal (PIP) joints are formed by the articulations between the proximal and middle phalanges of each finger, whereas the distal interphalangeal (DIP) joints are formed by the articulations between the middle and distal phalanges. The joint between the proximal and distal phalanx of the thumb is simply known as the interphalangeal (IP) joint of the thumb.

Motions

Classified as a true hinge joint, the elbow is able to flex 145°, with extension occurring as the elbow returns to the anatomical position (Fig. 12.3). Whereas soft tissues prevent other hinge joints, such as the knee, from hyperextending, elbow hyperextension is prevented by the olecranon process as it enters the olecranon fossa during extension. This bony block, unique to the elbow, predisposes this joint to bony injury from acute trauma.

The PRUJ and DRUJ are pivot joints, because their only movement is rotational. The unique terms of *supination* and *pronation* are used to describe forearm rotation (Fig. 12.4). These actions are produced by the radius rotating around the fixed ulna. With the forearm in a in a neutral, thumbs-up position (i.e., handshake position) and the elbow flexed 90°, the forearm can both supinate and pronate 90°, giving the PRUJ and DRUJ a combined 180° of motion. In contrast, the RCJ is a condyloid joint, allowing for the motions of flexion (85°), hyperextension (75°), abduction (20°), and adduction (35°) (Fig. 12.5). The specialized terms of radial and ulnar deviation are used to describe the motions of wrist abduction and adduction, respectively.

As with the RCJ, the MCP joints are condyloid in nature, whereas the PIP and DIP joints of the fingers, as well as the IP joint of the thumb, are all hinge joints (Fig. 12.6). Though the CMC joints of the fingers can flex and extend, as previously mentioned these joints maintain very little motion. However, the CMC joint of the thumb is classified as a saddle joint because it can perform the action of opposition (touching its distal phalanx with the distal phalanx of the fingers) in addition to being able to flex, extend, abduct, and adduct.

Ligaments, Bursae, and Nerves

Remember from Chapter 1 that medial and lateral joint stability for all hinge and condyloid joints is provided by collateral ligaments. Thus, the elbow is supported by the

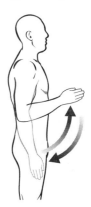

FIGURE 12.3 Elbow flexion and extension.
Adapted from Lippert: *Clinical Kinesiology and Anatomy*, 4th ed. 2006. Philadelphia: F.A. Davis Company, Fig. 10-2, pg 122, with permission.

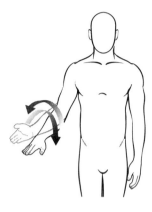

FIGURE 12.4 Forearm supination and pronation. Adapted from Lippert: *Clinical Kinesiology and Anatomy*, 4th ed. 2006. Philadelphia: F.A. Davis Company, Fig. 10-4, pg 122, with permission.

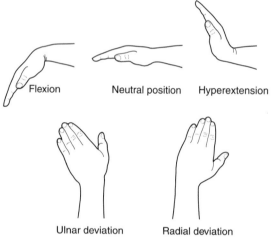

Flexion   Neutral position   Hyperextension

Ulnar deviation   Radial deviation

FIGURE 12.5 Motions of the wrist (radiocarpal joint). Adapted from Lippert: *Clinical Kinesiology and Anatomy*, 4th ed. 2006. Philadelphia: F.A. Davis Company, Fig. 11-2, pg 134, with permission.

medial, or ulnar, collateral ligament (UCL) and by the lateral, or radial, collateral ligament (RCL) (Fig. 12.7). Named for their respective distal attachments on the ulna and radius, the UCL originates from the medial epicondyle, whereas the RCL originates from the lateral epicondyle. Other collateral ligaments in this region include the UCL and RCL of the RCJ (Fig. 12.8) and the medial collateral (MCL) and lateral collateral (LCL) ligaments associated with each MCP and IP joint. Remember, each MCL prevents valgus forces from injuring its associated joint, whereas each LCL protects its joint from varus force injury.

Supporting the PRUJ is the annular ligament (Fig. 12.7). Unique in the fact that both its attachment points are on the ulna, this ligament wraps around the head of the

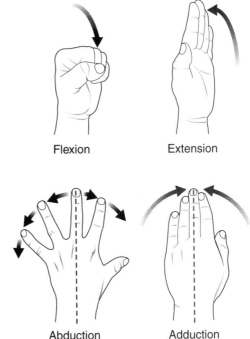

Flexion   Extension

Abduction   Adduction

FIGURE 12.6 Flexion/extension of the metacarpophalangeal and interphalangeal joints and abduction/adduction of the metacarpophalangeal joints. From Lippert: *Clinical Kinesiology and Anatomy*, 4th ed. 2006. Philadelphia: F.A. Davis Company, Fig. 12-5, pg 145, with permission.

radius, effectively holding the radial head next to the ulna. As a group, the ligaments supporting the IC joints are termed *IC ligaments*. These ligaments attach specific carpal bones together, creating a vast network of ligamentous tissue on both the dorsal and ventral aspects of the carpals (Fig. 12.8). Of note is the scapholunate ligament (SLL), connecting the scaphoid and lunate bones, and the ventrally located transverse carpal ligament, because it is this structure that forms the roof of the **carpal tunnel** (Fig. 12.9).

Though many bursae are located throughout this region, the olecranon bursa is the one injured most often. Located between the skin and the olecranon process,

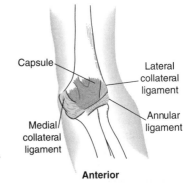

Capsule

Lateral collateral ligament

Annular ligament

Medial collateral ligament

Anterior

FIGURE 12.7 Ligaments of the elbow and proximal radioulnar joints. From Lippert: *Clinical Kinesiology and Anatomy*, 4th ed. 2006. Philadelphia: F.A. Davis Company, Fig. 10-11, pg 125, with permission.

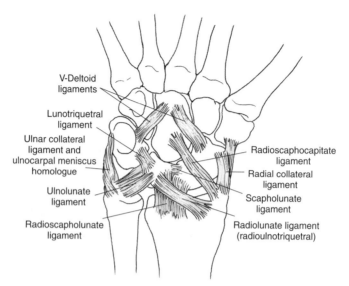

FIGURE 12.8 Radial collateral and ulnar collateral ligaments of the wrist. The intercarpal ligaments, of which the scapholunate is one, are also shown. Adapted from Levangie and Norkin: *Joint Structure and Function: A Comprehensive Analysis*, 4th ed. 2005. Philadelphia: F.A. Davis Company, Fig. 9-7, pg 311, with permission.

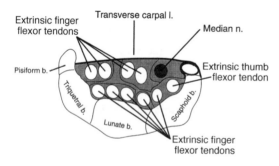

FIGURE 12.9 The carpal tunnel. Patients experience carpal tunnel syndrome when the median nerve becomes entrapped within this tunnel. Adapted from Starkey and Ryan: *Evaluation of Orthopedic and Athletic Injuries*, 2nd ed. 2002. Philadelphia: F.A. Davis Company, Fig. 15-8, pg 528, with permission.

this bursa protects the olecranon from direct trauma. The three primary nerves in this region—ulnar, radial, and median—provide the hand with its sensory distribution, as shown in Figure 12.10. The ulnar nerve is passed from the wrist to the hand through Guyon's canal, whereas the median nerve is passed to the hand through the carpal tunnel (Fig. 12.9). In addition to providing sensory distribution to the hand, these two nerves provide motor function to the hand's intrinsic muscles. Realize, however, that all three nerves provide motor function to the extrinsic muscles of the wrist and hand.

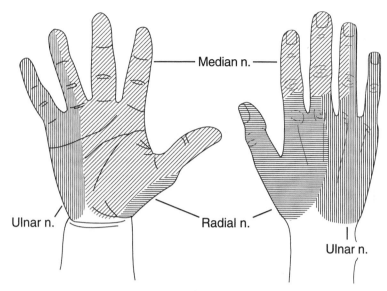

FIGURE 12.10 Sensory nerve distribution of the hand.
From Starkey and Ryan: *Evaluation of Orthopedic and Athletic Injuries*, 2nd ed. 2002.
Philadelphia: F.A. Davis Company, Fig. 15-9, pg 528, with permission.

Muscles and Tendons

The primary muscles that flex the elbow, the biceps brachii and brachialis, are located on the anterior aspect of the arm. The biceps brachii, which lies superficial to the brachialis, is also a major forearm supinator, whereas the pronator teres, a minor elbow flexor, is primarily responsible for forearm pronation (Fig. 12.11). Another elbow flexor, the brachioradialis, runs the length of the forearm after originating just superior to the lateral epicondyle (Fig. 12.12). The triceps, the prime elbow extensor, is located on the posterior aspect of the arm.

Muscles that move the hand are classified as either intrinsic or extrinsic based on where the muscles attach proximally. This site for all intrinsic hand muscles occurs entirely within the hand, whereas an extrinsic muscle originates from one or more of the following: humerus, radius, ulna, or interosseous membrane. All of these muscles maintain a distal attachment on one or more carpals or phalangeals. Muscles that solely attach to a carpal only move the RCJ, whereas those which attach to a phalanx act on both the wrist and the digit associated with the distal attachment.

The extrinsic muscles are located in two forearm compartments: anterior and posterior (Figs. 12.11 and 12.12). The posterior compartment muscles, which primarily extend the RCJ and/or fingers, originate from the lateral epicondyle via a common extensor tendon. The anterior compartment muscles originate from the medial epicondyle, ulna, and/or radius. This group is commonly referred to as the *flexor-pronator group,* because muscles within this compartment flex the wrist and fingers and, in the case of the pronator teres, pronate the forearm. Furthermore, when acting together, the medially located muscles within each compartment cause ulnar deviation, whereas the laterally positioned muscles radially deviate the RCJ.

Anterior view
Right arm

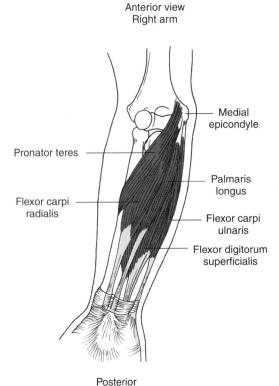

Pronator teres

Flexor carpi
radialis

Medial
epicondyle

Palmaris
longus

Flexor carpi
ulnaris

Flexor digitorum
superficialis

FIGURE 12.11 The anterior forearm muscles. The pronator teres pronates the forearm, whereas all others flex the wrist and/or the fingers. Note that some of these muscles attach to the medial humeral epicondyle.
From Levangie and Norkin: *Joint Structure and Function: A Comprehensive Analysis,* 4th ed. 2005. Philadelphia: F.A. Davis Company, Fig. 8-11A, pg 281, with permission.

Posterior
Right arm

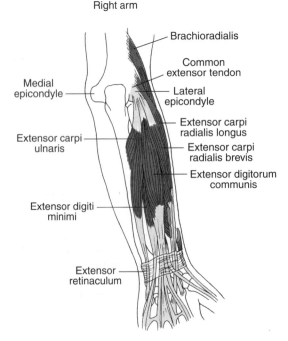

Brachioradialis

Common
extensor tendon

Medial
epicondyle

Lateral
epicondyle

Extensor carpi
radialis longus

Extensor carpi
ulnaris

Extensor carpi
radialis brevis

Extensor digitorum
communis

Extensor digiti
minimi

Extensor
retinaculum

FIGURE 12.12 The posterior forearm muscles, which contain the wrist and finger extensors, attach to the lateral humeral epicondyle via a common extensor tendon. Note that the brachioradialis muscle originates just above the lateral epicondyle. Adapted from Levangie and Norkin: *Joint Structure and Function: A Comprehensive Analysis,* 4th ed. 2005. Philadelphia: F.A. Davis Company, Fig. 8-11B, pg 281, with permission.

The extrinsic muscles of the thumb also originate from both compartments, the tendons of which form the borders of the **anatomic snuffbox**, a key anatomical landmark (Fig. 12.13). The tendons of the extrinsic muscles that flex the fingers and thumb pass through the carpal tunnel, as shown in Figure 12.9.

Intrinsic muscles of the hand are located in the **thenar eminence**, in the **hypothenar eminence**, and between the metacarpal bones (Fig. 12.14). The muscles located within the thenar eminence move the thumb and are innervated by the median nerve, whereas those within the hypothenar eminence act on the little finger and are innervated by the ulnar nerve. These nerves are also responsible for innervating the intrinsic muscles located between the metacarpals.

Examination of the Elbow, Forearm, Wrist, and Hand

As with most body regions, work proximal to distal when examining the elbow, forearm, wrist, and hand. Make sure to combine this information with what is presented in Chapter 7, because doing so ensures that all essential aspects of the evaluation are covered.

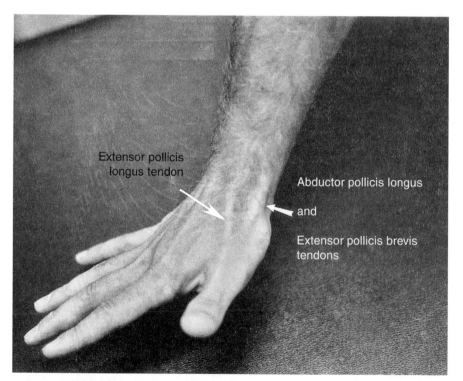

FIGURE 12.13 The anatomic snuffbox and its borders formed by the extrinsic thumb muscles. From Starkey and Ryan: *Evaluation of Orthopedic and Athletic Injuries*, 2nd ed. 2002. Philadelphia: F.A. Davis Company, Fig. 15-16, pg 535, with permission.

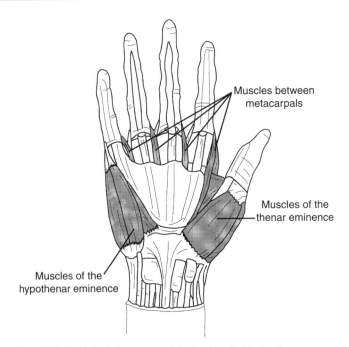

Muscles between
metacarpals

Muscles of the
thenar eminence

Muscles of the
hypothenar eminence

FIGURE 12.14 Intrinsic muscles of the hand located in the thenar eminence, in the hypothenar eminence, and between the metacarpal bones. Adapted from Starkey and Ryan: *Evaluation of Orthopedic and Athletic Injuries*, 2nd ed. 2002. Philadelphia: F.A. Davis Company, Fig. 15-7, pg 523, with permission.

History

As with any orthopedic evaluation, it is very important that a thorough history of how the injury occurred is obtained when examining the patient. This is particularly true when evaluating people with overuse injuries, because arriving at a differential diagnosis for these patients is mainly based on this portion of the assessment. Be aware that some injuries that occur in these areas, particularly those of the wrist and hand, have a poor outcome if they go unrecognized.[1]

Injuries that occur in the wrist and hand have a poor outcome if they
go unrecognized.

Start the history portion of the assessment by asking the patient whether the condition he or she is experiencing occurred over a period of days, weeks, or months or whether it resulted from something more traumatic, such as a direct blow or a fall. Regardless of how the injury happened, it is important to ask the patient where the pain is located, because this information, along with understanding the mechanism of injury (MOI), directs the ensuing physical examination. If the patient was injured by a fall, ask the patient to demonstrate how the injury occurred by having him or her reproduce the MOI by using the uninjured extremity for demonstration purposes. Usually, the patient reports falling on the outstretched arm, as shown in Figure 11.12 on page 324, because this mechanism hyperextends the wrist and elbow, a common way for these structures to be injured. The hand is also commonly injured from axial compression, torsion, and crushing forces. For example, a finger subjected to an axial compression force may result in a dislocated PIP or MCP joint or a fractured phalanx.[2,3]

For suspected overuse conditions, ask the patient whether he or she participates in activities that require repetitive use of the upper extremity, because this is the most common way to cause chronic conditions of these body parts. Ask whether the patient has recently changed the frequency, duration, or intensity of performing activities he or she is used to doing, such as playing tennis, and ask about any modifications in playing technique made recently. Have the patient point to the area that hurts most and indicate whether the pain stays localized or radiates. Radiating pain to the hand is indicative of median or ulna nerve damage or to the brachial plexus as described in Chapter 11. Be sure to determine whether the patient has incurred a previous injury to the region, because an occurrence of pain may be an indication of an old, undetected injury. Note the patient's age, because many patterns that cause overuse conditions are age dependent. For example, elbow pain in an adult is usually caused by soft tissue trauma, whereas the same pain in a child may be caused by an irritation to an ossification center or from an avulsion fracture.[2,4–6]

Physical Examination

Begin the physical examination with observation and palpation, followed by range-of-motion (ROM) and strength testing. Complete the examination by applying stress and special tests designed to evaluate these areas.

Observation

With the patient in the anatomical position, note how the upper extremity is aligned compared with the axial skeleton. In a healthy person, the elbow assumes a valgus position as the forearm angles away from the midline. Known as the **carrying angle**, this angle is naturally larger in females (10° to 15°) than males (5° to 10°) and becomes exaggerated when a person uses the hand to pick up a heavy object (Fig. 12.15). Increases (**cubital valgus**) and decreases (**cubital varus**), otherwise known as *gunstock deformity*, of this angle are indicative of elbow pathology such as a fracture. Ask the patient to abduct the shoulder 90° with the palm up and the elbow extended. Though elbows do not normally hyperextend, many females typically maintain 5° to 10° of **cubital recurvatum**, which is easily demonstrated with the elbow in this position. Next, observe the wrist and hand to determine whether these regions maintain the normal **position of function** (Fig. 12.16). Ask the patient to make a fist, and observe the height of the person's knuckles. Notice that the third MCP joint normally rides higher than the others. Any deviation from this relationship or from the normal position of function indicates that the hand or wrist has been traumatized. Some patients with an acute injury may support the entire upper extremity in the sling position, as shown in Figure 6.1 on page 129, making it challenging for the elbow's carrying angle and the position of function to be evaluated.[5–7]

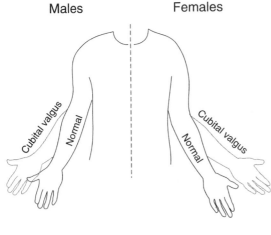

Males   Females

FIGURE 12.15 The normal carrying angle of the elbow and cubitus valgus, an increase in this angle. The normal female carrying angle is greater than that of the male.
From Starkey and Ryan: *Evaluation of Orthopedic and Athletic Injuries*, 2nd ed. 2002. Philadelphia: F.A. Davis Company, Fig. 14-9, pg 499, with permission.

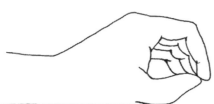

FIGURE 12.16 Position of function for the hand and wrist. The wrist is in slight extension, the metacarpophalangeal and proximal interphalangeal joints are in some degree of flexion, and the thumb is in opposition.
From Lippert: *Clinical Kinesiology and Anatomy*, 4th ed. 2006. Philadelphia: F.A. Davis Company, Fig. 12-30, pg 161, with permission.

After grossly observing the region for structural abnormalities, inspect the area for deformity, swelling, discoloration, masses, or other asymmetry, signs almost exclusively associated with acute, versus chronic, injury. If elbow swelling is present, determine whether it is extracapsular, which typically concentrates around the olecranon, or intracapsular, which is usually more diffuse and encompasses the entire joint. Look for irregularities of the bony contour of the elbow, as an elbow dislocation is usually easy to recognize because of the deformity that usually accompanies this injury. Be aware, though, that a fracture may or may not be visible to the naked eye. Check the wrist for a **ganglia cyst**, a common occurrence about the dorsal aspect of this joint. Caused by fluid leaking from either the wrist's joint capsule or the tendon sheath of the wrist extensor muscle, a wrist ganglion in many instances maintains an idiopathic onset and resolves spontaneously within a year's time. In cases where the presence of such a cyst is identified, instruct the person to observe how it acts over the course of several months, as long as it does not limit function or cause undue pain. When observing the hand, be sure to consider the possibility of a metacarpal or phalangeal fracture when significant swelling is present around the digits.[1,4,8]

Palpation
Begin palpation of the elbow by feeling the olecranon process as well as the medial and lateral epicondyles. Doing so checks bone integrity, evaluates the health of the olecranon bursa, and assesses the humeral attachment sites of the forearm muscle groups and elbow collateral ligaments. Palpate the entire lengths of the RCL and UCL and of the anterior and posterior forearm muscle compartments. Be sure to

feel for the annular ligament, located just distal to the radial head. With the patient's elbow extended, place your thumb on one epicondyle, your middle finger on the other epicondyle, and your index finger on the olecranon process. Note that when observed from medial to lateral, these bony landmarks form a straight line. Keeping your fingers on these structures, instruct the patient to flex the elbow. Note that the olecranon process moves distally, whereas the epicondyles remain stationary, causing these structures to now form an isosceles triangle. Any deviation from these normal bony alignments is indicative of elbow pathology. Next, palpate the area anterior to the elbow. Known as the cubital fossa, this region, outlined by the pronator teres medially and brachioradialis laterally, contains the distal tendon of the biceps brachii and the neurovascular bundle supplying the forearm, wrist, and hand.[5,6]

Palpate the patient's wrist by first finding the pisiform bone, a pea-shaped structure located just proximal to the hypothenar eminence. With your thumb placed over this bone and pointing toward the patient's index finger, instruct the patient to flex the wrist. This moves the hook of the hamate under your thumb, a common area of contusion and fracture. Working medial to lateral, continue to palpate both rows of carpal bones, because doing so assesses bony integrity and the health of the IC ligaments. In particular, note any pain, tenderness, crepitus, or deformity, particularly over the area of the scapholunate joint. Next, instruct the patient to extend the thumb as if he or she were hitchhiking. This highlights the extrinsic thumb extensor and abductor muscles that outline the anatomic snuffbox (Fig. 12.13). Palpate deep into this box for pain, because the scaphoid bone, the most commonly fractured carpal, makes up the floor of the snuffbox.[7,8]

Complete this portion of the assessment by palpating each metacarpal bone individually, starting proximally at the CMC joint and ending at the bone's corresponding MCP joint. Do the same for each digit, starting at the MCP joint and ending at the distal phalanx. Because these bones are so superficial, palpating them when they are injured causes the patient great discomfort. Using Figure 12.10 as a guide, evaluate the health of the patient's afferent nerves in the region. Check for the absence of moisture on the fingertips, because this signifies nerve injury to the digits. Finally, assess the health of the upper extremity's distal circulation by blanching the patient's fingertips. Circulation should return within 2 seconds; capillary refill that takes longer is indicative of circulatory pathology.[4,7]

Range-of-Motion and Strength Testing

Check the patent's active elbow and forearm ROM by having him or her flex, extend, supinate, and pronate, as illustrated in Figures 12.3 and 12.4. Next, perform these actions passively by moving the patient's elbow and forearm joints through these ranges. Do the same for motions of the wrist and hand, as shown in Figures 12.5 and 12.6, respectively. Understand that swelling of the hand for more than a few days can cause adhesions to develop in the region, resulting in decreased motion.[4-9]

To test the strength of the patient's elbow, perform a manual muscle test (MMT) by applying resistance to the anterior and posterior portions of the distal forearm as the patient flexes and extends the joint. To test the strength of the supinators and pronators, instruct the patient to place the forearm in the handshake position as previously described. Grasp the patient's hand as if to shake it. From this position, resist the patient's attempts to supinate and pronate the forearm. Using Figure 12.5 as a guide, test the strength of the RCJ by applying resistance as the patient moves the wrist through its ROM. All of these motions can be tested by asking the seated patient to place the forearm on a table with the wrist and hand dangling off the table's edge.

Because most hand and some wrist pathologies produce grip strength weakness, test hand strength by having the patient grip your hand as hard as he or she can. Next, test the integrity of the ulnar nerve–associated finger abduction strength by instructing the patient to resist attempts to adduct the MCP joints while the patient holds these joints in abduction. Test finger adduction strength by placing a piece of paper between the patient's fingers and instructing the patient to resist your attempts to remove the paper from the patient's hold. Underlying ulnar nerve pathology may exist if the MCP joints are weak. Test the integrity of the median nerve by trying to separate the patient's tightly opposed thumb and little finger. The median nerve is most likely injured if the patient's little finger can be separated from the thumb.[4]

Stress and Special Testing

Stress and special tests used to evaluate specific conditions of the elbow, forearm, wrist, and hand are described and discussed concurrently with the relevant musculoskeletal conditions covered in this chapter. Two tests, the percussion test and **Tinel's test**, can be used to examine multiple conditions in this region.

As discussed in Chapter 8, a percussion test is used to determine the presence of fracture in a long bone. Thus, when performed on the hand, this test evaluates the integrity of the metacarpals and phalanges. To perform a percussion test in this region, tap the end of each of the patient's digits. Begin with little force, gradually increasing the magnitude of each tap until the bones vibrate. Remember that vibration can also be achieved by applying a tuning fork to the end of the digit being tested. If the patient experiences localized pain anywhere along the bone, the test is positive for a possible fracture. This test is much more sensitive for a phalangeal fracture than it is for a metacarpal fracture.

Tinel's test, otherwise known as *Tinel's sign*, is used to determine the health of a superficial nerve. Indeed, the symptoms produced by this test can be elicited from any nerve that is easily palpable. In the wrist, this test is primarily used to evaluate the health of the median nerve as it passes through the carpal tunnel. In the elbow, Tinel's test is used to assess the condition of the ulnar nerve as it passes behind the medial aspect of the elbow, also referred to as the *funny bone*. This test is also used to assess the health of the ulnar nerve as it passes through Guyon's canal. To perform Tinel's test, use the tip of the middle or index finger to tap over the top of a superficial nerve (Fig. 12.17). As with the percussion test, start with little force, gradually increasing the magnitude of each tap. If positive, the symptoms produced by this test include tingling, burning, and paresthesia along the nerve's distribution distal to the tap site.

Musculoskeletal Imaging

As is the case with most body regions, standard plain-film radiograph views of the elbow and forearm include anteroposterior (AP) and lateral. Obtain these views in all cases of trauma and in instances where congenital abnormalities and developmental disorders are suspected. Add an oblique view of the elbow in cases of acute trauma and when injury is present in children and adolescents. Order stress radiographs when the clinical evaluation reveals elbow joint instability. Use magnetic resonance imaging

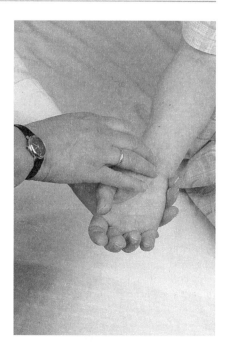

FIGURE 12.17 Tinel's test for injury to the median nerve as it passes through the carpal tunnel. From Dillon: *Nursing Health Assessment: A Critical Thinking, Case Studies Approach.* 2003. Philadelphia: F.A. Davis Company, Fig. 18-9, pg 633, with permission.

(MRI) to evaluate soft tissue injury to the elbow, such as a sprain to the UCL, and to identify the presence of loose bodies within the joint.[6,10]

In addition to obtaining posteroanterior (PA) and lateral x-rays for patients with a suspected wrist and/or hand injury, order an oblique view of the region, because this view, along with the lateral, is particularly helpful in identifying carpal fractures and dislocations. Also order a PA view of the carpals with the wrist in ulnar deviation after traumatic injury to this area. Known as the *scaphoid view*, this image helps to identify injury to the scaphoid, the carpal bone most commonly fractured. It also provides a better view for all carpal bones located on the wrist's radial side. Obtain a PA view with the patient's hand in a clenched position, because doing so helps to identify injury to the IC joints, the scapholunate joint in particular. Add a carpal tunnel view, a tangential, inferosuperior view of the wrist, to rule out injury to the bony structures associated with the carpal tunnel. Realize, however, that even after obtaining this battery of x-rays, it can be difficult to diagnose a carpal fracture, because these bones are small and line up closely to each other, making them overlap on film. Thus, in instances where initial x-ray findings are negative for a hand or wrist fracture but clinical findings indicate that a fracture exists, obtain follow-up plain-film radiographs 7 to 10 days later.[1,8,9,11,12]

Though not used often during the initial stages of musculoskeletal evaluation of the wrist and hand, MRI or computed tomography (CT) scans are appropriate to order in certain instances. This chapter highlights the conditions for which these tests should be ordered. Recognize that when patients are referred to another specialist, such as an orthopedist, MRI and CT scanning becomes more involved in the diagnostic process.

Conditions of the Elbow

Elbow conditions occurring from sports participation include injury to the collateral ligaments, ulnar nerve involvement, dislocation, bursitis, and epicondylitis. The majority of elbow injuries affect people who participate in throwing sports, such as baseball and softball. This is particularly true for younger people, whose immature musculoskeletal system is not developed enough to stand the repetitive stresses caused by constantly repeating an overhand throwing motion. When an acute injury does occur, it is usually caused by direct trauma or from a fall on the outstretched arm, as shown in Figure 11.12 on page 324, resulting in severe bony and soft tissue damage.

Collateral Ligament Sprains

Like the collateral ligaments of the knee, the elbow's collaterals are susceptible to acute injury from outside stresses. Fortunately, these external forces do not injure the UCL or RCL as often as they injure the knee's collaterals, because, in contrast to the lower extremity, the upper extremity is rarely planted firmly on the ground at the time external forces are applied to the body. In addition, when playing contact and collision sports, such as football and soccer, most contact is directed toward a player's lower extremities. However, certain sports, such as wrestling, require the participant's hands to be fixed on the ground during competition. In these instances, sprains to the UCL and RCL occur as the result of externally applied valgus, varus, and hyperextension forces.

Though not injured often by being struck by another person, the elbow's collateral ligaments are frequently exposed to external forces when a person attempts to prevent a fall by landing on the outstretched arm. The collateral ligament injured from this MOI directly relates to the path the force takes as it travels through the upper extremity. The UCL is also exposed to injury when a person participates in repetitive overhand throwing activities, because this action places valgus stresses on the medial aspect of the elbow. Though this MOI is almost exclusively associated with baseball pitchers, athletes who participate in other activities, such as javelin throwing and tennis, also injure the UCL in this fashion. Commonly referred to as **ulnar collateral insufficiency** (UCI), these activities cause a stretching, rather than a tearing, of the UCL. Indeed, this is the most common way this ligament is injured, whereas the RCL is rarely injured in this fashion.[13–17]

⬡PEARL⬡

Ulnar collateral insufficiency or a stretching of the UCL occurs when valgus stresses are repetitively placed on the medial side of the elbow, such as what happens during the overhand motion associated with throwing a baseball or javelin.

History and Physical Examination

The patient with RCL instability presents with a history of falling on the outstretched arm or being hit on the medial side of the elbow. These patients report localized pain over the lateral portion of the joint and report hearing and feeling popping within the elbow during motion. In more severe cases they relate that the elbow occasionally "locks" when they move it. The amount of swelling and pain the person presents with directly relates to the condition's severity. Elbow strength and ROM are not affected in patients with a first degree sprain, but these are decreased in people with second and third degree injuries. Because RCL injury is closely associated with annular ligament pathology (discussed later in this chapter), the integrity of this structure must also be evaluated when an injury to the RCL is suspected.[13,15]

Unlike patients with an RCL sprain, the person with UCI usually reports a long history of steadily increasing medial elbow pain that initially improves with rest. At times, this injury does occur as the result of a person performing one repetition of the offending activity, such as throwing a ball hard or hitting a tennis serve with a lot of force. When UCI is caused by this mechanism, the patient reports feeling a "pop" on the medial side of the elbow at the time of injury. When UCI is caused by microtrauma, the throwing athlete usually states that pain is worse during the early portion of the throwing phase and is significant enough to interfere with his or her throwing velocity. Regardless of cause, the anterior portion of the UCL in people with UCI is typically painful near the ligament's ulna attachment. This indicates that the ligament is torn. When associated with an insidious onset of symptoms, the patient's ROM and strength may or may not be greatly affected. However, people who experience an acute onset of UCI maintain decreases in both ROM and strength.[15-17]

As with the collateral ligaments of the knee, the presence of elbow joint instability can be verified by applying the valgus (UCL) and varus (RCL) stress tests[13,15] To perform the valgus stress test (Fig. 12.18):

• Position yourself laterally to the seated or standing patient.
• Grab the patient's distal forearm with one hand, and place your other hand on the lateral aspect of the elbow.
• With the elbow flexed 20° to 30°, apply a valgus force by pushing the joint medially with your proximal hand and pulling the forearm laterally with your distal hand.
• Watch the medial joint line for the presence of excessive motion or joint "opening" between the distal humerus and proximal ulna.

After completing the valgus stress test, reverse hand positions and perform the varus stress test by pushing the joint laterally with your proximal hand and pulling the forearm medially with your distal hand. In cases where minimal movement occurs with either of these tests, a first degree sprain probably exists. However, if the valgus or varus stress test produces excessive movement, note the type of end-feel present. A hard end-feel is indicative of a second degree collateral sprain, whereas a soft end-feel confirms the presence of a third degree injury.

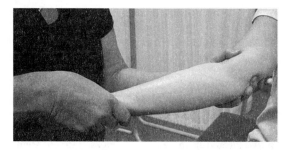

FIGURE 12.18 The valgus stress test is used to test the integrity of the ulnar collateral ligament. Reverse hand positions to test the integrity of the radial collateral ligament.

Management

Treat all patients with isolated first degree UCL and RCL sprains symptomatically with relative rest and cryotherapy and prescribe elbow rehabilitation exercises as outlined in Patient Teaching Handout (PTH) 12.1. Order x-rays for people with suspected UCI and second and third degree ligament sprains. Include valgus and varus stress radiographs to assess the extent of joint opening. Immobilize and refer all with suspected second and third degree collateral ligament sprains and UCI injuries to an orthopedist. People with a ligament sprain are treated with immobilization and sometimes surgery, whereas patients with UCI are initially treated conservatively, with a minimum of 6 weeks' rest from throwing accompanied by the implementation of an extensive rehabilitation program. It is also suggested that these patients receive an expert in biomechanical analysis to evaluate their technique (e.g., throwing, serving) to ensure that they avoid placing too much stress on the medial side of the elbow during the offending activity.[15,16]

Elbow Ulnar Nerve Neuropathies

Remember that at the level of the elbow, the ulnar nerve is located in the cubital tunnel. This nerve is exposed to direct trauma and, much like the UCL, it is at risk for injury when valgus stresses are placed on the elbow. Indeed, **ulnar nerve neuropathies** at the elbow frequently occur in conjunction with UCL instability.[14,16]

Neuropathies of the ulnar nerve at this level are caused by one of the following: contusion, stretching, subluxation, or entrapment. A contusion happens when the medial epicondyle receives a direct blow or when continuous pressure is applied to it, such as when a person rests the elbow on a hard surface for an extended period. This is a fairly common injury because the nerve lies superficially within the cubital tunnel and is relatively unprotected. A stretching neuropathy occurs as a result of repetitive overhand throwing, because this mechanism places a traction stress on the ulnar nerve, ultimately causing it to stretch over time. This stretching can lead to the nerve subluxating over the medial epicondyle, a condition that can lead to the development of friction neuritis. An entrapped ulnar nerve occurs deep within the cubital tunnel and is usually associated with hypertrophy of the flexor-pronator muscle group, which maintains its primary origin from the medial epicondyle.[5,14,17,18]

History and Physical Examination

Regardless of the specific condition causing the patient's symptoms, a person with an elbow ulnar nerve neuropathy reports posteromedial elbow pain and intermittent paresthesia along the area of the nerve's sensory distribution (Fig. 12.10). In the throwing athlete, these symptoms are aggravated by throwing and improve with rest. When compared with the contralateral side, the patient's involved elbow typically does not produce visible signs of injury. The person with a subluxating nerve may describe feeling a popping sensation over the medial epicondyle every time the elbow is flexed and extended. This is caused by the nerve exiting and entering the tunnel during elbow movement and may be felt when palpated. Placing direct pressure over the medial epicondyle and cubital tunnel while the patient flexes and extends the elbow may cause pain and paresthesia. In addition, the patient's wrist flexors may be weak, but realize that pain and sensory deficits occur before muscle weakness can be detected. People with this pathology usually have a positive Tinel's test when the portion of the ulnar nerve located in the cubital tunnel is tapped. Remember to always consider injury to the UCL in the throwing athlete who presents with ulnar nerve symptoms, because a similar mechanism injures these structures.[5,16,17]

A patient with an ulnar nerve neuropathy reports posteromedial elbow pain, has a positive Tinel's test, and experiences intermittent paresthesia along the area of the nerve's sensory distribution.

Management
Manage an elbow ulnar nerve neuropathy with rest, making sure the patient avoids both participating in the offending activity and placing pressure on the exposed elbow. Prescribe a nighttime extension elbow splint for a period of 4 weeks, because this immobilizes the nerve during sleep, allowing it to heal. Use cryotherapy treatments cautiously, remembering that the ulnar nerve, because of its superficial location, can be injured by the improper application of ice (discussed in Chapter 6). Refer people who do not respond to these conservative measures to an orthopedist. Surgical decompression and an anterior transfer of the nerve are often necessary for these patients.[5,16]

Dislocation
Elbow dislocations are classified by the direction the ulna and radius move in relation to the humerus. When a dislocation occurs in response to someone participating in sports, these bones most commonly move backward, resulting in a posterior dislocation. This usually happens when a person falls on the outstretched arm and injures, among other structures, the joint capsule and UCL. This injury is a frequent occurrence in sports and is seen in children as well as in adults. Indeed, the posterior elbow dislocation is the most common dislocation seen in children younger than 10 years and is second only to shoulder dislocations in frequency in adults. When accompanied by fractures to the coracoid and radial head, a common occurrence, a *terrible triad* injury of the elbow has occurred. The prognosis for patients with this condition is poor because it is difficult to treat these three injuries at the same time.[5,13,16–18]

The posterior elbow dislocation is the most common dislocation seen in children younger than 10 years and, in adults, is second only to shoulder dislocations in frequency.

History and Physical Examination
The patient with a posterior elbow dislocation presents by holding the upper extremity in the sling position, as shown in Figure 6.1 on page 129. However, in these instances, the elbow may be not be flexed as much as what is usually seen in people supporting the upper extremity this way. When inspected, noted deformity exists because the involved forearm typically looks shorter than the uninvolved forearm, owing to the posteriorly positioned olecranon process. In these cases, be sure to check the patient's distal circulation, sensation, and grip strength, because there may be neurovascular compromise resulting from either swelling or from the anteriorly situated humerus placing pressure on the neurovascular bundle located in the cubital

fossa. Once a preliminary diagnosis of a posterior elbow dislocation is made, there is no need to perform additional tests, such as determining strength and ROM levels, because doing so only causes the patient undue discomfort and pain.[5]

Management

Immediately immobilize the elbow of a patient with a suspected dislocation. Constantly monitor the patient's neurovascular status, because prolonged compromise of blood supply and nerve function distal to the dislocation could lead to the development of a **Volkmann's contracture**. Promptly refer the patient to an orthopedist or a medical facility that has the ability to treat this condition promptly, because an elbow dislocation is a medical emergency that requires immediate reduction. After x-rays confirm the diagnosis and reduction is complete, patients are treated with a hinged brace, allowing for limited joint motion during the healing process. This helps avoid prolonged elbow stiffness and a permanent loss of elbow extension.[5,16]

PEARL

An elbow dislocation is a medical emergency that requires immediate reduction.

Olecranon Bursitis

Because of its superficial location between the skin and the olecranon process, the olecranon bursa is extremely vulnerable to direct trauma. It can also become irritated by activities that require a person to perform repetitive elbow flexion and extension movements and by rubbing the elbow against an immovable surface. Indeed, chronic bursitis is the condition most commonly associated with this bursa. People with acute bursitis usually seek treatment soon after the injury incident, whereas patients with chronic bursitis may only decide to seek medical attention to determine why the area around the olecranon has become painful and swollen.[5,17,19,20]

History and Physical Examination

Patients with olecranon bursitis caused by direct trauma report that the elbow quickly swelled after being struck, whereas patients with chronic bursitis state that swelling accumulated around the joint over a period of time (Fig. 12.19). When compared, the swelling produced by an acute injury, generally located over the olecranon process, is much greater than what is associated with a chronic condition. In addition, though the swelling related to acute bursitis interferes with elbow motion and restricts activity, chronic swelling does not normally cause these complications.[20]

When palpated, the bursa of a person with acute bursitis is hot and causes great discomfort, whereas the chronically injured bursa is not nearly as warm or painful. Be aware that in instances of acute bursitis, the underlying olecranon may be fractured. Clinically, these patients present with a considerable amount of pain and swelling, are limited in their ability to flex the elbow, and report symptoms consistent with an ulnar nerve neuropathy.[5,17,19,20]

Management

Immobilize and apply a compression bandage to patients who have acute olecranon bursitis. Advise patients to apply an ice bag to the region, because this form of

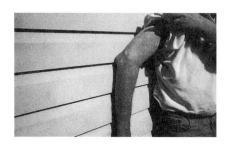

FIGURE 12.19 Olecranon bursitis.
From Dillon: *Nursing Health Assessment: A Critical Thinking, Case Studies Approach.* 2003. Philadelphia: F.A. Davis Company, pg 625, with permission.

cryotherapy can be used in conjunction with compression and elevation. Obtain x-rays and refer cases of bony injury to an orthopedist. If x-ray findings are negative, continue treating the patient with a compression wrap and cryotherapy. Introduce a period of relative rest by telling the patient to avoid the offending activity until the swelling subsides. If swelling does not subside in a timely fashion, refer the patient to an orthopedist so the bursa can be aspirated. Repeated aspirations over a period of a few weeks may be necessary to completely remove all of the fluid.[20]

When treating a patient with chronic olecranon bursitis, follow the same initial treatment plan as for someone with acute bursitis. Consider bursa aspiration only if symptoms persist in spite of conservative treatment or if the person desires a quicker resolution of the swelling. Though advocated by some, injection of corticosteroids into the bursa to aid the healing process is controversial and not necessarily needed during the initial stages of treatment.[20]

If a lasting reduction in swelling cannot be obtained with conservative measures, refer the patient to an orthopedist. Surgical intervention includes bursa excision, but this course of action, like most surgical decisions, is a treatment of last resort and is only considered after conservative treatment has failed. Regardless of treatment option, when a patient is ready to return to sports after a bout of olecranon bursitis, recommend that he or she protect the area with an elbow pad when participating in any activity that exposes the olecranon to direct trauma.[19,20]

Epicondylitis

The term *epicondylitis* is a general term used to encompass many overuse conditions of the medial and lateral elbow epicondyles. This condition is primarily caused by overloading either the common extensor tendon or the tendons of the flexor-pronator muscle group from their respective attachment points on the lateral and medial epicondyles. The result is tendinosis and/or a partial or complete tear of the affected tendon.[13,17]

Lateral epicondylitis (LE) usually occurs in patients who are involved in sports that require them to perform repetitive and excessive wrist extension activities, because these irritate the common extensor tendon's epicondyle attachment. Both males and females aged between 35 and 50 years who participate in sports such as tennis are at most risk of developing this condition. This gives rise to the condition's common name of *tennis elbow*, owing to the fact that to hit a backhand tennis stroke, the wrist must extend against the resistance produced by the ball as it contacts the racket. Though playing tennis certainly causes this injury, partaking in other activities, such as bowling, racquetball, and squash, also lead to its development. Indeed, this is the most common elbow problem seen in those who participate in sports.[5,13,15–18]

Much less common than LE, **medial epicondylitis** (ME), also known as *golfer's
elbow*, is caused by overusing the flexor-pronator muscle group. This condition is more
predominant in males than in females and, in addition to occurring in golfers, javelin
throwers, swimmers, and bowlers are also at risk of developing ME.[5,13,16,18]

History and Physical Examination

Regardless of which epicondyle is irritated, patients with epicondylitis almost
always relate an insidious onset of elbow pain, with pain descriptors ranging from
sharp to achy. This almost always coincides with the person's involvement in some
activity requiring extensive use of the wrist extensors or flexors. Patients with LE
report pain over the lateral aspect of the elbow, which sometimes radiates down the
lateral forearm, whereas patients with ME report pain over the medial elbow and
proximal forearm, which, at times, radiates down the medial forearm. Also, patients
with LE report pain when performing any motion requiring contraction of the wrist
extensors, such as typing or opening a door with a knob, whereas patients with ME
report a weak grasp that is noticeable when trying to complete activities such as
producing a firm handshake and lifting heavy objects, which place great stress on
the flexor-pronator muscle group.[5,15,16]

When observed, the elbow of patients with epicondylitis rarely produces noticeable
swelling, ecchymosis, and/or redness over the injured area. People with LE, however, are
tender anterior, medial, and distal to the lateral epicondyle, because this is the site of
the common extensor tendon. In addition, the **tennis elbow test** is almost always positive when administered to patients with LE.[15,16] To perform this test (Fig. 12.20):

• Instruct the patient to flex the elbow, pronate the forearm, extend the wrist, and
  clench the fist.
• Place one of your hands on the epicondyles and the other hand on the dorsal aspect
  of the patient's hand.
• Instruct the patient to resist your attempt to force the wrist into flexion.
• Pain produced around the lateral epicondyle by contracting the wrist extensor muscle
  group in this fashion is positive for LE.

Like patients with LE, patients with ME are painful over the proximal forearm just
anterior to the medial epicondyle, because this is where the flexor-pronator muscle group
is located. Use the results of the forearm pronation and wrist flexor MMT, both described
earlier in this chapter, to document the presence of ME. When performed, these strength
tests, owing to the stress such tests place on the flexor-pronator muscle group, either
increase the patient's pain and/or reveal muscle weakness. Remember to closely evaluate
the health of the underlying UCL in patients with suspected ME, because pain over the
medial epicondyle can be confused with injury to this ligament.[5,13,15,16]

Management

Because these are primarily soft tissue conditions, plain-film radiographs do not
provide additional information to help diagnosis LE or ME. Thus, rely heavily on

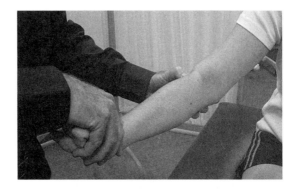

FIGURE 12.20 Tennis elbow test for lateral epicondylitis.

clinical findings to make a proper diagnosis. Once diagnosed, advise patients with these conditions to cease participation in the offending activity. Prescribe ice massage, because this form of cryotherapy works well in these instances. Advise people with LE to wear a resting short arm splint at night, because doing so rests the irritated common extensor tendon. Also, recommend that these patients wear a counterforce brace, otherwise known as a *tennis elbow strap*, when needed (Fig. 12.21). This brace, which can be purchased at any sporting goods store, reduces stress on the lateral epicondyle, diminishing the force the common extensor tendon places on the epicondyle. Though people with ME can also use a splint and strap, these devices do not work as well for these patients.[5,15,16]

As soon as pain and discomfort allow, implement a forearm strengthening and stretching exercise program, as described in PTH 12.1, for patients with LE and ME. Also, before returning the person to activity, have an expert evaluate the technique the patient uses when performing the offending activity. For example, if the cause of injury is hitting the backhand stroke in tennis, the person should have this psychomotor skill evaluated by a tennis professional to ensure that they are performing the stroke correctly. Though most patients respond well to conservative treatment, if pain does not subside or worsens within a 2- to 3-week period, refer the person to an orthopedist.

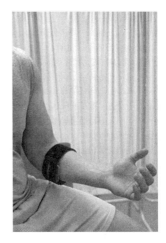

FIGURE 12.21 A tennis elbow strap is used as part of the management plan for lateral epicondylitis.
From Beam: *Orthopedic Taping, Wrapping, Bracing, and Padding.* 2006. Philadelphia: F.A. Davis Company, Fig. 9-23D, pg 301, with permission.

The next step in the treatment plan is the administration of a subaponeurotic corticosteroid injection directly over the origin of the common extensor tendon or in the area of the flexor-pronator muscle group. If needed, a second injection is administered 2 weeks after the first.[5,15,16]

Conditions of the Forearm

Fractures and dislocations are the most common acute forearm injures seen in sports. Fractures happen as a result of direct force trauma caused by contact with another player, a piece of sporting equipment, or an immovable object. For example, the forearm is vulnerable to fracture when it is struck by a lacrosse or hockey stick or when it collides with a soccer goalpost. As with many conditions, a fall on the outstretched arm, as shown in Figure 11.12 on page 324, also exposes the radius and ulna to fracture. Children maintain the highest risk for fracture in this area, because half of all fractures in this population occur in the forearm. Also, 75% of all childhood forearm fractures involve the distal radius, making this bone's distal growth plate vulnerable to injury.[17]

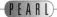
PEARL

Three out of four forearm fractures in children involve the distal radius, making this bone's distal growth plate vulnerable to injury.

In addition to causing the forearm to fracture, blunt-force trauma and falling on the outstretched arm can also cause the PRUJ and DRUJ to dislocate. Indeed, in most instances, a forearm dislocation occurs simultaneously with a fracture. Sometimes the PRUJ dislocates without the forearm fracturing. This injury is caused by a traction force, such as what happens when a parent, in great haste or out of frustration, grabs a child by the distal forearm and pulls. Otherwise known as a *pulled*, or *nursemaid's*, *elbow*, this forceful action tears the annular ligament, causing the head of the radius to separate from the ulna.

Overuse injuries of the forearm are caused by activities that eccentrically load the anterior and posterior muscle compartments. Though this mechanism leads to a variety of conditions, such as muscle strains and fasciitis, it also leads to compartment syndrome. Along with fractures and dislocations, compartment syndrome is one of the most common and potentially most serious conditions seen in the primary care setting.[16]

Fractures and Dislocations
Though usually managed in emergency medial facilities, it is not uncommon for people who fracture and/or dislocate the forearm to seek medical attention in the primary care setting. This is because these injuries commonly result in a nondisplaced or minimally displaced fracture or dislocation. At times, the lack of obvious deformity associated with these conditions causes the injured person to make an appointment to visit the primary care setting in lieu of going to the hospital emergency room immediately after the injury.[18]

History and Physical Examination
People with a forearm fracture and/or dislocation usually describe an MOI similar to what has already been described while reporting hearing sounds, such as cracking or popping, at the time of injury. Patients with a fracture usually support the forearm in

the sling position (Fig. 6.1 on page 129), whereas people with a PRUJ dislocation do not favor the injured extremity in any particular fashion. As with all fractures, signs that the person has broken a bone include swelling, deformity, and ecchymosis at the site of injury. The area is tender, and crepitus may be present. The patient's radial pulse and sensory status of the hand may be affected if the fracture has compromised the nerves and blood supply in the region. Although many types of forearm fracture exist, some of the more common are listed in Table 12.1. Though some of the fractures listed in this table, such as Colles' and Smith's fractures, are usually classified as wrist fractures, for completeness they are included here.

TABLE 12.1 Common types of forearm fractures

FRACTURE TYPE	MECHANISM OF INJURY	FRACTURE SITE(S)	ASSOCIATED DISLOCATION	NOTES
Monteggia's	Fall on the outstretched arm	Proximal ⅓ of ulna	PRUJ (anterior radial head dislocation)	Could involve injury to forearm nerves
Radial shaft (Galeazzi's)	Fall on the outstretched arm	Distal ⅓ of radius	DRUJ	Common in children; also known as a *reverse Monteggia's fracture*
Ulna shaft (nightstick)	Direct blow, as what occurs when people defend themselves from being struck	Distal ⅔ of ulna	None	None
Colles'	Fall on the outstretched arm	Distal radius; distal portion of fractured radius moves posteriorly	None	Most common in older women
Smith's	Fall on the outstretched arm	Distal radius; distal portion of fractured radius moves anteriorly	None	Also known as a *reverse Colles' fracture*
Olecranon	Direct blow, usually from falling directly on the olecranon	Olecranon of ulna	Posterior elbow dislocation	If associated with dislocation, the neurovascular bundle located in the cubital fossa may be affected

DRUJ = distal radioulnar joint; PRUJ = proximal radioulnar joint.

In cases of a PRUJ dislocation, where the head of the radius separates from the annular ligament, the radial head may be visible as it pushes laterally against the skin of the patient's forearm. In these instances, the head of the radius can be moved in an anterior/posterior fashion, a true sign that the integrity of the PRUJ has been disrupted. People with this condition are also unable to supinate and pronate the forearm, signs that a fracture in the region may also exist.

Use the compression (squeeze), traction, and percussion tests to clinically confirm the presence of a forearm fracture and/or dislocation. To perform these tests, instruct the patient to either stand or sit. Apply the compression test by encircling your hands around the distal end of the patient's forearm and gently squeezing the radius and ulna together. Increased pain with this maneuver is indicative of a fracture. Perform the traction test by pulling slightly down on the distal forearm. If this longitudinally applied stress decreases pain, a fracture may be present, whereas an increase in pain indicates soft tissue pathology. Finally, gently tap the forearm's superficial bony landmarks, causing vibrations to travel along the axis of the long bones. A fracture is indicated when the vibration stops at the fracture site, causing increased pain.

Management

Immobilize the forearm of patients with a suspected fracture or dislocation. To avoid complications, such as the development of a Volkmann's contracture, be sure to constantly monitor distal circulation and sensation. Order x-rays to verify the clinical diagnosis, and refer all confirmed cases to an orthopedist. Ultimately, the course of treatment depends on the type of fracture, the degree of displacement present, and whether the fracture is associated with a dislocation. Most patients are treated conservatively with casting, though surgical intervention is necessary in instances where the bones need to be aligned and/or secured. If the fracture disrupts one of the bone's growth plates, the orthopedist will monitor the patient for several years to ensure that growth proceeds normally.

Compartment Syndrome

When compared with those of the lower extremity, compartment syndromes of the upper extremity are rare. However, be aware that there are serious consequences of missing a case of forearm compartment syndrome.[21]

As with the anterior compartment of the leg, both chronic exertional compartment syndrome (CECS) and acute compartment syndrome (ACS) occur in the forearm. ACS typically occurs secondary to elbow dislocation or forearm fracture, whereas CECS is usually caused by repeated static contractions of the forearm muscles. Indeed, because of its overuse injury mechanism, CECS is seen in the primary care setting far more often than ACS is. Primarily affecting the wrist extensor muscle group, CECS most commonly occurs in sports such as gymnastics and weight lifting that require participants to use the hands to grasp for extended periods. These activities cause muscles in the forearm's posterior compartment to hypertrophy, ultimately increasing intracompartmental pressure.[21]

History and Physical Examination

People with CECS of the forearm report an insidious onset of forearm, wrist, and hand pain. This pain is usually described as a dull ache, which accompanies a feeling of firmness in the affected compartment. Patients state that, initially, these symptoms subsided with rest but reoccurred with activity. As the intensity of these symptoms increase, they also start occurring before, during, and after activity. Ultimately, the patient experiences hand and wrist weakness, which typically affects the person's activity level. It is at this point that the person usually seeks medical treatment.[21]

In most instances of CECS, the affected person's forearm looks perfectly normal, making the observation portion of the examination unremarkable. Palpation usually increases pain over the affected compartment, though no definitive area of point tenderness exists. However, the area may be warm because of the increased pressure building in the compartment. Distal circulation and sensory nerve patterns are normal in the early stages of CECS but become affected as the condition worsens. Passive flexion and hyperextension of the patient's fingers may cause paresthesia to the dorsal or palmar aspects of the hands and fingers, a telltale sign of CECS. Strength testing of the involved muscles causes the patient pain and, ultimately, reveals weakness of the affected muscles.[21]

Management
Initially treat patients with CECS conservatively with rest, ice, and elevation. Do not apply a compression wrap, because this may increase intracompartmental pressure. As with CECS of the leg, choose ice massage as the form of cryotherapy, because applying an ice bag to the region, even without using an elastic wrap to secure the bag, may increase pressure to the region. Though no definitive guidelines exist with regard to when it is appropriate to refer such cases to an orthopedist, err on the side of caution, because any increase in intracompartmental pressure can lead to forearm, wrist, and hand complications from neurovascular compromise. Be sure to immediately refer to an orthopedist or to an emergency medical facility those patients whose distal circulation and sensation have been affected, if symptoms worsen, or if a conservative course of treatment is ineffective. Surgical intervention includes compartment fasciotomy.[21]

Conditions of the Wrist

The incidence of wrist problems occurring in people who participate in athletic activities is relatively high. However, the wrist is injured much less often in younger people than in adults, because of the pliability of the wrist ligaments and the relatively thick layer of cartilage in this population. Though wrist injuries occur as a result of many factors, acute injury in this region is usually the result of the person falling on the outstretched arm, as shown in Figure 11.12 on page 324. This MOI forces the wrist into hyperextension, resulting in carpal fractures and IC joint sprains and dislocations. A common misconception when evaluating injury to this region is that all wrist pain is caused by a sprain of the wrist ligaments. Indeed, traumatic injuries involving the carpals are frequently missed, in part because these conditions can be difficult to view with standard x-rays. Also, though in many instances injuries of the wrist are obvious, some are subtle, requiring the examiner to be methodical when assessing the area.[1,7,9,22–24]

Carpal Fractures
Though any carpal bone is prone to injury, the scaphoid is the one by far most commonly fractured, because it accounts for up to 70% of all carpal fractures. This bone is particularly vulnerable to a fall on the outstretched arm, because the scaphoid

bridges the two rows of carpal bones, transmitting force from the wrist to the forearm. Unfortunately, this fracture is also the carpal fracture most commonly misdiagnosed. Even when diagnosed quickly and cared for properly, a fractured scaphoid can cause lifelong disability, because, when injured, this bone maintains a high incidence of nonunion, an outcome directly related to its poor blood supply at its proximal end. This means that delayed diagnosis of this injury only increases the chance of nonunion and the development of avascular necrosis. Thus, always suspect a scaphoid fracture when a patient reports with wrist pain, particularly if the person participates in collision or contact sports.[1-3,7-9,11,16,18]

(PEARL)

Always suspect a scaphoid fracture when a patient reports with wrist pain, because this is the most commonly fractured carpal bone, it is the most commonly undiagnosed fracture of the carpal bones, and, even when cared for properly, it maintains a high rate of nonunion.

Other carpal bones that typically fracture include the triquetrum, the second most commonly fractured carpal, the hamate, and the pisiform. Common types of triquetral fractures include chip and avulsion, though the body of this bone can also fracture. Most hamate fractures occur in the bone's hooked portion, a condition frequently seen in people who participate in sports.[9,16,11,18,25,26]

History and Physical Examination

People who report with a wrist fracture state that they fell on the hyperextended wrist in an attempt to break a fall (Fig. 11.12 on page 324). In these instances, immediately suspect a scaphoid fracture and, potentially, a fracture of the triquetrum. Differentiate between these injuries by determining where the patient's pain is located. People who injure the scaphoid have pain in the anatomic snuffbox, whereas those with triquetral fractures experience pain on the dorsal aspect of the wrist.[1,3,7-9,16,24,25]

When a patient states that the ulnar aspect of the palm absorbed most of the force from a fall, consider that they might have injured the hamate or pisiform, particularly if they report falling while holding an object, because this MOI causes the object to land between the hand and the ground on impact. Also consider a hamate fracture if the person reports a compression-type injury to the hypothenar eminence, such as what happens when the wrist is compressed by an implement, such as a golf club, when the implement makes contact with an immovable object, such as the ground. Patients who report placing repetitive stresses on this region, as what happens when a person plays tennis for an extended period, may also have fractured the hamate. Regardless of injury mechanism, the initial signs of a fractured hamate usually do not include extreme pain. Rather, these patients report a feeling of constant pressure over the bone. Because severe pain is not typically present, in many instances people with a fractured hamate do not have the condition evaluated right away, seeking medical attention only when the ill-defined, chronic pain they ultimately experience on the ulnar aspect of the wrist does not go away.[1,3,7,9,11,16,18,25,27]

The wrist of a patient with a carpal fracture usually has minimal swelling at the site of injury. This is particularly true for people who fracture the scaphoid. Thus, palpating around and directly into the anatomic snuffbox is the best way to diagnose a fractured scaphoid, because doing so causes the patient extreme pain. In these instances, applying an axial force to the patient's first metacarpal also causes pain, because this maneuver applies a compressive force on the scaphoid. Be aware that though many patients with a fractured scaphoid can move the affected wrist through its full ROM, the motions of wrist extension and radial deviation are the ones most likely to be affected by this condition.[1,3]

Pain in the anatomic snuffbox is a telltale sign of a scaphoid fracture.

In contrast to a scaphoid fracture, a triquetral fracture causes discomfort to the patient when the dorsal aspect of the wrist is palpated, whereas a hamate or pisiform fracture causes tenderness on the ventral aspect of the injured bone. Because the hamate is responsible for protecting the ulnar nerve at this level, patients with an injured hamate may display signs of paresthesia that follows the distribution of this nerve, as shown in Figure 12.10. People who have fractured this bone also experience increased discomfort when grip strength is tested.[1,9,11,16]

Management

Treat all patients with tenderness over the anatomic snuffbox as if they have a scaphoid fracture until proven otherwise. Do this by immobilizing the patient's wrist and thumb with a thumb spica splint and referring the person for x-rays. Order a scaphoid view in addition to the standard wrist views because, in many instances, standard views do not identify the fracture. At times, patients participating in competitive sports require a more urgent diagnosis, because the presence or absence of a scaphoid fracture can directly affect the return-to-play decision for these athletes. In these cases, consider ordering a CT or an MRI so an early definitive diagnosis can be made.[1,7–9,11]

Order a scaphoid x-ray view for all suspected cases of scaphoid fracture, because standard wrist views do not always identify the fracture.

Ultimately, the treatment of a person with an acute scaphoid fracture depends on the location and stability of the fracture. Most acute nondisplaced fractures occurring at the bone's distal portion respond well to simple immobilization. Thus, treat these patients with a short arm thumb spica cast with the wrist in slight radial deviation for 4 to 10 weeks. Obtain follow-up x-ray views every 2 weeks to monitor healing and so radiograph union can be documented, which typically occurs within 6 to 8 weeks. In some cases, clinical evidence of bone union, such as an absence of pain and full wrist function, precedes plain-film radiographic evidence by months. Thus, trust clinical findings as much as the results of x-ray evidence when determining the best course of action when treating a patient with a nondisplaced fracture of the scaphoid's distal pole.[1,7–9,11,16]

⬤ PEARL ⬤

Trust clinical findings to determine the best course of action when treating a patient with a nondisplaced fracture of the scaphoid's distal pole.

In contrast to patients who have an acute nondisplaced distal scaphoid fracture, refer to an orthopedist patients presenting with distal fractures more than 3 weeks old, acute distal fractures that are displaced, and fractures to the bone's middle or proximal portions, because all of these fractures maintain high incidences of nonunion.[16,28]

Even when x-ray findings for people with anatomic snuffbox pain are negative, this does not necessarily mean that the scaphoid is healthy, because this type of false-negative finding is common. Thus, in cases where x-ray findings are negative but pain in the snuffbox persists as a result of a traumatic event, treat the patient as if the bone is fractured by placing the patient in a thumb spica splint or cast. Obtain a second set of x-rays within 2 weeks of doing this. If at that time the patient is asymptomatic and the second set of x-rays are negative, allow the patient to resume pain-free activity. Instruct the patient to cease activity and report back immediately if pain returns. If the snuffbox is still tender after 2 weeks of immobilization, refer the patient to an orthopedist, regardless of the results of the second set of x-rays.[1,3,7–9,25]

⬤ PEARL ⬤

In cases in which x-ray findings are negative but pain in the snuffbox persists as a result of a traumatic event, treat the patient as if the scaphoid is fractured.

Treat the patient who has a potential hamate fracture by obtaining a carpal tunnel x-ray view, because the diagnosis for a hook of the hamate fracture is often delayed and sometimes goes undiagnosed because it does not always appear on standard plain-film radiographs. Even if x-ray findings are negative, obtain an MRI or CT scan if a strong clinical suspicion for a fracture exists. As with a scaphoid fracture, delayed diagnosis of a hamate fracture can lead to necrosis and nonunion. Once a hamate fracture is confirmed, apply a volar splint to the wrist and hand of the patient and refer him or her to an orthopedist. The initial treatment for a patient with this injury is casting for 4 to 6 weeks or until union is achieved. If this is not successful, more aggressive management includes surgical removal of bone chips located in the region.[1,3,7,8,11,25,27]

⬤ PEARL ⬤

A hook of the hamate fracture diagnosis is often delayed, and sometimes goes undiagnosed, because it does not always appear on standard plain-film radiographs.

Refer patients with a confirmed fracture of the body of the triquetrum to an orthopedist, because these patients require surgical repair. Treat patients with a triquetral chip or avulsion fracture with cast or splint immobilization for 4 to 6 weeks, because these conditions have a much better outcome with conservative treatment than do fractures to the triquetral body. Apply a short arm cast for 3 to 6 weeks for patients with a pisiform fracture, because these patients also heal well with conservative treatment.[1,9,16,26]

Wrist Sprains

A wrist sprain occurs when one or more of a person's IC ligaments become injured. As with most acute wrist injuries, a fall on the outstretched arm (Fig. 11.12 on page 324), forcing the joint into hyperextension and, in some instances, into ulna deviation is the most common MOI for a wrist sprain. Because there are so many ligaments in this region, a multiple ligament injury is a frequent result of such a traumatic event. When this occurs, the outcome is usually some degree of IC instability.[1,3,11]

Remember that the SLL, because it absorbs much of the force when a person falls on the outstretched arm, is the IC ligament most commonly involved in wrist sprains. Although small tears of this ligament result in pain, they do not usually affect SLJ stability. In contrast, large tears almost always cause instability. Also, be sure to consider the presence of avascular necrosis of the lunate when SLJ injury is suspected, because the signs and symptoms for these conditions are similar. Otherwise known as **Kienböck's disease**, this condition is seen in the young adult population aged between 30 and 40 years and occurs over time from repetitive stress wrist activities, such as those caused by swinging a golf club. Its cause can also be idiopathic, making this condition challenging to diagnose.[1,3,7,26,29,30]

History and Physical Examination

Patients with a sprained wrist primarily report point tenderness at the site of injury. For example, people with instability of the SLJ report specific discomfort over the wrist's dorsoradial aspect. Though all who injure the wrist report pain, patients with SLL involvement report the most discomfort. Indeed, the amount of pain reported by a patient with an SLJ sprain is often disproportional to the amount of force that caused the injury.[3,7,11,23,30]

Unlike carpal fractures, people with a wrist sprain, particularly those who injure the SLJ joint, present with swelling on the wrist's dorsoradial side. Extreme tenderness over the area, an audible popping sound occurring when the patient actively moves the wrist through its ROM, and a decrease in grip strength are all signs of SLL and SLJ injury. If the lunate has dislodged from the scaphoid, the patient's third MCP joint appears equal in height with the other knuckles when the patient makes a fist. Known as **Murphy's sign**, this finding is indicative of a lunate dislocation commonly associated with an instable SLJ.[1,11]

PEARL

Murphy's sign, where the patient's third MCP joint appears equal in height with the other knuckles when the patient makes a fist, is indicative of a dislocated lunate.

Management

Order standard wrist x-rays for patients with suspected ligamentous injuries of the wrist. Be sure to order a PA view with the hand in a clenched position, because this is the best way to document the presence of SLJ widening. Make a diagnosis of SLJ instability if PA views reveal more than a 3-mm gap between the scaphoid and lunate. Apply a thumb spica splint to all patients with suspected SLJ instability, and refer them to an orthopedist. If left untreated, the instability may widen, causing the capitate to shift down into the gap formed by the dislocation. Ultimately, this results in the carpal rows collapsing on one another. Patients whose x-rays confirms the presence of IC instability, lunate dislocation, or Kienböck's disease are best treated by an orthopedist. As long as neither fracture nor instability is present, treat all other patients with a sprained wrist by splinting the region for up to 6 weeks. Be sure to schedule the patient for follow-up visits at 2-week intervals to ensure that proper healing occurs. During this time prescribe stretching and strengthening rehabilitative exercises as shown in PTH 12.1 as the patient's pain and discomfort allow.[1,2,7,11,25,30]

Carpal Tunnel Syndrome

Carpal tunnel syndrome (CTS) is the most common compressive neuropathy occurring in people who participate in sports. This condition occurs when the median nerve becomes entrapped in the carpal tunnel as it passes from the forearm to the hand (Fig. 12.9). This usually happens when people perform repetitive grasping motions or when they do activities, such as typing on a keyboard, that require the wrist to stay in a flexed position for prolonged periods.[1,3,22]

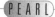

PEARL

Carpal tunnel syndrome, caused by an entrapment of the median nerve in the carpal tunnel, is the most common compressive neuropathy occurring in those who participate in sports.

History and Physical Examination

Patients with CTS report hand pain and numbness that follows the distribution of the median nerve, as shown in Figure 12.10. They report that these symptoms occur most often after performing the offending activity and intensify at night. People who have CTS symptoms for a long time usually present with atrophy of the thenar muscles, a by-product of the median nerve's inability to innervate these muscles. In most instances, this affects the patient's grip and thumb strength. Tinel's test is positive (Fig. 12.17), as is Phalen's test, the definitive clinical diagnostic test for CTS.[1,3,22] To perform this test (Fig. 12.22):

• With the patient seated, instruct him or her to flex both wrists to 90°, placing the backs of the hands against each other.
• Tell the person to hold this position for at least 1 minute.
• Pain and paresthesia after the distribution of the median nerve occurring at any time during this test is indicative of CTS.

Management

Initially treat patients with CTS by obtaining a carpal tunnel x-ray view and by getting standard plain-film radiographs of the wrist. After bony injury has been ruled out, treat people with CTS by modifying their activity and by advising them to wear a night splint to hold the wrist in a position of slight hyperextension during sleep. In severe cases and in instances in which symptoms become worse while the patient is being treated, expand this extension splinting technique to include daytime hours. Prescribe stretching exercises as outlined in PTH 12.1 for the anterior forearm muscles, because doing so increases flexibility and enlarges the space within the carpal tunnel. Though it may take months for the symptoms of CTS to subside, most people heal with these

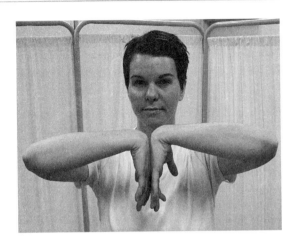

FIGURE 12.22 Phalen's test for carpal tunnel syndrome.

conservative measures. Refer patients who do not respond within 12 weeks of conservative treatment to an orthopedist. In these cases, the orthopedist may decide to treat the patient with a course of oral and/or local corticosteroid injection. If this does not work, surgical intervention in the form of carpal tunnel decompression is indicated.[1,12,22]

Wrist Ulnar Nerve Neuropathy

In addition to being at risk for injury at the level of the elbow, the ulnar nerve is also vulnerable to trauma at the wrist. Known as **Guyon's canal syndrome** or *ulnar nerve palsy*, ulnar nerve injury at this level is a compressive neuropathy of the nerve as it passes in Guyon's canal. Here, the ulnar nerve is subjected to compressive forces when both repetitive and continuous pressure are placed on the ulnar aspect of the palm, such as what happens when someone maintains a firm grasp on a handlebar while riding a bicycle. Thus, this condition is also known as *cyclist palsy*, though it can occur in anyone who participates in a sport in which the person must grasp an implement, such as a tennis racket, during play.[1,3,22]

History and Physical Examination

Patients with this condition report a gradual onset of numbness over the distribution of the ulna nerve, as shown in Figure 12.10. Some report this symptom as transient; others relate that it is more permanent. Patients who report chronic symptoms usually present with atrophy of hypothenar muscles, a by-product of the ulnar nerve's inability to innervate these muscles. In most instances, this affects the patient's ability to grip, adduct the fingers, and oppose the thumb and little finger. Tinel's test is positive, because tingling and numbness are produced over the distribution of the ulna nerve in the hand when the area over Guyon's canal is tapped.[1,3,22]

Management

Initially treat patients with this condition by ruling out the presence of a bony abnormality such as a hook of the hamate fracture. Do this by ordering standard x-rays for the wrist and hand. As mentioned previously, refer all people with a fracture to an orthopedist. Treat all other patients with relative rest, and relieve pressure in the region by telling the patient to pad the palmar aspect of the wrist during activity. This can be done by purchasing padded gloves such as those commonly used by cyclists. Also tell cyclists affected by this condition to readjust bicycle handlebars to lessen pressure on the injured area and to continually change hand positions when riding.[1,22]

de Quervain's Syndrome

de Quervain's syndrome, or tenosynovitis of the tendons that form the radial border of the anatomic snuffbox, is the most common tendinopathy of the wrist seen in the athletic population. This condition occurs when people forcefully grasp an implement, such as a golf club or tennis racket, while they repetitively move the thumb and wrist. It also has a high occurrence in females who provide child care, because these tendons commonly become irritated from carrying infants and small children for extended periods.[1,3,4,11,22]

History and Physical Examination

Patients with de Quervain's syndrome report localized radial side wrist and thumb pain that, at times, extends proximally into the forearm. In certain instances, numbness radiates to the distal aspects of the thumb. Signs that normally indicate the presence of injury, such as swelling, are usually absent in this condition, though the affected tendons are very painful when touched. Also, because the tendons that surround the snuffbox connect to extrinsic muscles that move the thumb, the actions of thumb extension and abduction usually increase the patient's pain and may be weak. **Finkelstein's test** is typically positive when performed on people with de Quervain's syndrome.[1,3,4,11,22] To perform this test (Fig. 12.23):

- Instruct the patient to place the thumb inside the closed fist.
- Support the patient's forearm with your hand.
- Tell the patient to ulnarly deviate the wrist.
- Tenosynovitis is present if this test produces pain.

Management

Treat a patient with de Quervain's syndrome by immobilizing the region with a wrist and a thumb spica splint. Instruct the patient to keep the area immobilized until pain subsides. Once this happens, tell the patient to gradually increase thumb activity until full function is restored. Advise the patient to initiate forearm stretching and strengthening exercises as outlined in PTH 12.1. In instances in which immobilization and activity are not enough to alleviate pain, refer the patient to an orthopedist. Injecting the affected tendon sheath with corticosteroids is usually the next step in the treatment process.[1,3,4,11,22]

Conditions of the Hand

Participation in sports readily exposes the hand to trauma, and injuries to this region account for a high percentage of primary care office and emergency department visits. Indeed, sports injuries are the most common etiology of hand fractures in the younger age groups, with the many ligaments supporting the IP and MCP joints, regardless of the person's age, also injured often. Be aware, however, that patients may not initially

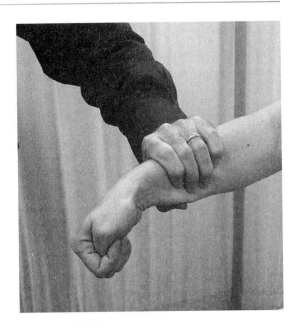

FIGURE 12.23 Finkelstein's test for de Quervain's syndrome.

appreciate how severe an injury in this region is. This means that people are as likely to seek treatment in the primary care setting, sometimes days or even weeks after the injury occurred, as they are to pursue immediate care through emergency medical means.[2,7,11]

Though the hand can be acutely injured by a variety of mechanisms, such as from a twisting-type force, it is most commonly traumatized when compression forces are delivered to the area with the fingers in one of the following positions[8,11,25]:

- hyperextended;
- closed in a clenched fist position, as when a person uses the fist to strike an immovable object; or
- extended, where the force is delivered to the tips of the fingers.

Traumatic Metacarpal Fractures

The metacarpals are the most commonly fractured bones in the hand. Most such fractures are the result of low-impact trauma, making conservative treatment in the form of immobilization the preferred course of treatment. However, people who fracture these bones as a result of high-impact trauma may not respond well to conservative methods, necessitating that they be referred to a specialist for further treatment and possible surgical intervention. Be sure to take extra care when evaluating a potential fracture of the metacarpal of the thumb, because this condition requires special attention.[11]

History and Physical Examination

The person presenting with a metacarpal fracture almost always relates a history of a traumatic event. In these instances, a visual deformity is clearly evident, particularly when a **boxer's fracture** occurs. This fracture, which involves the fourth and fifth metacarpals, typically results from an axial compression mechanism, because these bones are the first to come into contact with an object when the fist is clenched. Be aware that when the proximal end of a metacarpal fractures, it often dislocates from the CMC joint, a condition that often goes undetected. In the thumb, this injury is referred to as a **Bennett's fracture**. Thus, when evaluating a patient for a possible metacarpal fracture, be sure to verify the stability of each CMC joint during the assessment. In some instances of metacarpal fracture, the percussion test, as described previously, is positive, but remember that this test is not overly sensitive for trauma to these bones. If a metacarpal is fractured, it is not necessary for ROM and strength be evaluated, because doing so provides little additional information and causes the patient undue pain and discomfort.[4,8,9,11,25]

Management

Obtain standard plain-film radiographs for all patients presenting with a suspected metacarpal fracture. Treat patients with singular, simple fractures conservatively with a splint or a cast. Treat all others, including patients with multiple metacarpal, boxer's, and Bennett's fractures, by immobilizing the person's wrist and hand in a position of function and referring the patient to an orthopedist. Treatment for these patients includes reduction, immobilization, and, if necessary, internal fixation through surgical intervention. When a metacarpal fracture is detected early, manual reduction, if needed, is easily obtained, helping to prevent future instability of the CMC joint.[4,8,9]

Traumatic Metacarpal Sprains and Dislocations

If a macrotrauma event does not cause the metacarpals to fracture, it may cause the CMC or MCP joint to sprain or dislocate. In other instances, a sprain or dislocation occurs in conjunction with a fracture. For example, in the previous section, the possibility of a CMC dislocation occurring as a result of a metacarpal fracturing at its proximal end is mentioned. Indeed, the CMC joints are fairly stable structures, making them susceptible to injury only when a related structure is injured at the same time. In contrast, the MCP joints are highly vulnerable to traumatic injury with or without other structure involvement. Furthermore, sprains and dislocations of the MCP joints can be very subtle. Consequently, it is not uncommon for a person to report to the primary care setting with an unreduced MCP dislocation. Thus, be sure to take extra care when evaluating MCP joint injury, always considering the possibility that the joint is dislocated, even if the patient reports days or weeks after the date of injury.[2,9]

History and Physical Examination

The person who presents with an MCP sprain or dislocation most commonly states that the affected "knuckle" was "bent backward" or "to the side" at the time of injury. These mechanisms stretch the joint's capsule and collateral ligament arrangement, resulting in tears of these soft tissues. If a simple dislocation occurs, it usually does so dorsally, with the proximal phalanx hyperextending approximately 60°. This makes the dislocation noticeable because the proximal phalanx becomes lodged in front of its associated metacarpal. If a complex dislocation occurs, the proximal phalanx becomes positioned parallel to the metacarpal's shaft. This causes the metacarpal head to shift laterally, winding up between the intrinsic hand muscles. This arrangement makes a complex dislocation less noticeable than a simple dislocation. In either case, the patient with an MCP dislocation reports great discomfort when the injured area is palpated. In contrast, the joint of the person with a sprain is not nearly as painful. Also, a patient with an MCP dislocation is unable to make a fist and abduct the involved joint, whereas a patient with a sprain is usually able to perform these actions, albeit with pain.[2]

As with the knee and elbow, valgus and varus stress tests are used to confirm MCP joint pathology. However, people with an unreduced dislocation may not be able to tolerate the pain caused by these tests. Thus, do not perform these tests on patients with a suspected dislocation.[2] To perform MCP joint valgus and varus stress tests (Fig. 12.24):

- Instruct the patient to place the hand in a forearm-pronated, elbow-flexed position.
- While stabilizing the patient's wrist and metacarpals with one hand, grasp the proximal phalanx of the involved finger with your other hand.
- Perform the valgus and varus stress tests by abducting and adducting the MCP joint.
- Excessive movement in either direction is indicative of an MCP joint sprain.

Management

Obtain standard hand plain-film radiographs for all suspected MCP joint injuries. Immobilize and refer to an orthopedist all documented cases of unreduced dislocation or fracture within the joint. Ultimately, the dislocated MCP joint is treated with closed reduction. Treat patients with an MCP joint sprain with dorsal finger splint immobilization for 6 to 8 weeks. After this splint is removed, teach the person how to "buddy tape" the injured finger to an uninjured finger, because this provides stability for the healing joint. Do this by showing them how to tape the proximal, middle, and distal phalanges of the injured finger to the same bones on an adjacent finger, keeping the joints free of tape to allow full finger function. Be sure to place some padding between the fingers, because this prevents skin irritation. Though discomfort and stiffness can last for months, people with an MCP joint sprain usually heal without complication.[2,4,8]

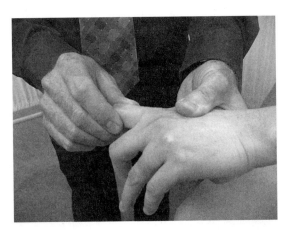

FIGURE 12.24 Valgus and varus stress tests for metacarpophalangeal joint sprain.

Ulnar Collateral Ligament Sprain of the Thumb's Metacarpophalangeal Joint

Gamekeeper's thumb, also referred to as *skier's thumb*, is a sprain of the UCL of the thumb's MCP joint. This is a particularly disabling injury because it occurs in the digit that allows the hand to grasp items. As a result, patients usually seek medical attention soon after the injury occurs. A UCL thumb sprain is typically caused by forced abduction and extension of the MCP joint, as what happens when a skier, with the wrist and hand secured in a ski pole strap, places the hand out to break a fall. In certain instances, this injury occurs in conjunction with a Bennett's fracture, so always consider both of these conditions as part of the differential diagnosis when a patient presents with pain in the area of the thumb's MCP joint.[4,8,25]

PEARL

Gamekeeper's thumb commonly occurs in conjunction with a Bennett's fracture, so consider both of these conditions as part of the differential diagnosis when a patient presents pain in the area of the thumb's MCP joint.

History and Physical Examination

A patient with this condition relates experiencing immediate thumb pain and swelling after landing on the thumb in an attempt to break a fall. Within a week, the area appears ecchymotic, and the patient presents with an inability to grip things normally, owing to weakness of the thumb's intrinsic muscles. This presence of gamekeeper's thumb can be confirmed by performing the **thumb abduction stress test**, because this is the definitive clinical diagnostic test for this injury.[4,8,11,25] To perform this test (Fig. 12.25):

• Instruct the patient to place the hand in a forearm-supinated, elbow-flexed position.
• While stabilizing the patient's wrist with one hand, grasp the proximal phalanx of the thumb with your other hand.
• Abduct the thumb's MCP joint.
• Excessive movement is indicative of a UCL sprain.
• If this test opens the joint greater than 30°, a third degree sprain exists.

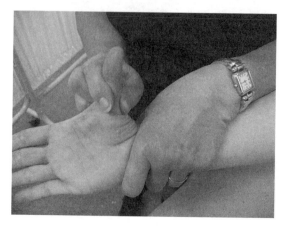

FIGURE 12.25 Abduction stress test for ulnar collateral ligament instability of the thumb's metacarpophalangeal joint.

Management

Order an MCP abduction stress x-ray to confirm this diagnosis. Refer the patient immediately to an orthopedist if a complete ligament tear is suspected, because surgical intervention is necessary in these cases. For all other patients, immobilize the MCP joint with a thumb spica splint and re-examine the patient after 2 weeks. If gapping still occurs with the abduction stress test, refer the patient to an orthopedist. If improvement is noted at the 2-week follow-up, continue with thumb spica immobilization for another 4 weeks, making sure to monitor healing at regular intervals. If needed, surgical repair of the ligament can occur up to 8 weeks after injury without affecting the final outcome. Thus, as long as the condition progressively improves, there is room to try conservative treatment for a period of time.[2,4,8]

Traumatic Fractures of the Finger Phalanges

Finger phalangeal fractures are common occurrences in people who participate in sports such as basketball and football, which expose these digits to injury. Fractures to the proximal and middle phalanges are usually caused by a direct blow applied to the dorsum of the hand, whereas crushing forces are most responsible for distal phalanx fractures. Regardless of cause, people who fracture a finger do not always seek treatment through emergency medical means, requiring that this condition be evaluated in the primary care setting.[2,4,9]

History and Physical Examination

The patient with a fractured phalanx always relates a traumatic episode that damaged the finger. Typical signs of a fractured finger include obvious swelling and noted deformity. In instances of a nondisplaced fracture, the injured digit points in the same direction as the healthy ones, whereas in cases of displaced fractures, the finger appears bent toward the palm, causing the injured digit to assume a claw-like position. Though any fractured finger produces a significant amount of pain, fractures to the distal phalanx are especially tender from the soft tissue trauma that accompanies this crush injury. There is little need to test ROM and strength of the finger when a fracture is suspected, because performing these tests provides little useful information and causes the patient undue discomfort. Use the percussion test, as described previously, to help clinically confirm the presence of a phalangeal fracture.[2,4,8,9]

Management

Order standard hand x-rays for all people with a suspected phalangeal fracture. Apply a dorsal splint and refer patients with a displaced fracture to an orthopedist. Treatment for patients with a displaced proximal and/or middle phalangeal fracture includes reduction, internal wire fixation, and splinting. Whereas splinting is discontinued after 2 to 3 weeks, the wire fixation is removed at 4 weeks.[2,9]

Treat patients with nondisplaced proximal and middle phalangeal fractures with a dorsal splint. Be sure to splint the joints above and below the fracture in 30° flexion. Also treat patients with a distal phalanx fracture and its associated DIP joint with a dorsal splint. Instruct the patient to keep the splint on for 3 to 4 weeks. After this, teach the patient how to buddy tape the injured finger, as previously described. Tell patients recovering from a distal phalanx fracture to expect prolonged tenderness of the finger tip, a direct result of the accompanying soft tissue damage.[2,4,8,9]

Traumatic Phalangeal Sprains and Dislocations

Of all the hand joints, the DIP and PIP joints are the ones at greatest risk of traumatic injury. The resulting condition, usually a sprain or dislocation, typically occurs in people who participate in sports such as basketball and volleyball, because the fingertips of these athletes are at high risk of being struck by a ball traveling at a significant speed. When this happens, an axial compression load is applied to the digit, resulting in a sprain to the DIP joint and a hyperextension injury to the PIP joint. If the force is great enough, the middle phalanx moves dorsally in relation to the proximal phalanx, causing the PIP joint to dislocate. Though the proper way to care for a dislocation is to allow properly trained medical personnel to reduce the dislocation, typically the person with this injury, or a bystander such as an athletic coach, performs the reduction by "pulling" on the digit immediately after injury occurrence. These are the patients who are most likely to report to the primary care setting for evaluation and treatment.[2,4,8,11]

History and Physical Examination

The finger of a patient with a recent sprain or reduced PIP dislocation presents with visible swelling over the affected joint. The injured site is also painful when touched. The patient is unable to make a fist, because these conditions limit the motion of the affected joint. Performing a valgus and varus stress test of the DIP and PIP joints, first in full extension and then in 35° flexion (Fig. 12.26), confirms the presence of injury. A complete MCL rupture exists if laxity occurs with the valgus stress test, whereas a complete LCL rupture exists if laxity occurs with the varus stress test. If ligament laxity is absent but the MOI and signs produced by the injury indicate that the joint has been injured, a partial ligament tear probably exists.[2]

Management

Treat patients with a PIP or DIP joint injury by applying a dorsal splint to the injured finger and by obtaining standard plain-film radiographs to rule out a fracture. Refer people with any bony involvement to an orthopedist. Manage all other patients with a dorsal finger splint with the finger in 30° flexion for 4 weeks. After removing the splint, instruct the patient to use the buddy taping technique, as previously described, because this helps prevent the joint from hyperextending.[2,4,8]

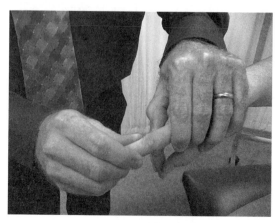

FIGURE 12.26 Valgus and varus stress tests for the interphalangeal joints of the digits.

Traumatic Distal Interphalangeal Joint Tendon Injuries

Traumatic injuries to the DIP joints of the fingers typically involve the joint's extensor or flexor tendon. The most common of these injuries, **mallet finger**, otherwise known as *baseball finger* or *drop finger*, occurs when this joint's extensor tendon avulses from its attachment on the distal phalanx. This occurs when the DIP joint is suddenly hyperflexed when the joint is either at rest or actively extending. The result is a flexion deformity, owing to the inability of the extensor tendon to extend the DIP joint. This frequently occurs in those who play the position of catcher in baseball, because the fingertips of these athletes are constantly struck by balls that ricochet off the ground. Because of its increased length, the middle finger is most affected.[2,4,8,11]

Whereas mallet finger is an extension tendon injury, **jersey finger** is an avulsion of the DIP joint's flexor tendon from its attachment on the distal phalanx. The term *jersey finger* is derived from its usual MOI, which is a forceful extension of a flexing DIP joint, such as what happens when a football player, in an attempt to make a tackle, grabs an opposing player's jersey as the player races by him. Though this condition can affect any digit, it most commonly occurs in the ring and little fingers.[2,4,8,11]

History and Physical Examination

Whereas patients who present with mallet finger commonly states that they "jammed" their finger against a hard object, those who have jersey finger relate feeling a "tearing" sensation in the area of the DIP joint at the time of injury. In either case, the affected DIP joint is swollen and disfigured, with the joint of the patient with mallet finger stuck in a flexed position, whereas the joint of the patient with jersey finger looks extended. Patients with mallet finger are unable to actively extend the involved joint, whereas patients with jersey finger cannot flex the injured joint. In the case of mallet finger, the affected DIP joint can be passively extended by returning the distal phalanx to its proper position. The ability to move the distal phalanx in this manner commonly leads to this injury being misdiagnosed in the primary care setting. As with mallet finger, jersey finger also goes unnoticed because, even in the acute stages of DIP joint injury, the person is still able to flex the PIP joint of the involved finger. Thus, it is common for the patient with jersey finger to seek medical attention only after the initial pain and swelling subside, at which time the person realizes that he or she cannot flex the injured DIP joint.[2,4,8,11]

> The DIP joint of a patient with mallet finger appears to be stuck in a flexed position, whereas the joint of the patient with jersey finger looks extended.

Management

Immobilize the DIP joint of the patient with mallet or jersey finger, and obtain standard hand x-rays to rule out bone involvement. Immediately refer all patients with suspected jersey finger to an orthopedist so the torn tendon can be surgically reattached, preserving function of the DIP joint. Ideally, surgery occurs within 10 days after injury so as to avoid a retraction of the injured tendon. Thus, do not delay in referring these patients for follow-up care.[2,4,8]

Also refer patients with mallet finger to an orthopedist if radiographs reveal the presence of a fracture. For all others, apply a dorsal splint to the DIP joint for 6 to 8 weeks. Convey to the patient the importance of not removing the splint during this time, because doing so results in extending the splinting time by an additional 6 weeks to ensure healing. Avoid splinting the digit's associated PIP joint, because this unnecessarily causes finger stiffness. In cases where the patient presents with a nonacute mallet finger, advise the person to keep the splint on for up to 3 months, but realize that these injured joints rarely regain full extension.[2,4,8,11]

Traumatic Proximal Interphalangeal Joint Tendon Injuries

The most common traumatic PIP joint tendon injury, a **boutonnière deformity**, otherwise known as a *buttonhole deformity*, is a flexion contracture condition of this joint. It is caused by blunt-force trauma to the tip of a finger, causing the digit's PIP joint to flex forcefully, such as what happens when a volleyball hits the tip of a player's finger at a high rate of speed. This results in a rupture of the digit's extensor tendon near its attachment site on the middle phalanx. In some instances, this MOI causes a **pseudoboutonnière deformity**, where DIP hyperextension occurs along with the PIP flexion contracture. This occurs when the outer portions of the finger's extensor tendon "slip" out of place, placing a flexion traction on the DIP joint.[4,8,11]

History and Physical Examination

Patients presenting with a boutonnière deformity state that they "jammed" the finger, resulting in their not being able to move it. The involved PIP joint is swollen, and the associated DIP joint is hyperextended, with this hyperextension deformity greater in pseudoboutonnière than in boutonnière deformity. Though these patients are unable to actively extend the PIP joint, passive full extension is easily obtained.[4,8,11]

Management

After ruling out bony involvement through standard hand x-rays, use a dorsal finger splint to immobilize the PIP joint in an extended position for patients with a boutonnière deformity. Be sure to allow full function of the DIP joint so as to avoid the development of joint adhesions and contractions. Immobilize for a minimum of 4 weeks, realizing that it may take up to 8 weeks for full healing to occur. Refer patients with a pseudoboutonnière deformity to an orthopedist.[8,11]

Lifespan Considerations

Though elbow pathology can occur in either gender and in any age group, the youngest athletes who participate in overhand throwing sports are most susceptible to injury. Indeed, elbow pain is the most common injury symptom in young baseball players. As with the adult, the medial side of the younger athlete's elbow is most likely to become injured as a result of valgus stresses associated with overhand throwing activities.

Whereas these stresses in adults cause injury to the ulnar nerve and UCL, when placed on the young elbow they injure bone and growth plates instead of soft tissue. This is because at this stage of physical development, growth plates are weaker than soft tissue attachment sites in the region. In younger people, these valgus forces concentrate around the medial epicondyle, placing the child's distal humeral apophysis and surrounding structures at risk for development of **little league elbow** (LLE).[6,14,31]

PEARL

Elbow pain is the most common injury symptom in young baseball players.

Little League Elbow

Historically, the term *little league elbow* has been used to describe medial apophysitis of the distal humeral growth plate in the skeletally immature person. Though this condition is still the primary cause of medial elbow pain in this population, today the definition of LLE has expanded to include avulsion of the medial epiphysis, articular changes to the capitulum and radial head (such as osteochondritis desiccans), and avulsion of the olecranon's posterior epiphysis. It typically occurs in skeletally immature pitchers, usually encompassing those aged 9 to 12 years, who throw overhead for extended periods. It happens most often during the acceleration phase of pitching, because this is when most force is placed on the elbow's medial side. This usually results in a partial separation of the medial apophysis from the humerus, or a Salter-Harris type 1 fracture. Because of its high rate of incidence in children, always consider LLE as part of the differential diagnosis when evaluating medial elbow pain in this population, even if symptoms are minimal.[14,17,31-34]

PEARL

Always consider LLE as part of the differential diagnosis when evaluating medial elbow pain in children who are involved in heavy throwing activities.

Patients with LLE state that the first indication that something was wrong was when they experienced an insidious onset of arm fatigue. This symptom coincides with a reported presence of general soreness on the anterior aspect of the proximal forearm. Indeed, these are the first signs of impending injury. Next, patients state that this presence of general soreness developed into medial elbow and proximal forearm pain a few days after pitching or participating in a like activity, such as throwing excessively from shortstop to first base. They report that this pain initially subsided between practice sessions, only to have it reappear when they resumed throwing. Patients typically state that they decided to seek medical treatment when this medial elbow pain affected their throwing, and sometimes batting, performance.[14]

When questioned, people with LLE report throwing many pitches in a short period of time, which usually corresponds with a loss in velocity. The medial aspect of the patient's elbow, distal arm, or proximal forearm is visibly swollen, a telltale sign of this injury. The person's medial epicondyle is tender, because this is the origin for the pronator and anterior forearm compartment muscles. These symptoms may be accompanied by a decrease in elbow ROM, particularly in extension, and paresthesia of the elbow and forearm. Elbow and forearm muscle weakness is present, and pain occurs with resisted pronation. Though a valgus stress test of the elbow is negative, performing this test, normally used to check the integrity of the UCL, produces medial elbow tenderness of the patient with LLE.[14,17,31,34,35]

Because this condition affects the child's growth plate, obtain AP, lateral, and oblique x-rays to confirm the diagnosis and to determine the degree to which the medial apophysis has separated from the distal humerus. Plain-film radiographs also reveal changes of the capitellum and radial head, avulsions of the olecranon and/or medial epicondyle, hypertrophy of the medial epicondyle, bony fragmentation, loose cartilage bodies, and osteochondral lesions. Refer the patient to an orthopedist if x-rays document any of the above conditions. Realize, however, that plain-film radiographs may be normal even in instances where LLE is present. Thus, even in the absence of positive x-ray findings, rely on the clinical findings to make a diagnosis of LLE.[6,14,31,35]

Initially treat patients with LLE with 6 to 8 weeks of rest. In most instances, this means the child should not pitch for the rest of the competitive baseball season. However, these patients may be able to play other positions, such as first base, which requires minimal throwing. Recommend that the child do this only if he or she can compete with minimal discomfort. Once pain has subsided, instruct the patient to stretch and strengthen the forearm and elbow muscle groups, as shown in PTH 12.1, and initiate a gradual return to throwing and pitching activities. Use follow-up x-ray studies to gauge healing and to make return-to-play decisions. Most patients can return to competitive pitching and throwing 12 weeks after injury. If conservative treatment fails, refer the patient to an orthopedist. Surgical intervention involves pinning the medial apophysis.[6,14,31,34,35]

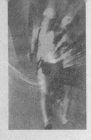

CASE STUDY
Conditions Involving the Elbow, Forearm, Wrist, and Hand

SCENARIO
A 35-year-old female office worker comes to your practice reporting ongoing right elbow pain. Though she cannot identify an exact date of injury, she states that the pain started after she joined a women's racquetball league 3 months previously. League participation requires that she play two nights a week for an hour at a time. The pain started as a dull ache, which originally disappeared quickly after she played. Eventually, the pain became sharper and more intense, and though its intensity decreased after playing, it was constantly present. A few weeks ago, the level of pain increased to the point that she was forced to stop playing. At that time, the pain was waking her at periodic intervals throughout the night and was affecting her ability to do her job because she could not type without severe discomfort. Since this time, the pain has subsided but is still present.

This patient is a novice racquetball player who joined the league to increase the amount she exercised and for the social interaction that being a part of a league offers. She wants to return to league play as soon as possible so she can resume exercising and so the social ties she has developed can be maintained.

PERTINENT HISTORY
Medications: Currently taking ibuprofen, 200 mg tid for the elbow pain. Ortho Tri-Cyclen Lo × 10 years.
Daily multivitamin.

Family History: Mother has high blood pressure; father has congestive heart failure. No sisters or brothers.

PERSONAL HEALTH HISTORY
Tobacco Use: Smoker until age 30.

Recreational Drugs: Denies use.

Alcohol Intake: 1 to 2 drinks after playing racquetball twice per week. 2 to 4 drinks on the weekend.

Caffeinated Beverages: Consumes 5 to 6 cups coffee throughout the day.

Exercise: Racquetball twice per week. Occasionally walks on the weekends for 15 to 20 minutes at a time.

Past Medical History: Body mass index during a physical examination at age 34 indicated borderline obesity. The same physical examination revealed that the patient had dyslipidemia. Had the normal childhood diseases of mumps and chickenpox.

(case study continues on page 408)

CASE STUDY
Conditions Involving the Elbow, Forearm, Wrist, and Hand (continued)

PERTINENT PHYSICAL EXAMINATION*
The patient's elbows appear symmetrical, and there is no visual sign of injury to the right elbow. ROM and strength are normal, though flexing and extending the elbow actively, passively, and with resistance produces pain. The lateral epicondyle and the area just distal to this bone are extremely tender. The tennis elbow test is positive.

RED FLAGS FOR THE PRIMARY HEALTH CARE PROFESSIONAL TO CONSIDER
A young, obese person with high cholesterol levels is at risk for cardiovascular disease. A lack of being able to play racquetball is also affecting this patient's social well-being.

RECOMMENDED PLAN
- Advise the patient not to play racquetball until the elbow pain totally subsides.
- Implement a tennis elbow treatment program, including ice and anti-inflammatory medication (ibuprofen 600 mg tid), and provide the patient with stretching and strengthening exercises for the forearm and elbow.
- Prescribe a resting short arm splint to be worn at night.
- Recommend that the patient wear a counterforce brace (tennis elbow strap) at work and when performing rehabilitation exercises. Tell the patient that this strap should also be worn when she returns to playing racquetball.
- Advise her to seek advice from a racquetball professional regarding her racquetball playing technique.
- Review the patient's eating habits, recommending ways to improve her diet.
- Advise the patient to join a fitness center that hires qualified staff and offers formal cardiovascular and resistance training exercise programs. This will help the patient incorporate exercise into her daily routine and can act as a conduit for additional social interaction.
- So you can monitor the patient's elbow treatment, diet and exercise routines, and social well-being, insist that she sees you for a follow-up visit 2 to 3 weeks after the initial visit.

*Focused examination limited to key points for this case.

REFERENCES

1. Parmelee-Peters K, Eathorne SW. The wrist: common injuries and management. *Prim Care* 2005;32:35.
2. Goitz RJ, Tomaino MM. Traumatic hand injuries: evaluation and management. *J Musculoskelet Med* 2002;19:204.
3. Howse C. Wrist injuries in sport. *Sports Med* 1994;17(3):163.
4. Hong E. Hand injuries in sport. *Prim Care* 2005;32:91.
5. Budd GM, Piccioni LH. Identifying and treating common problems in the elbow. *Am J Nurs Pract* 2005;9(2):41.
6. Klingele KE, Kocher MS. Little league elbow: valgus overload injury in the pediatric athlete. *Sports Med* 2002;32(15):1005.
7. Daniels JM, Zook EG, Lynch JM. Hand and wrist injuries, part I: nonemergent evaluation. *Am Fam Physician* 2004;69:1941.
8. Dingle SR, Connolly JF. Hand and wrist injuries in athletes: 20 clinical pearls. *J Musculoskelet Med* 2003;20:394.
9. Altizer L. Hand and wrist fractures. *Orthop Nurs* 2003;22:232.
10. American College of Radiology Practice Guideline for the Performance of Radiography of the Extremities, 2003 (Res. 11). Effective October 1, 2003. Retrieved from: http://www.acr.org. Accessed 8/30/08.
11. Rosner JL, Zlatkin MB, Clifford P, et al. Imaging of athletic wrist and hand injuries. *Semin Musculoskelet Radiol* 2004;8:57.
12. McKinnis LN. *Fundamentals of Musculoskeletal Imaging*, 2nd ed. Philadelphia, PA: FA Davis Co., 2005.
13. Chung CB, Kim HJ. Sports injuries of the elbow. *Magn Reson Imaging Clin N Am* 2003;11:239.
14. Whiteside JA, Andrews JR, Fleisig GS. Elbow injuries in young baseball players. *Phys Sportsmed* 1999;27(6):87.
15. Sellards R, Kuebrich C. The elbow: diagnosis and treatment of common injuries. *Prim Care* 2005;32:1.
16. Rettig AC. Elbow, forearm and wrist injuries. *Sports Med* 1998;25(2):115.
17. Andrews JR, Whiteside JA. Common elbow problems in the athlete. *J Orthop Sports Phys Ther* 1993;17(6):289.
18. Rettig AC, Patel DV. Epidemiology of elbow, forearm, and wrist injuries in the athlete. *Clin Sports Med* 1995;14:289.
19. McFarland EG, Gill HS, Laporte DM, et al. Miscellaneous conditions about the elbow in athletes. *Clin Sports Med* 2004;23:743.
20. McFarland EG, Mamanee P, Queale WS, et al. Olecranon and prepatellar bursitis: treating acute, chronic, and inflamed. *Phys Sportsmed* 2000;28(3):2000.
21. Wasilewski SA, Asdourian PL. Bilateral chronic exertional compartment syndromes of forearm in an adolescent athlete: case report and review of the literature. *Am J Sports Med* 1991;19:665.
22. Rettig AC. Wrist and hand overuse syndromes. *Clin Sports Med* 2001;20:591.
23. Huurman WW. Injuries to the hand and wrist. *Adolescent Med* 1998;9:611.
24. Schaffer TC. Common hand fractures in family practice. *Arch Fam Med* 1994;3:982.
25. Resnik CS. Wrist and hand injuries. *Sem Musculoskelet Radiol* 2000;4(2):193.
26. Geissler WB. Carpal fractures in athletes. *Clin Sports Med* 2001;20:167.
27. Morgan WJ, Slowman LS. Acute hand and wrist injuries in athletes: evaluation and management. *J Am Acad Orthop Surg* 2001;9:389.
28. Langhoff O, Anderson JL. Consequences of late immobilization of scaphoid fractures. *J Hand Surg (Br)* 1988;13:77.
29. Lewis DM, Osterman AL. Scapholunate instability in athletes. *Clin Sports Med* 2001;20:131.
30. Hester PW, Blazer PE. Complications of hand and wrist surgery in the athlete. *Clin Sports Med* 1999;18:811.
31. Cassas KJ, Cassettari-Wayhs A. Childhood and adolescent sports-related overuse injuries. *Am Fam Physician* 2006;73:1014
32. Brogdon BG, Crow NE. Little leaguer's elbow. *Am J Roentgenol* 1960;83:671.

33. American Academy of Pediatrics. Policy statement: risk of injury from baseball and softball in children. *Pediatrics* 2001;107:782.
34. Adirim TA, Cheng TL. Overview of injuries in the young athlete. *Sports Med* 2003;33:75.
35. Behr CT, Altchek DW. The elbow. *Clin Sports Med* 1997;16:681.

SUGGESTED READINGS

Mastey RD, Weiss AP, Akelman E. Primary care of hand and wrist athletic injuries. *Clin Sports Med* 1997;16:705.
Rettig AC. Athletic injuries of the wrist and hand, part II: overuse injuries of the wrist and traumatic injuries of the hand. *Am J Sports Med* 2004;32:262.
Rudzki JR, Paletta GA. Juvenile and adolescent elbow injuries in sports. *Clin Sports Med* 2004;23:581.

WEB LINKS

http://aappolicy.aappublications.org/cgi/content/full/pediatrics;107/4/782. Accessed 8/30/08. American Academy of Pediatrics policy statement on baseball and softball injuries in children.

http://www.ninds.nih.gov/disorders/carpal_tunnel/detail_carpal_tunnel.htm. Accessed 8/30/08. National Institute of Neurological Disorders and Stroke Web site containing information about diagnosis, treatment, and prevention of carpal tunnel syndrome.

http://www.cdc.gov/niosh/docs/97-141/ergotxt5a.html. Accessed 8/30/08. National Institute for Occupational Safety and Health publication that discusses musculoskeletal disorders of the hand and wrist.

3

CONDITIONS INVOLVING OTHER SYSTEMS

13

Conditions Involving the Head and Face

● Brian J. Toy, PhD, ATC

The fact that injuries involving the head and face range from minor to life threatening makes these regions challenging to evaluate. Frequently, minor head injuries go unnoticed or are taken too lightly by coaches, parents, and primary health care providers. Athletes themselves may regard symptoms such as a recurring headache or an inability to concentrate on a task as normal consequences of participating in contact and collision sports. These symptoms may signal the development of a condition that can threaten the athlete's life.

Anatomy of the Head and Face

The head (skull) is divided into two discrete portions: cranial and maxillofacial. Though a comprehensive review of the anatomy of these regions is beyond the scope of this text, relevant anatomical information is presented here.

Bones and Joints

The cranium is composed of eight flat bones whose primary function is to protect the brain (Fig. 13.1). These bones are connected by a series of suture joints that transform from slightly moveable during infancy and early childhood to immovable in late childhood and young adulthood. Except for the mandible (lower jaw bone), the 14 bones of the facial region attach to one another or to one or more of the cranial bones. The mandible articulates with the temporal bones to form the right and left temporomandibular joints (TMJs), whose primary function is to open and close the mouth. Each TMJ is supported by a joint capsule, a temporomandibular ligament, and an articular disk.

Scalp

The scalp is the well-vascularized covering of the cranium. Figure 13.2 illustrates its five tissue layers, from the outermost skin to the periosteum directly covering the cranial bone. The scalp helps protect both the bones of the cranium and the brain.

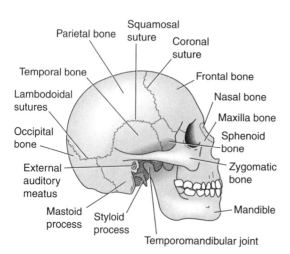

FIGURE 13.1 Lateral view of the bones and sutures of the skull.

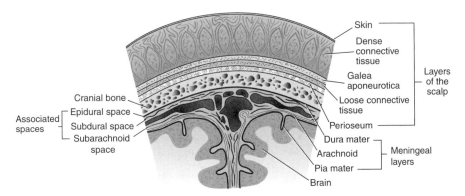

FIGURE 13.2 Layers of the scalp, meninges, and associated spaces.

Brain

The brain is divided into three distinct regions: cerebrum, cerebellum, and brainstem (Fig. 13.3). The largest of the three, the cerebrum, is divided as follows: one frontal lobe, two temporal lobes, two parietal lobes, and one occipital lobe. The names of these lobes correspond to the cranial bones superficial to them. The cerebrum is responsible for all higher functions, including conscious thought, speech, movement, memory,

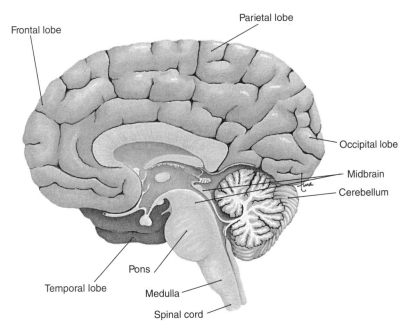

FIGURE 13.3 Midsagittal section of the brain showing lobes of the cerebral cortex, the cerebellum, and portions of the brainstem.
Adapted from Scanlon: *Essentials of Anatomy and Physiology*, 5th ed. 2007. Philadelphia: F.A. Davis Company, Fig. 8-6A, pg 177, with permission.

hearing, vision, interpretation of somatic sensory data, cognition, and reasoning. At the posterior base of the cerebrum is the cerebellum, a cluster of tissue responsible for coordinating complex motor skills such as walking, balance, posture, and coordination. The brainstem includes the midbrain, pons, and medulla. It connects motor and sensory pathways between the brain and the spinal cord and maintains respiratory and cardiac life-sustaining functions.

The vulnerable tissue of the brain is protected by three meningeal layers (Fig. 13.2). These soft tissue structures are located between the inner aspect of the cranium and the brain's surface. The most superficial layer, the dura mater, or *tough mother*, consists of highly vascular fibrous connective tissue. Though this layer lines the inner aspect of the cranial bone, a potential epidural space exists between the dura mater and the cranium. This space is realized if fluid, such as blood, invades the area. The middle meningeal layer, the arachnoid mater, or *spidery mother*, is an avascular, web-like structure. The subdural space, located between the arachnoid and the dura mater, can also become infiltrated by fluid. The innermost layer, the pia mater, or *gentle mother*, is a delicate layer of connective tissue nourished by minute blood vessels and is physically attached to the underlying brain. The subarachnoid space, the area between the arachnoid and the pia mater, maintains cerebrospinal fluid that acts to cushion the brain when an external force is applied to the head.

Eye

The 2.5-cm-diameter eye, or globe, comprises many parts, several of which are protective (Fig. 13.4). The upper and lower eyelids protect the eye from foreign body invasion and distribute tears produced by the lacrimal glands equally across the eye's surface. The transparent conjunctiva lines both eyelids and covers the sclera, the eye's outer, dense, white portion. The sclera provides structure for the eye and is the attachment point for six extrinsic muscles that move the eye in all planes. Anteriorly, the cornea is continuous with the sclera. It provides protection for the underlying pupil and iris and transmits light to the retina. The circular, colored iris surrounds the pupil and is responsible for controlling the pupil's diameter, which regulates the amount of light entering the eye. The iris also divides the eye's anterior cavity into anterior and posterior chambers. These chambers are bathed in aqueous humor, a fluid constantly produced and reabsorbed by the body. This process is responsible for maintaining intraocular pressure. Immediately posterior to the iris is the lens. This structure is responsible for bending and refracting light rays before they are transmitted to the retina. The posterior cavity lies immediately behind the lens and is composed of vitreous humor, a gelatinous substance that maintains the normal shape of the eye. Images from incoming stimuli are formed on the retina, a light-sensitive layer of tissue that lines the back of the eye. It maintains rods, which detect light, and cones, which detect color. The macula, located on the retina in an area directly opposite the lens, maintains an abundance of cones. The fovea, located in the center of the macula, is composed only of cones. The retina converts visual images into nerve impulses, which are transmitted to the cerebral cortex for processing via the optic nerve (cranial nerve [CN] II). The optic nerve connects to the retina in the area of the optic disk.

Ear

Divided into outer, middle, and inner portions, the ear enables us to hear and helps maintain balance (Fig. 13.5). The outer ear includes auricle and canal (external auditory

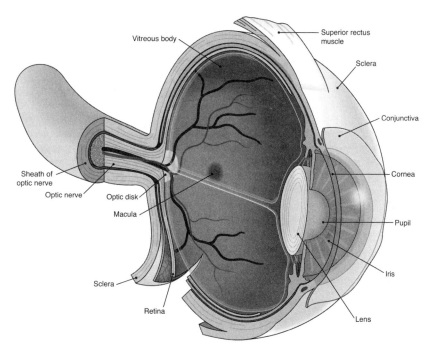

FIGURE 13.4 Cross section of the eye.
Adapted from Dillon: *Nursing Health Assessment: A Critical Thinking, Case Studies Approach.* 2003. Philadelphia: F.A. Davis Company, Fig. 10-4B, pg 247, with permission.

meatus) portions and consists mostly of cartilage. It is divided from the middle ear by the tympanic membrane, or *eardrum*, a flat tissue that collects and transmits sound to the middle ear. The eustachian tube connects the middle ear to the nasopharynx, which allows air to enter and leave it. By compressing and decompressing entering air, the middle ear passes sound to the inner ear through the three tiniest bones in the body: the malleus, incus, and stapes. Located within the temporal bone, the inner ear comprises the cochlea, which is responsible for hearing, and the semicircular canals, which are responsible for balance. The cochlear branch of the vestibulocochlear (acoustic) nerve (CN VIII) transmits sound information to the brain, whereas the vestibular branch of this nerve relays head position.

Nose

The razor-thin nasal bone composes the upper portion of the nose, whereas the lower nasal area consists of cartilage (Fig. 13.6). The nasal septum divides the nose into right and left nasal cavities, with the lateral wall of each cavity maintaining upper, middle, and lower conchae and an associated meatus. Air enters the nose through the nasal vestibule and passes through the nasopharynx as it makes its way to the oropharynx. Odor molecules stimulate olfactory receptors in the epithelium of the upper nasal cavity, allowing for the sense of smell. Impulses are transmitted to the brain along the olfactory nerve (CN I).

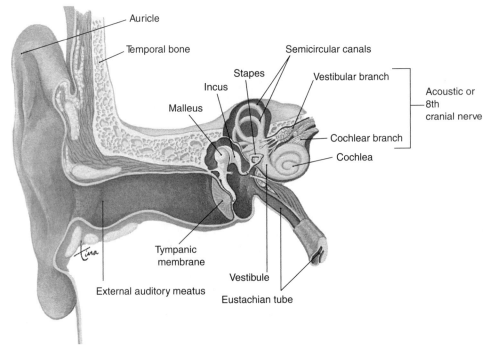

FIGURE 13.5 External, middle, and inner ear anatomy.
From Scanlon: *Essentials of Anatomy and Physiology*, 5th ed. 2007. Philadelphia: F.A. Davis Company, Fig. 9-7A, pg 211, with permission.

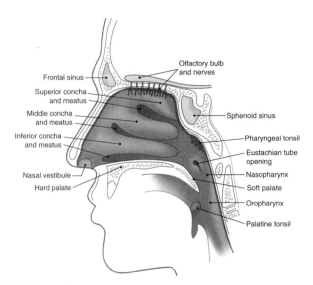

FIGURE 13.6 Internal nose.
Adapted from Dillon: *Nursing Health Assessment: A Critical Thinking, Case Studies Approach.* 2003. Philadelphia: F.A. Davis Company, Fig. 9-4, pg 197, with permission.

Mouth

The mouth, or *oral cavity*, contains the tongue, tonsils, glossopalatine and pharyngopalatine arches, uvula, posterior pharyngeal wall, teeth, gums, lips, and cheeks (Fig. 13.7). The roof of the mouth is composed of the hard palate anteriorly and the soft palate posteriorly. A total of 32 adult teeth are normally present, though many people have four wisdom teeth removed in adolescence or early adulthood. Each tooth has three parts: the crown, the neck, and the root. The core of each tooth is made up of the pulp and associated nerves and blood supply. Being the first segment of the digestive system, the mouth takes in, chews, and exposes food to salivary enzymes, beginning its mechanical and chemical digestion. Taste buds located in the tongue's papillae allow us to recognize sweet, bitter, sour, and salty substances.

Cranial Conditions

Of the estimated 1.5 million head injuries that occur in the United States each year, 20% are sports related. Fortunately, the past decades have brought a significant decrease in reported fatal and nonfatal head injuries in interscholastic and intercollegiate athletes. This decrease has been attributed to rule changes in certain sports, player education, and implementing and upgrading standards for playing equipment designed to protect the head from injury. A heightened awareness among health care providers and patients regarding the dangers involved in returning to participation too quickly after a head injury has also contributed to the reduction in sports-related head injuries. Because the consequences of misevaluating head injuries could be fatal, it is imperative that every primary health care provider be skilled in head injury assessment and make sound decisions regarding initial treatment, follow-up care, and return to participation (RTP)[1-4]

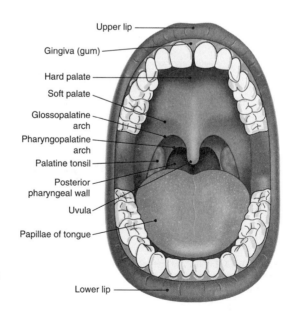

FIGURE 13.7 Structures of the mouth.
From Dillon: *Nursing Health Assessment: A Critical Thinking, Case Studies Approach.* 2003. Philadelphia: F.A. Davis Company, Fig. 9-5, pg 197, with permission.

Labels in figure:
Upper lip
Gingiva (gum)
Hard palate
Soft palate
Glossopalatine arch
Pharyngopalatine arch
Palatine tonsil
Posterior pharyngeal wall
Uvula
Papillae of tongue
Lower lip

Mechanisms of Injury

Brain injury occurs as a result of a blow to a stationary or moving head (Fig. 13.8). The mechanism that causes a **coup injury** occurs at the site of impact and usually results from a direct blow to a stationary, unprotected head. For example, a golf ball hitting the head at a high rate of speed results in a coup injury. This mechanism causes **focal brain lesions**, cerebral contusions, and depressed skull fractures.[4,5]

A blow to a protected, moving head against an unyielding object causes the brain to accelerate and travel in a linear fashion away from the site of impact (Fig. 13.8). When it reaches the area directly opposite the impact site, the brain decelerates abruptly as it makes contact with the cranium. The outcome of such an injury mechanism is a **contrecoup injury**, in which the brain is traumatized opposite the impact site. The result is usually a diffuse brain injury such as a cerebral concussion. This linear acceleration-deceleration mechanism, which sometimes occurs in combination with a coup mechanism, is responsible for most sports-related brain injuries. A diffuse brain injury also results from a series of repeated subconcussive forces, much like those a boxer experiences during a competitive bout or those a football player receives from the constant helmet-to-helmet collisions that occur during the course of a football game. These repetitive subconcussive forces also have a cumulative affect on a person's brain across a playing season or an athlete's career.[4,5]

PEARL

A linear acceleration-deceleration mechanism of injury, which commonly causes a diffuse contrecoup injury, is responsible for most sports-related brain injuries.

A rotational mechanism of injury (MOI), by which the brain is twisted in some fashion, can also cause an acceleration-deceleration brain injury. Though not as

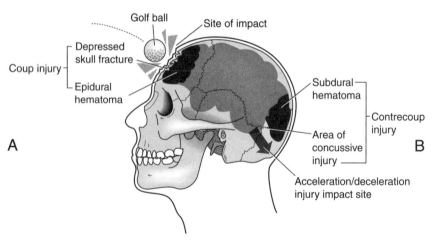

FIGURE 13.8 Coup and contrecoup injury showing an epidural hematoma and depressed skull fracture occurring at the site of impact (A) and a subdural hematoma and concussive injury occurring at the site opposite of impact (B).

common as a linear mechanism, a rotational MOI produces the most severe brain tissue damage. In football, grabbing an opponent's face mask and violently twisting the head and neck is an example of how a rotational brain injury may occur.[4,5]

Mild Traumatic Brain Injury (Concussion)

Though universal agreement for the definition of a **concussion** does not exist, the term is derived from the Latin *concutere*, meaning violent agitation or shaking of the brain. Classified as a **mild traumatic brain injury** (MTBI), a concussion is a trauma-induced clinical syndrome characterized by alteration of mental status that may or may not involve loss of consciousness (LOC).[4,6-8]

Sport-related MTBI represents a substantial percentage of head injuries in the pediatric population and is the most common cranial condition encountered when working with children and adolescents. It is also the most common athletic head injury experienced across the life span. The highest incidence of MTBI occurs in people who participate in football, with ice hockey, rugby, boxing, basketball, baseball, soccer, and softball players also affected. When compared with males, females maintain an increased risk for MTBI in the sports listed in Box 13.1.[6,9-12]

Unfortunately, during many scholastic and collegiate practice sessions and games, health care providers trained to recognize MTBIs and determine their severity and management are not available. Even when a health care provider is present, he or she may not recognize that a concussion has occurred, because student athletes often do not report symptoms. This failure to report concussion symptoms is particularly disturbing because, when compared with older athletes, high school athletes are more vulnerable to MTBI, demonstrate prolonged memory dysfunction after a concussion, and are three times more likely to experience a second episode after an initial MTBI incident. It also takes longer for pediatric patients to recover from MTBI events. By gaining an appreciation of the complexities associated with MTBI, health care providers are able to make sound judgments when treating the concussed pediatric patient.[4,6,9,13-15]

(PEARL)

When compared with adults, younger athletes are more vulnerable to MTBI, demonstrate prolonged memory dysfunction after a concussion, are three times more likely to experience a second episode after an initial MTBI incident, and take longer to recover from MTBI events.

BOX 13.1
SPORTS IN WHICH FEMALES HAVE A HIGHER INCIDENCE OF MILD TRAUMATIC BRAIN INJURY THAN MALES

Softball (when compared with baseball for males)*	Basketball†
	Lacrosse‡
Soccer†	

*High school. †High school and college. ‡College.

Powell JW, Barber-Foss KM. Traumatic brain injury in high school athletes. *JAMA* 1999;282:958; Dick RW. *NCAA Injury Surveillance System: 1984-1991*. Overland Park, KS: National Collegiate Athletics Association, 1999.

Signs and Symptoms

Although no two incidences of MTBI present the same way, the most common signs and symptoms include those listed in Box 13.2. In some instances, noticeable clinical manifestations of an MTBI may disappear within minutes after the injury incident. On other occasions, signs and symptoms may appear only after several minutes to several hours have elapsed. The variability of the symptoms, their onset, and their resolution makes each MTBI situation unique.[4]

As the history of the injury is obtained, be aware that it is common for athletes to report that they "got their bell rung" or received a "ding" to the head. Athletes may use this terminology because head injury is typically accompanied by an episode of tinnitus, otherwise known as *ringing in the ears*. Unfortunately, using these terms leads to a false assumption by players, coaches, and parents that a concussive injury is not a serious medical condition. Thus, health care providers should avoid using these terms, and educate coaches and other colleagues not to use them when describing a sports-related concussion.[4,15]

Diagnosing

Because head injuries can cause confusion, disorientation, impaired memory, and poor concentration, when questioned the patient may be unable to provide adequate information about the injury. This may hinder your ability to determine the full extent of the injury and the best course of action. Collecting a description of the incident from the patient's parents, the school's certified athletic trainer, or, in the absence of such a professional, the patient's coach, can help fill in the details needed to make a proper diagnosis.

Traditionally, an LOC incident, with or without the presence of amnesia, has been the determining factor when making an MTBI diagnosis. The current school of thought, however, is that neither LOC nor amnesia has to occur for a head injury to be classified as a concussion. Rather, it is generally agreed on that a diagnosis of MTBI is made if a person presents with one or more of the clinical features listed in Box 13.2. Keep in mind that, among these symptoms, dysfunction of memory is a more sensitive indicator of MTBI than is LOC and that something as simple as a headache might be the only indication that a patient has a concussion.[6,8,16,17]

BOX 13.2
CLINICAL FEATURES OF MILD TRAUMATIC BRAIN INJURY

Transient confusion	Lethargy
Disorientation	Vomiting
Impaired consciousness	Headache
Dysfunction of memory	Dizziness
Loss of consciousness (<30 minutes)	Fatigue
Seizures	Poor concentration
Irritability	

Department of Health and Human Services, Centers for Disease Control and Prevention. *Heads Up: Facts for Physicians About Mild Traumatic Brain Injury (MTBI)*. Retrieved from: http://www.cdc.gov/ncipc/tbi/Facts_for_Physicians_booklet.pdf. Accessed 9/5/08.

The examination of a patient who has sustained a head injury includes checking for the person's orientation to time, place, person, and situation, because this helps to assess transient confusion and level of consciousness. Asking the person to count backward and to relate the months of the year in reverse order evaluates the patient's ability to concentrate. To check memory function, have the patient recall recent events, and ask him or her to repeat three words and three objects at 5-minute intervals. Strength, coordination, sensation, and pupil function all should be assessed as part of the neurological examination, as should balance via the administration of Romberg's test (Fig. 13.9).[8,16]

One of the most challenging aspects of head injury management is determining when to order radiograph and/or neuroimaging testing. With an array of traditional and newer imaging methods available, it would seem prudent to order some form of testing to help in making clinical decisions. Unfortunately, skull radiographs, magnetic resonance imaging (MRI), computed tomography (CT), and electroencephalography (EEG) play a very limited role in evaluating MTBI, because these tests cannot[4,16,18,19]

• measure the subtle effects of concussion,
• identify a concussion or determine its severity,
• indicate when complete recovery has occurred after a concussion, or
• contribute to the RTP decision.

Thus, obtaining neuroimaging for patients with MTBI is reserved for those instances in which a focal brain lesion is suspected. This is discussed later in this chapter.

Grading

Grading MTBI severity is one of the biggest challenges primary health care providers face when managing the health of a concussed patient. With approximately 20 different published methods used to determine concussion severity, universal agreement on how to grade MTBI severity does not exist. Furthermore, many of these grading

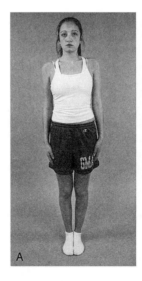
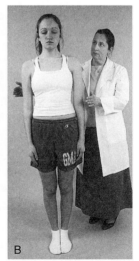

FIGURE 13.9 Romberg's test: eyes open (A) and eyes closed (B). From Dillon: *Nursing Health Assessment: A Critical Thinking, Case Studies Approach.* 2003. Philadelphia: F.A. Davis Company, Romberg test, A and B, pg 613, with permission.

methods rely on the occurrence of LOC and amnesia to determine degree of injury, but basing severity on these two findings alone is not wise. It is for these reasons that, in 2001, at the First International Conference on Concussion in Sport, experts in this field suggested abandoning all forms of concussion injury grading systems. In 2006, these and other experts further recommended that concussions be classified as either simple or complex based on how quickly a patient's symptoms disappear. According to these guidelines, a simple concussion resolves itself within 7 to 10 days, whereas in a complex concussion, symptoms linger for a longer period of time or become worse when the person exerts himself or herself. Patients who have multiple concussions over the course of time are also classified as having a complex concussion.[7,16,20,21]

(PEARL)

A simple concussion is one in which the patient's symptoms resolve in 7 to 10 days, whereas the symptoms of a patient with a complex concussion linger for a longer period of time.

Though it has been suggested that concussion grading systems be abandoned, many in the health care field still prefer to use a grading system to determine the extent of an MTBI. Two well-accepted methods used in the clinical setting include the one published by the American Academy of Neurology (AAN) (Table 13.1) and Cantu's Evidence-Based Grading System for Concussions (Table 13.2). The AAN's grading scale bases concussion severity on signs and symptoms that occur within the first 15 minutes after injury, whereas Cantu's scale emphasizes the presence and overall duration of patient symptoms, and waits for all symptoms to subside before grading the severity of the injury. Cantu's practical approach to concussion grading is supported by many who claim that the best way to determine concussion severity is only after all concussion symptoms have disappeared and the patient's neurological examination results are normal.[8,21,22]

Clinical Treatment

Though many health care providers prescribe prescription or over-the-counter (OTC) NSAIDs to MTBI patients, scientific evidence supporting this practice does not exist.

TABLE 13.1 American Academy of Neurology Concussion Grading Scale

Grade 1 (mild)	Transient confusion; no LOC; symptoms and mental status abnormalities resolve in less than 15 minutes
Grade 2 (moderate)	Transient confusion; no LOC; symptoms and mental status abnormalities last more than 15 minutes
Grade 3 (severe)	Any LOC

LOC = loss of consciousness.

Practice Parameter: the management of concussion in sports (summary statement). Report of the Quality Standards Subcommittee of the American Academy of Neurology. *Neurology* 1997;48:581 (with permission).

TABLE 13.2 Cantu's Evidence-Based Grading System for Concussion

Grade 1 (mild)	No LOC; posttraumatic amnesia* or postconcussion signs or symptoms lasting less than 30 minutes
Grade 2 (moderate)	LOC lasting less than 1 minute; posttraumatic amnesia* or postconcussion signs or symptoms lasting more than 30 minutes but less than 24 hours
Grade 3 (severe)	LOC lasting more than 1 minute; posttraumatic amnesia* lasting more than 24 hours; postconcussion signs or symptoms lasting more than 7 days

*Retrograde or anterograde.

LOC = loss of consciousness.

Cantu RC. Posttraumatic retrograde and anterograde amnesia: pathophysiology and implications in grading and safe return to play. *J Athl Train* 2001;36:244 (with permission).

Indeed, NSAIDs should not be prescribed, because they decrease platelet function and increase the chance for cranial bleeding. Acetaminophen in OTC strength can be prescribed as needed for pain relief, but patients should be advised to use this medication sparingly, because any pain reducer can mask MTBI symptoms.[4,23]

⬤ PEARL ⬤

Do not prescribe NSAIDs for an MTBI patient, and use oral pain reducers sparingly.

Home Care

After the patient has been evaluated and it is determined that it is safe for him or her to return home, the patient can be released to a caregiver who will commit to stay with and monitor the person. This is particularly important when MTBI symptoms disappear within minutes of the incidence of injury, because underlying pathology may still be present. Written instructions, as presented in Patient Teaching Handout (PTH) 13.1, should be given to the caregiver to help him or her monitor the health status of the patient during recovery.[4]

As noted in PTH 13.1 and in contrast to popular practice, there is no evidence supporting the value of waking a sleeping MTBI patient to monitor symptoms. In fact, constantly waking a recovering MTBI patient can increase symptoms during the waking hours because of sleep-pattern interruption. Thus, caregivers should be instructed to wake the patient only cautiously and on a case-by-case basis. In general, patients who have experienced LOC or prolonged periods of amnesia, as well as those who have significant symptoms at bedtime, should be wakened at 3- to 4-hour intervals throughout the night. Doing this allows the caregiver to determine whether symptoms have increased and whether the patient is experiencing a decreased level of consciousness. Both of these conditions suggest the presence of a more serious brain injury that requires immediate attention.[4]

Instruct caregivers to wake a sleeping **MTBI** patient only in cases of **LOC**, in prolonged periods of amnesia, or if the patient has significant symptoms at bedtime.

Return to Participation

When working with athletes, one of the most challenging decisions any health care provider has to make is determining when it is safe to return the patient to sports activities after MTBI. Unfortunately, the majority of professionals are forced to base their RTP decisions mostly on clinical experience, because there is little research to guide these decisions. Furthermore, RTP decisions can hinge on which functions are assessed before making a final decision. For example, a patient may be found fit to participate based on asymptomatic findings for confusion, disorientation, consciousness, memory dysfunction, and dizziness. However, the patient still may be experiencing other symptoms, such as fatigue, headaches, and trouble concentrating, that were not evaluated, or that the patient did not reveal in an attempt to return to participation earlier than would be prudent.[6,13,20]

Determining the amount of time a person should be prohibited from activity once symptoms have disappeared is an inexact science. What is known, however, is that a direct relationship exists between the severity and number of MTBI occurrences and the minimal duration of time a person should be excluded. This means that the patient's prior history of MTBI must be thoroughly reviewed to determine the amount of recovery time needed after MTBI. Table 13.3 provides guidelines for making RTP decisions. In general, an MTBI patient should not be cleared for participation until he or she is completely free of all symptoms listed in Box 13.2 for at least 7 days. Simply put, this means that a patient should be withheld from participation for 7 days starting with the first day he or she is symptom free. Doing so allows the patient to be monitored to ensure that symptoms do not reappear. This also minimizes the risk of recurrent injury.[4,8,13,22]

Do not clear an **MTBI** patient for participation until the person is completely symptom free for at least 7 days.

Because it may take days, weeks, or months for a person to become asymptomatic after an MTBI, implementing suggested RTP can be challenging, as athletes, parents, and coaches may not see the wisdom in withholding a symptom-free person from participation. In such situations, these people need to be educated about the dangers of returning a head-injured patient too soon to athletic activities. These dangers, which are later discussed in detail, include

• making a case of undiagnosed focal brain lesion worse,
• developing **postconcussion syndrome**, and
• predisposing the patient to an episode of **second impact syndrome**.

After the 7-day waiting period has elapsed, the MTBI patient can ease back into exercise and sports. Initially, patients can participate in light exercise activities, such as

TABLE 13.3 When to return to participation an MTBI patient who is symptom-free

GRADE OF CONCUSSION	TIME UNTIL RETURN TO PLAY*
Grade 1 concussion	15 minutes or less
Multiple grade 1 concussions	1 week
Grade 2 concussion	1 week
Multiple grade 2 concussions	2 weeks
Grade 3—brief LOC (seconds)	1 week
Grade 3—prolonged LOC (minutes)	2 weeks
Multiple grade 3 concussions	1 month or longer, based on clinical decision of evaluating physician

*Time after the patient is asymptomatic with normal neurologic assessment at rest and with exercise.

LOC = loss of consciousness; MTBI = mild traumatic brain injury.

Practice Parameter: the management of concussion in sports (summary statement). Report of the Quality Standards Subcommittee of the American Academy of Neurology. *Neurology* 1997;48:581 (with permission).

jogging, so long as they are reevaluated during and immediately after exercise sessions to see whether symptoms reappear. If symptoms do not return, patients can partake in non–concussion-producing, sport-specific activities. For example, a football player can participate in noncontact football drills during the regular football practice time. If the patient remains asymptomatic, he or she can return to full participation status. Anyone who has a return of any symptom at rest, with exertion, or during sport-specific activities should not be cleared.[4,8,20,22]

PEARL

Return-to-participation criteria should include the absence of all symptoms at rest, with exertion, and during non–concussion-producing sport-specific activities.

Disqualification

As challenging as it may be to determine when and for how long to exclude a symptom-free MTBI patient from participation, determining whether to recommend season or career disqualification can be much more difficult, because the number and degree of concussions necessary to cause permanent brain damage are unknown. It may help to bear in mind that people who have one MTBI maintain an increased risk for subsequent MTBIs and that failure to properly manage concussions may lead to the consequences identified earlier. So, it is prudent to follow the AAN's recommendation of disqualifying, for the remainder of the athletic season, a person who has a third concussion within that season. This does not mean, however, that the person is automatically cleared to participate in subsequent sports seasons. For example, if a high school male is disqualified from participating in football after a third concussion during the fall athletic season, he must receive clearance before participating in any winter sport. Also, use caution when using the term *athletic season*, because this can be defined as seasonal (fall, winter, spring), a semester (fall, spring), or year, depending on the competition level (e.g., high school, college, professional). These factors can increase the difficulty of determining the point at which patients can safely resume their athletic careers.[4,6,8,22]

If an athlete continues to experience MTBI incidents, he or she should be engaged in career disqualification discussions, particularly if the athlete participates in activities such as football, ice hockey, or lacrosse, which repeatedly expose the head to subconcussive forces. The more conservative experts in this field recommend career disqualification for athletes who have experienced three concussions within their athletic career. This arbitrary approach to disqualification is without scientific support and does not allow for consideration of the severity of MTBI incidents. In addition, career disqualifications usually do not specify whether the person is disqualified from all activities or just certain athletic endeavors. In consideration of the challenges of disqualification decisions, it is wise to refer athletes who have experienced multiple concussions for a neurological consultation.[4]

Refer those who have experienced multiple concussions for a neurological consultation.

Postconcussion Syndrome

Although MTBI symptoms usually subside over a period of a few hours to a few weeks, in some instances the symptoms do not resolve within the expected time frame. In other cases, initial symptoms disappear as expected, only to reappear at a later date. In either case, full symptom resolution may not occur for months or years. In instances in which the patient's symptoms persist for more than 6 weeks, a diagnosis of postconcussion syndrome is made.[13]

Though any concussive symptom could linger for an extended period of time, most postconcussion patients report experiencing one or more of the symptoms outlined in Box 13.3. For some patients, several or all of these symptoms are present at rest, whereas for other patients, these symptoms only occur during exertion. Regardless, postconcussion syndrome is often unresponsive to treatment and can lead to a lifetime of disability. This means that patients reporting postconcussive symptoms after an MTBI incident should not be cleared for participation, because doing so predisposes them to serious consequences, such as second impact syndrome (discussed later in this chapter). These patients must be referred for a neurological consultation.[24]

Returning an MTBI patient to sports participation before complete dissipation of symptoms can have serious consequences.

BOX 13.3
COMMON SYMPTOMS OF POSTCONCUSSION SYNDROME

Decreased attention span	Depression
Impaired memory	Blurred vision
Irritability	Vertigo
Persistent headache	Sensitivity to noise
Fatigue	Judgment problems
Dizziness	Anxiety

Adapted from: Cantu RC, Voy R. Second impact syndrome: a risk in any sport. *Phys Sportsmed* 1995;23(6):27; McCrea M, Guskiewicz KM, Barr W, et al. Acute effects and recovery time following concussion in collegiate football players: the NCAA Concussion Study. *JAMA* 2003;290:2556; Ryan LM, Warden DL. Post concussion syndrome. *Int Rev Psychiatry* 2003;15:310.

Second Impact Syndrome

Second impact syndrome occurs when the head receives a subsequent blow before the concussive symptoms from an initial blow have fully subsided. In most cases, this happens when an MTBI patient is cleared to participate prematurely. The second injury does not have to be severe or directly impact the head region but causes immediate swelling of the brain. Symptoms develop rapidly, and within seconds or minutes the person collapses from respiratory arrest. The mortality rate with second impact syndrome is extremely high, and although it can occur across the life span, mortality is more common among pediatric athletes.[24,25]

Ensure that a pediatric patient is completely asymptomatic from a previous head injury before clearing the person for participation.

Focal Brain Lesions

Because death or permanent disability can result from an untreated focal brain lesion, or *intracranial hemorrhage*, a lesion development must be ruled out during the initial and follow-up evaluations of any acute head injury. This assessment can be tricky because the signs and symptoms of a focal brain lesion are similar to those of an MTBI. A key difference is that the signs and symptoms of a focal lesion usually worsen as time passes. Thus, any patient with worsening symptoms should be referred for neurological consultation to rule out lesion development. Fortunately, focal brain lesions are not common among patients who participate in sports. Of those that do occur, the most common types are epidural and subdural hematomas.[4]

Rule out the presence of a focal brain lesion during the assessment of MTBI.

Epidural Hematoma

An **epidural hematoma** results from blood seeping into the epidural space. This lesion usually forms as a result of a coup injury, most commonly in the skull's temporal region. Hematoma development is typically a by-product of an external object striking the unprotected head with enough force to cause a depressed skull fracture (Fig. 13.8). Such an injury usually causes arterial bleeding, which prompts the epidural hematoma's signs and symptoms to occur within minutes. These include a quick decline in mental status, a state that directly relates to the increasing size of the hematoma; ipsilateral pupil dilation; and contralateral facial paralysis.[26]

Subdural Hematoma

Three times more likely to occur than an epidural hematoma, a **subdural hematoma** develops from bleeding into the subdural space and is the condition most responsible for postconcussion sports-related deaths. This lesion is usually caused by repeated blows to the protected or unprotected head, such as those that occur during a football game or boxing bout. This contrecoup, acceleration-deceleration mechanism causes the network of veins within the brain to tear, resulting in subdural bleeding (Fig. 13.8). Symptoms of an acute subdural hematoma can take up to 3 days to manifest, whereas symptoms of a chronic subdural hematoma can take weeks or months to develop. LOC is commonly associated with both the acute and chronic forms.[4,26]

Diagnostic Techniques for Focal Brain Lesions

Although diagnostic imaging techniques play a limited role in evaluating MTBI, MRI, CT, and EEG screenings maintain high sensitivity for diagnosing focal brain lesions. Thus, these neuroimaging tests should be used for any head injury case that involves[4,8,16,18]:

- LOC,
- severe amnesia,
- abnormal physical or neurological findings,
- increasing or intensified symptoms, or
- symptoms that last longer than 1 to 2 weeks.

Obtain neuroimaging screenings in **MTBI** cases that include **LOC**, severe amnesia, increasing symptoms, or symptoms that do not gradually subside.

Maxillofacial Conditions

Traumatic and chronic maxillofacial conditions occur in people across sports, life span, and gender. Once identified, most of these conditions require referral to an appropriate specialist.

Mechanisms of Injury

Though some maxillofacial conditions develop over a period of time and are chronic, most are caused by acute trauma. Indeed, the incidences of acute maxillofacial sports injuries far outnumber chronic conditions. Acute injuries occur when a person is struck with a piece of athletic equipment, such as ball, or by a body part of another person, such as an elbow, during competition. Because the proximity of the cranium to the maxillofacial bones also places the brain at risk during blunt-force trauma to this region, MTBI and focal brain lesions must be ruled out during the assessment of maxillofacial injury.

Conditions Involving the Eye

For obvious reasons, injury to the eye can have serious consequences if not handled properly. Most sports-related acute eye injuries occur when a person's orbit is struck by a ball or when the globe gets poked by an errant finger. At minimum, being struck by a ball results in an orbital hematoma, or *black eye*, but in some instances the patient experiences more serious damage. A finger that makes contact with the globe can damage any number of structures. Thus, any standard protocol for the evaluation and treatment for all serious traumatic eye conditions must include immediate referral to an ophthalmologist.

PEARL

Immediately refer all patients with serious traumatic eye conditions to an ophthalmologist for evaluation and treatment.

In response to the high incidence of serious eye trauma in sports, interscholastic and intercollegiate athletic governing bodies mandate the use of approved eye protection in activities such as ice hockey and lacrosse. However, because traumatic eye injury can occur as a result of participation in virtually any athletic activity, all patients should be encouraged to use proper eye protection during sports participation.[27]

Subconjunctival Hemorrhage

Bleeding in the sclera occurs when an object larger than the size of the eye's orbit strikes the area without making contact with the eye itself, as when a person is hit in the eye by a baseball. The resulting **subconjunctival hemorrhage** causes the white of the eye to become red and inflamed. Though any eye trauma should be considered serious, a subconjunctival hemorrhage does not affect vision and usually resolves itself spontaneously. Patients with signs of visual disturbance at the initial or any subsequent evaluation should be referred to an ophthalmologist.[28]

Hyphema

When an object small enough to invade the orbit makes direct contact with the eye, blood vessels in the iris can rupture. When this occurs, blood settles into the eye's anterior chamber (Fig. 13.10). The resulting **hyphema** causes the patient pain and blurred vision.[27,29]

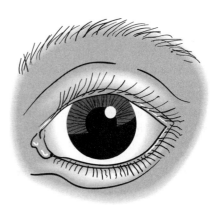

FIGURE 13.10 Fluid in the anterior chamber (hyphema).

Blood in the anterior chamber, which typically causes the chamber's aqueous fluid to assume a reddish tint, is a telltale sign of a hyphema. An ophthalmoscope can document the presence of blood too small to be detected with the naked eye. Though bleeding may be self-correcting and blood that is present may be naturally reabsorbed, a hyphema is a serious, sight-threatening condition, and these patients should be immediately referred to an ophthalmologist. Transporting the patient from your office to the ophthalmologist's should be done with the person's head erect, because this isolates bleeding to the inferior aspect of the chamber and helps prevent the area of blood infiltration from widening.[27,29]

Corneal Laceration

A **corneal laceration**, or *open globe*, is a serious ocular injury that usually occurs when a sharp object, such as a fingernail or ice skate blade, comes in contact with the cornea. Symptoms include pain, decreased visual acuity, photophobia, decreased eye movements, and bloody tears. Typically, a hyphema accompanies a corneal laceration. When visualized, the pupil looks tear-shaped and the anterior chamber appears shallow or flat. Bubbles may also be present in this chamber. The head of patients with a corneal laceration must be kept erect and immobile, and the affected eye should be covered by a protective shield. These patients should be immediately referred to an ophthalmologist for evaluation and possible surgical intervention.[29]

Detached Retina

A **detached retina** can be caused by blows to the head or result from disease. Risk factors for retinal detachment include nearsightedness, heredity, and aging. If caused by head or eye trauma, the detachment may not present until days or weeks after the date of injury. Though a retinal detachment is painless, if it is not treated quickly, it can cause permanent partial or total vision loss.[27]

A person with a detached retina presents with a history of blurred vision, seeing bright flashes of light, loss of the eye's central or peripheral field of vision, and the appearance of eye floaters. Patients may also report a "film" or "curtain" impairing their sight. Bed rest is the conservative treatment of choice, whereas more serious detachments are treated surgically. Patients with a suspected retinal detachment should be disqualified from participation until the person is evaluated by an ophthalmologist.[27]

Orbital Fracture

Sports-related orbital, or *blow-out*, fractures typically occur when the orbit is struck by a hard object (e.g., baseball, softball) traveling at a great rate of speed. The force generated by such objects can cause the eye to be displaced posteriorly (Fig. 13.11). The resulting increase in pressure causes the bones that form the floor of the orbit to fracture.[27,29,30]

Patients with this condition report pain with eye movement, diplopia, and cheek paresthesia. Asymmetry of the eyes is present, because the eye on the affected side rides lower than the noninvolved eye. Upward eye movement is decreased on the affected side. Radiographs confirm the fracture. People with a nondisplaced blow-out fracture are treated symptomatically with rest and careful monitoring. These patients are disqualified from sports that place the orbit at risk for a direct blow until the injury has fully healed, which usually takes 4 to 6 weeks. Patients with displaced fractures and those who experience visual disturbances that do not self-correct should be referred to an ophthalmologist.[28-31]

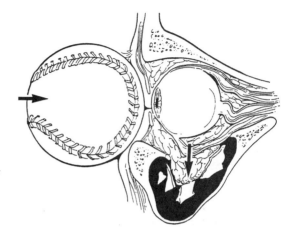

FIGURE 13.11 Blow-out fracture. From Starkey and Ryan: *Evaluation of Orthopedic and Athletic Injuries*, 2nd ed. 2002. Philadelphia: F.A. Davis Company, Fig. 16-11, pg 577, with permission.

Conditions Involving the Ear

Acute injuries to this region usually involve the external ear, whereas chronic conditions occur in both internal and external structures. Wrestling, football, and lacrosse organizations attempt to protect players from ear injury by requiring that they wear a helmet or ear guards. However, though this practice should be encouraged, realize that using such equipment does not guarantee that a person's ear will remain unharmed during sports participation.

Auricular Hematoma

An **auricular hematoma,** otherwise known as *cauliflower ear,* is caused by repetitive rubbing of the auricle against a nonyielding surface and is seen most frequently in wrestling (Fig. 13.12). The most common MOI occurs when a wrestler's ear is forced

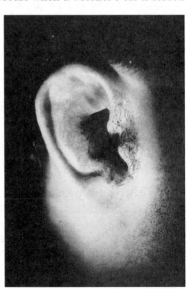

FIGURE 13.12 Auricular hematoma, or *cauliflower ear.* From Starkey and Ryan: *Evaluation of Orthopedic and Athletic Injuries*, 2nd ed. 2002. Philadelphia: F.A. Davis Company, Fig. 17-11, pg 592, with permission.

into and rubs along the surface of a wrestling mat. This friction injury leads to fluid buildup in the area.[30,32]

A patient who has an auricular hematoma usually reports pain and throbbing of the ear and has obvious swelling of the auricle. This swelling is easily palpated, and its presence causes the auricle's anatomic landmarks to disappear. Once an auricular hematoma is confirmed, the associated fluid should be drained with a needle and syringe. An ear compression bandage used for a week or two after drainage prevents edema return, as does instructing the patient to modify his or her activity until the condition subsides. Patients with this condition should be scheduled for multiple follow-up examinations because it is common for the hematoma to return. In these instances, the fluid may need to be redrained multiple times.[31,32]

If this condition is not treated quickly or properly, the hematoma eventually hardens, compromising the region's blood supply. Ultimately, this causes necrosis of the underlying tissue. The outcome is an auricle that is permanently disfigured, resembling the shape of a piece of cauliflower. Because the only way to repair this disfigurement is with surgery, many people who develop an auricular hematoma opt to leave the ear in the disfigured shape.[31,32]

Otitis Externa

Otitis externa is caused by wetness that is allowed to linger in the ear canal for an extended period of time, altering the canal's normal pH balance. Though referred to as *swimmer's ear* because of its prevalence in this population, otitis externa can occur in anyone who does not properly dry the ear canal after water and bathing activities. If left untreated, the infection may spread to the middle ear. Common symptoms include otalgia, itching, otorrhea, ear discomfort, and hearing loss. When inspected, the person's ear canal appears red and irritated, two common signs of this condition. Pulling on the patient's earlobe increases pain and discomfort, as does palpating the lymph nodes located around the mastoid process. These lymph nodes are also swollen.[33]

Otitis externa can be prevented and treated by teaching patients proper ear canal–drying techniques. People involved in water activities should also irrigate the ear canals on a regular basis by using an acidifying agent, such as white vinegar and alcohol mixed in equal parts. Doing this lowers the canal's pH level and prevents bacteria from forming in the region. In addition, patients should refrain from excessively cleaning the ears, because this activity removes cerumen, which, because of its acetic and antimicrobial properties, naturally protects the canals from bacterial infection. When these measures do not help, prescribing an ear drop solution containing 3% boric acid and alcohol may be necessary. In severe cases, a broad-spectrum antibiotic may be needed to combat the infection. Though some recommend the use of earplugs for people who are involved in extended water activities, if inserted improperly these plugs can cause problems, such as causing cerumen to become impacted within the canal.[33]

Conditions Involving the Nose, Mouth, and Jaw

Because of its location in the front of the face, the nose is highly susceptible to blunt-force trauma. Sports-related nasal injuries usually occur when an object or another player's body part, most commonly the elbow, strikes the nose. Because severe swelling and bleeding usually accompany acute nose trauma, the entire maxillofacial region must be thoroughly evaluated to rule out involvement of surrounding structures. In addition, blunt-force trauma also causes injury to the mouth and jaw. Thus, these injuries require a thorough evaluation of the maxilla and mandible and necessitate that the inside of the mouth be evaluated for possible injury to the teeth.

Rule out surrounding structure involvement when evaluating blunt-force trauma to the nose, mouth, and jaw.

Nasal Fracture

A nasal fracture is the most common facial fracture resulting from sports participation. This injury happens when a force is delivered to the face frontally, depressing the nose, or from the side, causing the nose to deviate laterally. Bleeding, immediate swelling, and noted deformity are typical signs, but a lack of deformity does not necessarily rule out a fracture.[31,34]

The patient with a nasal fracture reports having heard a "crunch" or "crack," described as the sound of biting into uncooked macaroni. Visual inspection reveals a swollen, sometimes ecchymotic nose that may or may not be deviated to one side. Because radiographic evaluation does not always confirm a fracture, these clinical findings are usually enough to make this diagnosis. Visualizing the nasal passages with an otoscope can determine whether a septal hematoma is present, a condition that may develop within hours after the injury. If present, the mass should be drained, because one that is not can lead to infection. Displaced nasal fractures should be referred to a head and neck surgeon for reduction. RTP can usually occur fairly quickly for nondisplaced fractures, with the limiting factors being pain and ability to breathe through the injured nasal passageways. To protect the nose from further injury, patients should wear a commercially produced face mask during activity until the condition fully heals.[31,34]

Mandible Fracture

The mandible is the second most common facial bone to fracture during sports activities. Resulting from a high-velocity direct blow, mandible fractures most commonly occur in the bone's body, condyle, and angle regions. In the majority of cases, at least two areas fracture. In some cases, the incidence of mandible fracture occurs in combination with TMJ dislocation.[30,31]

The chief concern of a patient with a mandible fracture is increased pain with mouth opening and closing. Obvious facial distortion and malocclusion of the teeth are also present. An inability of the patient to talk normally is apparent, particularly if the fracture is complicated by a dislocation. Palpating the area causes the patient pain, and touching the area produces abnormal motion at the fracture site. Patients with a fractured mandible typically have a positive tongue blade test (Fig. 13.13). Radiographs confirm the fracture. Initial treatment includes jaw immobilization, whereas long-term management calls for internal fixation of the jaw. Patients treated with internal fixation are disqualified from contact and collision sports for a minimum of 6 weeks. Noncontact sports can be played as tolerated.[30,31]

Temporomandibular Joint Dysfunction

The TMJ is injured by acute (direct blow), spontaneous (large yawn), chronic (grinding of teeth during sleep), and idiopathic means. Symptoms include considerable pain and discomfort in the area of the TMJ. Spasm may occur in the overlying facial muscles.[35]

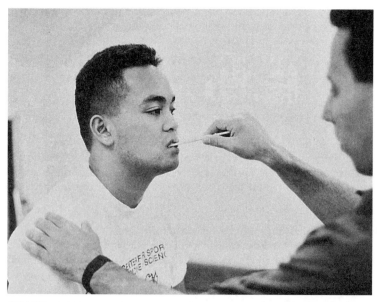

FIGURE 13.13 Tongue blade sign. As the patient attempts to hold a tongue depressor with a clenched mouth, the examiner rotates the depressor. A positive sign occurs if the patient is unable to maintain a firm bite or pain is elicited.
From Starkey and Ryan: *Evaluation of Orthopedic and Athletic Injuries*, 2nd ed. 2002. Philadelphia: F.A. Davis Company, Box 17-3, pg 603, with permission.

Patients with a TMJ injury typically present with a jaw that is pushed forward from its normal position. This abnormality is highlighted when the patient clenches the teeth. Dislocation on one side causes asymmetrical deviation of the chin, whereas bilateral dislocation causes the jaw to protrude. The patient may also report a popping or cracking feeling during jaw opening and closing, which can be verified by palpating the TMJ (Fig. 13.14). Conservative treatment for a patient with a TMJ injury includes jaw immobilization via a custom-designed removable mouthguard. Surgical intervention is indicated in certain situations. To protect the integrity of the TMJ, an athlete may need to wear an approved mouthguard during all future sports activities.[35]

Dental Conditions

Acute trauma to the teeth usually results in tooth fracture, luxation, or complete avulsion. Because dental trauma may also affect the mandible and/or TMJ, the condition of these structures must be assessed when evaluating dental injury. After initially evaluating and treating dental trauma, all patients must be immediately referred to a dentist or oral surgeon as indicated.[30]

Immediately refer patients with dental trauma to a dentist or oral surgeon as indicated.

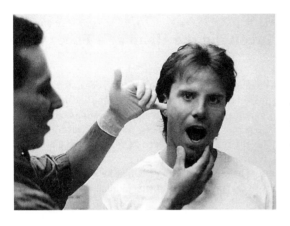

FIGURE 13.14 Temporomandibular joint palpation. While the examiner lightly presses the fifth finger in the outermost portion of the auditory canal, the patient opens and closes the mouth.
From Starkey and Ryan: *Evaluation of Orthopedic Injuries and Athletic Injuries*, 2nd ed. 2002. Philadelphia: F.A. Davis Company, Fig. 17-16, pg 595, with permission.

When a tooth fractures, the severity of injury is dependent on how much of the tooth's pulp is involved. Initially, these injuries are treated by instructing the patient to gently bite into gauze or a clean towel. Doing so helps to control bleeding and decreases pain by limiting nerve exposure to air, saliva, and temperature changes. All tooth fragments should be saved and sent with the patient to the dentist.[30,36,37]

If a tooth becomes luxated, it usually becomes extruded or intruded. The extruded tooth appears longer, whereas the intruded tooth appears shorter, than the surrounding teeth. In instances of tooth extrusion, it is safe to gently push the tooth back into its proper position. In contrast, the intruded tooth should not be repositioned. In either case, the patient's lower and upper jaws should be immobilized in preparation for transport to the dentist's or oral surgeon's office. This can be accomplished by inserting the patient's playing mouthguard into his or her mouth or by having the patient gently bite down on a clean towel or gauze pad.[30,36,37]

Treating a case of tooth avulsion correctly and in a timely fashion can lead to a favorable outcome for the patient. If properly replanted within 30 minutes of being dislodged, an avulsed tooth has a 90% chance of survival. However, the survival rate decreases as the amount of time the tooth remains out of its socket increases. When a tooth becomes avulsed, it should be handled only by its enamel portion and cleaned with sterile saline solution before its being reimplanted. Afterward, the patient's upper and lower jaws should be immobilized before sending or transporting the person for emergency dental care. If reimplantation is not possible, the tooth should be stored in milk, saline solution, saline-soaked gauze, or cold water or be placed in the athlete's cheek or under the tongue.[30,36,37]

An avulsed tooth that is reimplanted within 30 minutes has a 90% survival rate.

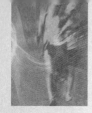

CASE STUDY
Conditions Involving the Head and Face

SCENARIO

A 17-year-old high school football player is brought in by his mother to be evaluated after sustaining a concussion 9 days ago. At the time of injury, signs and symptoms included no LOC and transient amnesia of about 15 minutes, with some disorientation lasting about 25 minutes. After initial evaluation by the school's certified athletic trainer, he was told that he could not return to play for at least 1 week and that he needed to be cleared to play by his primary health care provider. In 2 days, this patient wants to play in the state championship game. College recruiters will also be present at the game. He insists that he is fine and for the past week has been secretly practicing with teammates after official football practice has ended.

PERTINENT HISTORY

History and physical done without mother in room.

Medications: Albuterol metered-dose inhaler for mild asthma. Uses less than one time per month. No other medications. No known drug allergies.

Family History: Paternal grandfather with hypertension. Otherwise unremarkable.

PERSONAL HEALTH HISTORY

Tobacco Use: Nonsmoker. No history of oral tobacco use.

Alcohol Intake: Says has signed school athletic pledge and does not use any alcohol during the football season. Admits to drinking 2 to 3 beers on weekends during the off-season.

Recreational Drugs and Banned Substances: Tried marijuana once during the summer he was 15, but admits to no drug use since that time. Denies any steroid use.

Caffeinated Beverages: Has an occasional soft drink (1 to 2 per week); otherwise no caffeine.

Diet: Says he has a big appetite. Tries to eat lots of protein and carbohydrate loads before a game. To increase muscle mass, uses creatine powder mix.

Past Medical History: Frequent otitis media as a child. Childhood asthma triggered by respiratory infections. Rarely needs inhaler at present.

History of Present Illness: Sustained a concussion 9 days ago from a collision injury during football game. No LOC, amnesia for 15 minutes, and disoriented to time and place for 25 minutes. Had ongoing dizziness, headaches, fatigue, and inability to concentrate on school work for about 1 week. He says all of those symptoms resolved 3 days ago, and he is adamant about his readiness to play.

PERTINENT PHYSICAL EXAMINATION*

Neurological Examination: Oriented to time, place, and person. Cranial nerves II through XII: no deficits. Negative Romberg's test. Gait: smooth and easy without evidence of dizziness.

*Focused examination limited to key points for this case.

Cardiopulmonary: Lungs clear to auscultation; no crackles or wheezing. Blood pressure: 124/70 mm Hg resting, 120/68 mm Hg standing. Heart: no murmurs or clicks. Rate regular: 64 bpm resting, 66 bpm standing.

RED FLAGS FOR THE PRIMARY HEALTH CARE PROFESSIONAL TO CONSIDER

Although today's examination is within normal limits, by history, the patient's concussion symptoms resolved only 3 days ago. It is not safe for this athlete to return to play in 2 days because he must be symptom free for at least 1 week. Although this is no doubt an extreme disappointment to the athlete, his coaches, his teammates, and his parents, the cost of returning to participation too early must be considered and emphasized. Allowing the student to return to participation too quickly after MTBI increases the risk of second impact syndrome—a syndrome associated with a high mortality rate.

RECOMMENDED PLAN

- Because the patient is still a minor, get signed permission from his mother so that you can communicate your findings and recommendations to the school's certified athletic trainer.
- Provide a thorough explanation to the mother and the athlete about the risk involved if he continues to practice or returns to participation too early.
- Be aware that this might create a crisis for this athlete, and carefully assess the athlete's response to your decision.
- Problem solve with the school administrative personnel and certified athletic trainer to determine when another opportunity will present for the patient's performance to be observed.

REFERENCES

1. National Center for Injury Prevention and Control, Division of Injury and Disability Outcomes and Programs. *Traumatic Brain Injury in the United States: Emergency Department Visits, Hospitalizations, and Deaths, 1995-2001.* Atlanta, GA: Centers for Disease Control and Prevention, 2004.
2. Sosin DM, Sniezek JE, Thurman DJ. Incidence of mild and moderate brain injury in the United States, 1991. *Brain Inj* 1996;10:47.
3. Mueller FO, Cantu RC. *Twenty-Fifth Annual Report of the National Center for Catastrophic Sports Injury Research: Fall 1982-Spring 2007.* Retrieved from: http://www.unc.edu/depts/nccsi/AllSport.htm. Accessed 9/5/08.
4. Guskiewicz KM, Bruce SL, Cantu RC, et al. National Athletic Trainers' Association Position Statement: management of sport-related concussion. *J Athl Train* 2004;39:280.
5. Gennarelli T. Mechanisms of brain injury. *J Emerg Med* 1993;11(suppl 1):5.
6. Guskiewicz KM, Weaver NL, Padua DA, et al. Epidemiology of concussion in collegiate and high school football players. *Am J Sports Med* 2000;28:643.
7. Maroon JC, Lovell MR, Norwig J, et al. Cerebral concussion in athletes: evaluation and neuropsychological testing. *Neurosurgery* 2000;47:659.
8. Practice Parameter: the management of concussion in sports (summary statement). Report of the Quality Standards Subcommittee of the American Academy of Neurology. *Neurology* 1997;48:581.
9. McKeever CK, Schatz P. Current issues in the identification assessment, and management of concussions in sports-related injuries. *Appl Neuropsychol* 2003;10:4.
10. Leininger BE, Gramling S, Farrell AD, et al. Neuropsychological deficits in symptomatic minor head injury patients after concussion and mind concussion. *J Neurol Neurosurg Psychiatry* 1990;53:293.
11. Ommaya A, Salazar A. A spectrum of mild brain injuries in sports. In: *Proceedings of the Mild Brain Injury Sports Summit.* Dallas, TX: NATA, Inc., 1994:72.
12. Powell JW, Barber-Foss KM. Traumatic brain injury in high school athletes. *JAMA* 1999;282:958.
13. McCrea M, Guskiewicz KM, Barr W, et al. Acute effects and recovery time following concussion in collegiate football players: the NCAA Concussion Study. *JAMA* 2003;290:2556.
14. Field M, Collins MW, Lovell MR, et al. Does age play a role in recovery from sports related concussion? A comparison of high school and collegiate athletes. *J Pediatr* 2003;142:546.
15. Lovell MR, Collins MW, Iverson GL, et al. Grade 1 or "ding" concussions in high school athletes. *Am J Sports Med* 2004;32:47.
16. Aubry M, Cantu R, Dvorak J, et al. Summary and agreement statement of the First International Conference on Concussion in Sport, Vienna 2001. *Br J Sports Med* 2002;36:6.
17. Collins MW, Iverson GL, Lovell MR, et al. On-field predicators of neuropsychological and symptom deficit following sports-related concussion. *Clin J Sport Med* 2003;13:222.
18. Committee on Quality Improvement, American Academy of Pediatrics and Commission on Clinical Practice and Research, American Academy of Family Physicians. The management of minor closed head injury in children (AC9858). *Pediatrics* 1999;104:1407.
19. Johnston KM, Ptito A, Chankowsky J, et al. New frontiers in diagnostic imaging in concussive head injury. *Clin J Sport Med* 2001;111:166.
20. Theye F, Mueller KA. Heads up: concussions in high school sports. *Clin Med Res* 2004;3:165.
21. McCrory P, Johnston K, Meeuwisse W, et al. Summary and agreement statement of the 2nd International Conference on Concussion in Sport, Prague 2004. *Br J Sports Med* 2005;39:196.
22. Cantu RC. Posttraumatic retrograde and anterograde amnesia: pathophysiology and implications in grading and safe return to play. *J Athl Train* 2001;36:244.
23. McCrory P. New treatments for concussion: the next millennium beckons. *Clin J Sport Med* 2001;11:190.
24. Cantu RC, Voy R. Second impact syndrome: a risk in any sport. *Phys Sportsmed* 1995;23(6):27.
25. Saunders RL, Harbaugh RE. The second impact in catastrophic contact-sports head trauma. *JAMA* 1984;252:538.

26. Bailes JE, Hudson V. Classification of sport-related head trauma: a spectrum of mild to severe injury. *J Athl Train* 2001;36:236.
27. Zagelbaum B. Sports-related eye trauma: managing common injuries. *Phys Sportsmed* 1993;21(9):25.
28. Jeffers JB. Considerations of anatomy, physiology and pathology of sports related ocular injuries. *Athl Train J Natl Athl Train Assoc* 1985;20(3):195.
29. Rodriguez JO, Lavina AM, Agarwal A. Prevention and treatment of common eye injuries in sports. *Am Fam Physician* 2003;67:1481.
30. Mathews B. Maxillofacial trauma from athletic endeavors *Athl Train J Natl Athl Train Assoc* 1990;25:132.
31. Harmon KG, Rubin A. Facial injuries in sports: a team physician's guide to diagnosis and treatment. *Phys Sportsmed* 2005;33(4):56.
32. Davidson TM, Neuman TR. Managing ear trauma. *Phys Sportsmed* 1994;22(7):27.
33. Davidson TM, Neuman TR. Managing inflammatory ear conditions. *Phys Sportsmed* 1994;22(8):56.
34. Schendel SA. Sports-related nasal injury. *Phys Sportsmed* 1990;18(10):59.
35. Buescher JJ. Temporomandibular joint disorders. *Am Fam Physician* 2007;76:1477.
36. Honsik KA. Steps to take for dental injuries. *Phys Sportsmed* 2004;32(9):28.
37. Douglass AB, Douglass JM. Common dental emergencies. *Am Fam Physician* 2003;67:511.

SUGGESTED READINGS

Kelly JP. Loss of consciousness: pathophysiology and implications on grading and safe return to play. *J Athl Train* 2001;36:249.

McCrea M, Hammeke T, Olsen G, et al. Unreported concussion in high school football players: implications for prevention. *Clin J Sport Med* 2004;14:13.

Ryan LM, Warden DL. Post concussion syndrome. *Int Rev Psychiatry* 2003;15:310.

WEB LINKS

www.aan.com/professionals. Accessed 9/5/08.
American Academy of Neurology Web site providing extensive information related to the practice of, education on, and latest research in neurology.

www.biausa.org. Accessed 9/5/08.
Brain Injury Association of America Web site reviewing state resources, referral resources, and current legislation and policies related to brain injury and disability.

http://www.cdc.gov/ncipc/tbi/physicians_tool_kit.htm. Accessed 9/5/08.
Department of Health and Human Services Centers for Disease Control and Prevention Web site providing primary health care professionals with guidance in regard to diagnosing and managing patients with mild traumatic brain injury.

14

Conditions Involving the Thorax, Abdomen, and Genitalia

● **Brian J. Toy, PhD, ATC**

Though injuries of the thorax, abdomen, and genitalia do not happen nearly as often as those of the musculoskeletal system, trauma in these regions, particularly when incurred by the thorax and abdomen, can be catastrophic. This is especially true if the resulting conditions go unrecognized or if diagnosis and treatment are delayed. It is for these reasons that you must be thorough when evaluating trauma to these areas.[1]

Anatomy of the Thorax, Abdomen, and Genitalia

Maintaining a general anatomical knowledge of the thorax, abdomen, and male and female genitalia provides a basis with which you can develop a reasonable differential diagnosis when evaluating sports-related injury to these regions.

Bones and Joints

The thorax, or *rib cage*, is composed of 12 pair of ribs, costal cartilage, and the sternum, or *chest bone* (Fig. 14.1). These structures are responsible for protecting the underlying heart and lungs, and the lower ribs also protect some of the internal abdominal organs, such as the spleen and liver, from trauma.

The ribs are classified as one of three types: true, false, or floating. They are arranged in this fashion based on how they attach or do not attach to the sternum. For

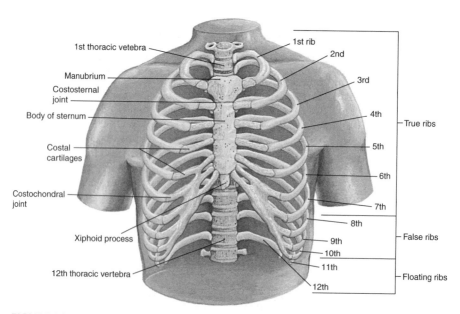

FIGURE 14.1 Anterior view of the rib cage.
Adapted from Scanlon: *Essentials of Anatomy and Physiology*, 5th ed. 2007. Philadelphia: F.A. Davis Company, Fig. 6-11, pg 123, with permission.

example, the first seven pairs of ribs, also known as *true ribs*, connect to the sternum at the costosternal joints by way of their own costal cartilage. In contrast, the costal cartilages of ribs 8 through 10, otherwise known as *false ribs*, indirectly attach to the sternum by first connecting to the coastal cartilage of rib 7. Each true and false rib attaches to its corresponding costal cartilage at an individual costochondral joint. Because it is more pliable than bone, costal cartilage allows the chest to expand during forceful inhalation, providing the body with more oxygen when needed. Instead of attaching to the sternum, the lower two pairs of ribs "float" within the surrounding musculature, giving rise to their designation as *floating ribs*.

Muscles and Ligaments

The primary thorax muscles include the intercostals, located between the ribs, the serratus anterior, and the pectoralis major, or *chest muscle* (Fig. 14.2). The pectoralis major protects the anterior portions of the upper ribs from blunt-force trauma, leaving the lower ribs exposed to injury. The abdominal wall is comprised of seven muscles. These include the vertically situated right and left rectus abdominis, the obliquely positioned external and internal obliques, and the transversus abdominis (Fig. 14.2)

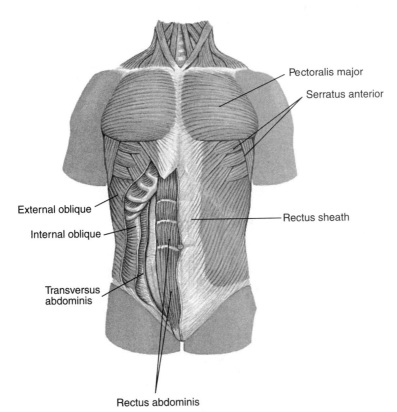

FIGURE 14.2 Muscles of the thorax and abdomen, anterior view.
Adapted from Scanlon: *Essentials of Anatomy and Physiology*, 5th ed. 2007. Philadelphia: F.A. Davis Company, Fig. 7–10A, pg 155, with permission.

Enclosed in a "rectus sheath," the two rectus abdominis muscles run from the pubis to the ribs as they pass on either side of the umbilicus. The external obliques are situated superficially as they run from the ribs to the iliac crest and the rectus sheath, whereas the deep-lying internal obliques arise from the iliac crest and attach to the ribs. The oblique muscles rotate the trunk and, working in unison with the rectus abdominis muscles, laterally flex the trunk. The most inferior portion of the external oblique helps to form the inguinal ligament, a structure that runs from the anterior superior iliac spine (ASIS) to the pubis (Fig. 14.3). As the external oblique forms this ligament, it rolls under itself, producing a passageway known as the **inguinal canal**. The opening of this canal near the ASIS is known as the *internal*, or *deep*, *inguinal ring*, whereas the opening near the pubis is termed the *external*, or *superficial*, *inguinal ring*. In men, this canal provides a passageway for the vas deferens and testicular artery and veins as they pass from the body to the scrotal sac. The inguinal region is an area of abdominal weakness, one that has the potential to cause problems in both the pediatric and adult populations. Finally, lying deep to the rectus abdominis and oblique muscles is the transversus abdominis, a structure that helps to keep the internal abdominal contents from protruding. Lower portions of this muscle also help form the inguinal canal.

Thoracic Cavity

The primary structures in the thorax, the heart and lungs, are protected from trauma by the rib cage. The lungs are encased in a thin, serous membrane known as the *pleura*, whereas the heart is surrounded by a fibrous pericardial sac. The diaphragm, a muscle

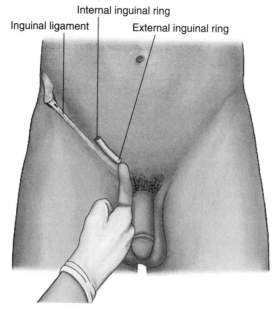

FIGURE 14.3 The inguinal region in the male.
From Dillon: *Nursing Health Assessment: A Critical Thinking, Case Studies Approach.* 2003. Philadelphia: F.A. Davis Company, pg 580, with permission.

involved in inspiration and expiration, forms the floor of the thoracic cavity and divides this region from the abdominal cavity.

Abdominal Cavity

The abdominal cavity is divided into four quadrants. These include the right upper (RUQ), left upper (LUQ), right lower (RLQ), and left lower (LLQ) quadrants (Fig. 14.4). Further subdivisions include the umbilical, the region around the umbilicus; and the epigastric and hypogastric, the areas above and below the umbilical region, respectively. Dividing the abdomen in this fashion allows for the location of intra-abdominal organs to be identified within each quadrant (Table 14.1). Portions of the small and large intestines are located in all four quadrants.

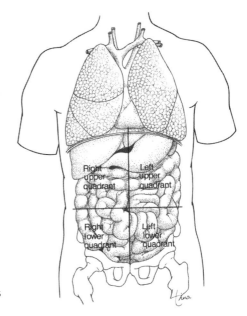

FIGURE 14.4 Abdominal quadrant system. From Scanlon: *Essentials of Anatomy and Physiology*, 5th ed. 2007. Philadelphia: F.A. Davis Company, Fig. 1-7A, pg 17, with permission.

TABLE 14.1 Location of abdominal organs

RIGHT UPPER QUADRANT	LEFT UPPER QUADRANT
Liver	Spleen
Right kidney	Left kidney
½ Pancreas	½ Pancreas
Gallbladder	Stomach

RIGHT LOWER QUADRANT	LEFT LOWER QUADRANT
½ Bladder	½ Bladder
Appendix	

Genitalia

The external male genitalia include the penis and scrotum, a skin-covered pouch that houses the testes, epididymis, and spermatic cord. In women, the term *vulva* is used to describe the female external genitalia. It consists of the labia majora, labia minora, clitoris, vestibule of the vagina, and vaginal opening.

Conditions of the Thorax

Thoracic injuries are divided into those affecting the chest wall, such as rib and sternal fractures, and those affecting the intrathoracic organs, such as **myocardial contusion, pulmonary contusion, pneumothorax**, and **hemothorax**. Thus, a primary goal when evaluating the thorax is to differentiate between these two injury types. This can be challenging, because patients with an injured heart or lung report injury mechanisms and symptoms similar to those of patients with a musculoskeletal injury. However, one symptom that differs between these conditions is the type of pain the person experiences. The pain of a person with a musculoskeletal problem is more likely to be vague and remain localized, whereas the pain experienced by someone with an internal organ injury may radiate to the jaw or to one or both shoulders. In the end, appreciate that any traumatic injury to the chest may disturb cardiopulmonary functions, ultimately proving fatal if not promptly diagnosed and corrected.[1-3]

Any traumatic injury to the chest may disturb cardiopulmonary functions, ultimately proving fatal if not promptly diagnosed and corrected.

Mechanisms of Injury

Traumatic injuries to the thorax occur from two primary mechanisms: blunt-force trauma and sudden deceleration forces. This places people who participate in collision sports, such as football and ice hockey, at a high risk of injuring the thorax, because these activities consistently expose participants to both injury mechanisms. Indeed, blunt-force trauma is the most frequently encountered type of thoracic injury in the pediatric athlete. Those involved in bicycling and skiing are also at risk, because high-speed deceleration forces commonly occur in these activities. In addition, recognize that as a result of the elastic and compliant nature of the child's thorax, blunt-forces may grossly deform the thorax of young people, only for it to return to its normal shape without leaving any sign of injury. Hence, any history of a compression injury in the pediatric patient should alert you to the possibility of extensive underlying thoracic pathology, even if the chest appears normal. Furthermore, it is not uncommon for a patient to present with an injured thorax without reporting any history of trauma to the region. This makes the resulting insidious onset of chest pain challenging to treat.[1,4]

Blunt-force trauma is the most frequently encountered type of thoracic injury in pediatric athletes.

Chest Wall Injury

Injuries to the chest wall are divided into two types: those that occur traumatically and those that have an insidious onset. These latter, painful conditions, otherwise known as *chest wall syndromes*, are of particular concern to athletes and must always be considered as a potential of chest wall pain in this population.[2,4]

Chest Wall Syndromes

Chest wall syndromes are thoracic soft tissue injuries that occur as a result of excessive twisting forces placed on the torso, such as what happens when a person serves a tennis ball, runs, or swims. These overuse rib cage injuries include **costochondritis**, **Tietze's syndrome**, and **slipping rib syndrome**. Though these conditions occur in patients of any age and gender, they most commonly occur in the young.[4-6]

In general, a patient who complains of nonspecific chest wall pain with no known etiology is usually diagnosed as suffering from costochondritis. This is particularly true when noncardiac pain is identified in those at risk for a cardiac etiology. Costochondritis most commonly occurs in the area of ribs 2 through 5, and patients who have it present with a history of chest pain accompanied by localized anterior chest wall tenderness on or near the costochondral or chondrosternal joints. This condition does not produce swelling, and, in most cases, pain can be reproduced by applying direct pressure over the affected costochondral or chondrosternal joint. Pain also increases when a patient adducts the shoulder on the affected side at the same time he or she rotates the head to the same side.[4,6]

As with costochondritis, Tietze's syndrome is a benign condition characterized by anterior chest wall pain with no history of trauma. It is distinguished from costochondritis by the presence of swelling in the area of pain at the affected costochondral or chondrosternal joint. Tietze's syndrome is most commonly seen in the area of the second and third ribs.[4,6]

PEARL

Tietze's syndrome is distinguished from costochondritis by the presence of swelling in the area of pain at the affected costochondral or chondrosternal joint.

Slipping rib syndrome, or *painful rib syndrome*, arises from hypermobility of the anterior ends of the false ribs, causing these ribs to slip under the superior adjacent rib. Unlike other chest wall syndromes, this condition is sometimes caused by blunt-force trauma, with the patient's pain starting many months after the initial trauma. Seen more in females than in males and occurring across the life span, people with slipping rib syndrome initially report sharp lower chest or upper abdominal pain that lasts for only a few seconds. This sporadic pain is followed by aching that may last for several days. The patient may also describe a "slipping" or "popping" feeling in the area of the affected ribs. Palpating the lower costal margin produces tenderness, and pushing on the affected rib produces pain.[4,6]

Though X-rays are not helpful in diagnosing a chest wall syndrome, plain-film radiographs help rule out the presence of a fracture in patients with any of these conditions. This means that diagnosing a person with a chest wall syndrome is usually based on clinical findings. In general, these conditions are self-limiting. That is, patients can participate in sports or exercise as long as the pain they are experiencing allows them to do so. However, even if the pain subsides for a period of time with rest and activity modification, it may reoccur at a later date. If rest and activity modification do not offer patients with slipping rib syndrome sufficient pain relief, surgical intervention is indicated. In these instances, the patient should be referred for surgical consultation because resection of the anterior end of the affected ribs is the treatment of choice.[2,4,5]

Rib Contusion and Fracture

Blunt-force trauma is the most frequent way to contuse or fracture a rib, with the fourth through ninth ribs being the most commonly affected across all age groups. However, the rib cage of the child is less likely to fracture, because of its elasticity, making a rib fracture in this age group a significant occurrence. Thus, additional injury, such as intrathoracic trauma, should be suspected when a rib fracture occurs in the pediatric patient.[1]

PEARL

Suspect the presence of intrathoracic trauma when a rib fracture occurs in a pediatric patient.

A contused or fractured rib is extremely painful and can restrict the patient's ability to fully inhale and exhale during respiration. Because the ribs are fairly superficial, the area that is injured becomes elevated after it is traumatized. In the case of fracture, this elevation presents as a hard mass that develops as a result of swelling and the injured ribs pushing against the overlying skin. Indeed, in instances of fracture, usually more than one rib is involved. A displaced rib fracture can lead to the development of a pneumothorax or hemothorax, both discussed later in the chapter. Also, at times lower rib fractures are also associated with splenic, hepatic, and renal injury, so the abdomen should be evaluated when a fracture of one or more of these structures is suspected. Clinically, the **sternal compression test** is used to differentiate between a contusion and a fracture. To perform this test, instruct the patient to inhale as you compress the chest by placing one hand over the sternum and one hand over the thoracic spine. Little to mild pain caused by this test indicates the presence of a contusion, whereas moderate to extreme pain is indicative of a fracture.[1]

Though obtaining plain-film radiographs of the injured patient is a standard course of action following a traumatic rib injury, x-rays do not always show a fracture. Furthermore, even if a fracture is documented, a rib cage contusion and a fracture are managed similarly by reducing the patient's pain and protecting the area from further injury. This is done by prescribing oral analgesics, such as acetaminophen, by instructing the patient to apply ice to the area, and by advising the person to avoid offending activities until pain subsides. The application of a commercial rib belt may also offer the patient some relief (Fig. 14.5). Realize that a contusion heals quicker than a fracture does, though patients with either condition can take weeks to recover. Patients with a fracture should not return to participation too soon, because doing so places the person at risk for developing a more serious condition, such as a pneumothorax or hemothorax. Once the patient is fully healed, rib padding should be used to protect the area during participation.[1]

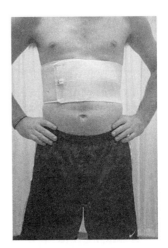

FIGURE 14.5 A commercial rib belt helps with patient comfort for those with an injured thorax.
From Beam: *Orthopedic Taping, Wrapping, Bracing, and Padding.* 2006. Philadelphia: F.A. Davis Company, Fig. 12-7B, pg 394, with permission.

Rib Stress Fracture

Because the ribs are not weight-bearing bones, it may seem that the chest is an unusual location for a stress fracture to occur. However, this is not the case. Indeed, stress fractures account for much of the thorax pain occurring in athletes. Usually affecting ribs 4 through 8, rib stress fractures most commonly happen to those who participate in rowing, particularly when rowers change their rowing technique or increase their training load.[4,6]

Patients with rib stress fractures present with an insidious onset of vague chest pain that is difficult to localize. Though it does not initially prevent patients from participating in their chosen activity, most report that the injury started as low-level chest pain for days or weeks. Left untreated, the pain becomes sharp, ultimately affecting athletic performance and prohibiting participation. When ribs 4 through 8 are affected, the patient's pain is usually located in the posterior thoracic wall, near the spinal border of the scapula. The injured rib is point tender, and the patient reports pain with deep breathing and with rolling over in bed. In the later course of healing, a callus formation may be palpable over the site of injury.[4,6]

Because plain-film radiographs do not show a stress fracture unless callus formation has started, obtaining a bone scan is the proper course of action for patients suspected of having this injury. Once confirmed, the patient with a stress fracture is treated with rest for 4 to 6 weeks, which is followed by a gradual return to activity. Ultimately, it can take as few as 6 weeks and up to 10 weeks to return the patient to full sports participation.[4,6]

Sternal Contusion and Fracture

Usually resulting from blunt-force trauma, sports-related sternal contusions and fractures are uncommon occurrences. This is because the sternum is fairly well protected by the equipment worn by athletes who participate in collision activities. Nonetheless, when these injuries occur, they often accompany an intrathoracic injury, discussed later in this chapter. This means that a patient with a traumatized sternum may also have a more serious, underlying condition.[1]

Rule out the presence of an intrathoracic injury whenever the sternum has been traumatized.

Patients with an injured sternum report localized sternal pain and tenderness. A sternal view plain-film radiograph can confirm the presence of a fracture, though sternal fractures do not always appear on a standard x-ray. Patients with a contused or fractured sternum are treated with oral analgesics and ice. The person should also avoid the offending activity until pain subsides.[1]

Intrathoracic Injury

Intrathoracic injury includes those conditions occurring in the heart and lungs, such as a myocardial contusion, pulmonary contusion, pneumothorax, and hemothorax.

Myocardial Contusion

Otherwise known as a *cardiac bruise*, a myocardial contusion most commonly results from blunt-force trauma to the sternum. It also results when a rapid deceleration force is applied to the body, such as what happens in collision sports and high-speed activities such as football, cycling, and skiing. This mechanism causes the heart to strike against the ribs and sternum, ultimately resulting in a contusion. Fortunately, significant cardiac events are rare after blunt-force trauma in children.[1]

When the heart is bruised, most signs and symptoms occur within 24 hours of injury, making it imperative that patients who sustain a blow to the chest be carefully monitored during this period. When they do occur, symptoms of a bruised heart resemble those of an acute myocardial infarction, usually manifesting in the form of dysrhythmias, chest pain, and shortness of breath. Any case of suspected myocardial contusion should be immediately referred to a cardiologist so the patient's cardiac rhythm and vitals can be monitored. This condition is self-limiting, and the patient can resume activity as pain and discomfort allow.[1,3]

Pulmonary Contusion

A pulmonary contusion, or *bruising of the lung*, commonly occurs as a result of a non-penetrating deceleration injury mechanism. Damage occurs as a result of the lung banging against the chest wall, which causes the lung to compress. A pulmonary contusion can also be a consequence of a displaced rib fracture. Because a child's rib cage is more flexible than an adult's, the young are more prone to this injury. Thus, instead of causing a rib fracture, a compressive blow delivered to the chest of the pediatric patient often causes the rib cage to contuse a lung.[1,3]

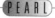

Blunt-force trauma to the chest of a child is more likely to contuse a lung than fracture a rib.

Patients with a pulmonary contusion present with a cough, hemoptysis, shortness of breath, and respiratory difficulty. Diminished breath sounds, rales, or both are present when the lungs are auscultated. Patients with a suspected pulmonary contusion should be referred to a pulmonary specialist. Recognize, however, that pulmonary contusions, much like chest wall injuries, are usually self-limiting, with no long-term consequences. Once diagnosed, these patients gradually return to activity as symptoms subside.[1]

Pneumothorax and Hemothorax

A pneumothorax is a collection of air between the chest wall and lung in the pleural space, whereas a hemothorax is a collection of blood in this area. These injuries result from sudden compressive forces delivered to the chest wall. They also occur when a fractured rib pierces the pleura. In addition to puncturing the pleura, in many cases a fractured rib is also responsible for lacerating a lung, ultimately causing the bleeding associated with a hemothorax. Unfortunately, these conditions are commonly encountered in pediatric chest trauma, making it vital that they are quickly recognized in the clinical setting.[1,3]

Patients with a pneumothorax and hemothorax report with sudden chest pain, tachypnea, and dyspnea. Breath sounds are decreased on auscultation, and a tracheal shift to the opposite side of the injury occurs. Bleeding from the mouth may occur in cases of hemothorax. A chest x-ray confirms the presence of either of these conditions. All patients with confirmed and suspected cases of either a pneumothorax or hemothorax should be referred for advanced medical care. Treatment usually includes surgical intervention to drain fluids from the pleural space. In most instances, the patient can return to participation within a few days after surgery.[1,3]

Conditions of the Abdomen

When compared with injuries to the extremities, injuries to the abdomen do not occur as often in sports. When they do happen, they are often subtle in presentation, making it challenging at times to come to a definitive diagnosis. Indeed, abdominal pain is difficult to evaluate, because what appears to be a fairly harmless condition may turn out be an internal organ injury, a scenario that is particularly likely in children. It is for these reasons that abdominal injuries often go unrecognized or are poorly treated by health care providers, a disturbing fact because visceral injury can result in a life-threatening situation. Thus, every report of abdominal pain should be taken seriously.[3,7,8]

PEARL

An abdominal injury can be difficult to evaluate because what appears to be a fairly harmless condition may turn out be an internal organ injury, a scenario that is particularly likely in children.

Abdominal injuries are divided into two types: musculoskeletal conditions of the abdominal wall and intra-abdominal injuries, those that involve one or more internal organs. Recognize that differentiating between abdominal wall injury and intra-abdominal injury is an extremely challenging task because the chief concern of patients with any abdominal trauma is pain. This makes it difficult to distinguish patients with a minor medical condition from those with a serious internal injury.

Finding out what aggravates and what makes the condition less painful can help develop an accurate differential diagnosis. For example, patients with a musculoskeletal condition are often able to relieve pain by continually changing body positions, whereas this is not always the case for those in pain from an intra-abdominal injury. Also, muscular pain is usually tender only over the area where the trauma occurred, whereas intra-abdominal injury is more diffuse. Thus, it is extremely important to obtain a detailed patient history and complete a thorough physical examination for those with abdominal trauma.[7-9]

Mechanisms of Injury

Regardless of injury type, blunt-force trauma is the most common way the abdomen is injured, but realize that conditions of the abdominal wall can also occur as a result of microtrauma. When a traumatic event does occur, both the abdominal musculature and the internal organs are at risk for injury. The damage caused by such a mechanism is usually more severe if the athlete is unprepared for the external blow, such as what happens when a football receiver reaches overhead to catch a pass at the same time an opposing player contacts the abdomen in an attempt to make a tackle. Intra-abdominal injuries also occur as a result of sudden deceleration forces, such as what happens in whiplash injuries commonly associated with automobile accidents. Other ways to injure the abdominal muscles include abrupt movements of the torso and forceful contractions of the muscles as they are being stretched. Thus, sports that require a person to repeatedly rotate the trunk, like golf, tennis, racquetball, and baseball, and the repetitive activities of running and jumping expose abdominal muscles to injury.[1,3,5,7,9]

PEARL

Blunt-force trauma is the most common way the abdomen is injured.

Abdominal Wall Injury

Injuries to the abdominal wall usually result in contusions, strains, and herniations. When these occur, the rectus abdominis muscles, due to their vulnerable location and responsibility for supporting the internal organs, are usually involved to some extent. In general, abdominal wall pain is usually aggravated by specific postures and is more discrete and well localized than the more diffuse pain associated with intra-abdominal injury. Also, unlike herniations in this region, abdominal wall contusions and strains rarely affect a person's performance in sports for a long time, though the patient's symptoms can persist for weeks.[1,5,9]

Abdominal Wall Contusion

As with any contusion, blunt-force trauma is the cause of most abdominal wall contusions. People with this condition present with pain and swelling at the site of injury, which is usually located at the lower portion of the rectus abdominis, just distal to the umbilicus. If this injury is evaluated more than 72 hours after it occurred, the area may be ecchymotic due to hematoma development, otherwise known as *Cullen's sign.*[1,9]

As long as an intra-abdominal injury has been ruled out, an abdominal wall contusion or hematoma is treated conservatively by advising the patient to avoid activities that cause pain or expose the abdomen to trauma. A computed tomography (CT) scan

can rule out intra-abdominal injury when it is difficult to differentiate between abdominal wall injury and a more serious condition. A CT scan can also confirm the presence of a hematoma.[9]

Abdominal Wall Strain

As with the abdominal wall contusion, the rectus abdominis muscles are the ones most often affected in an abdominal wall strain. These injuries are caused by abrupt movements of the torso and forceful muscle contractions when the muscles are stretched. They also occur in people who participate in activities such as golf and tennis, which require extensive amounts of trunk rotation during activity.[5,9]

Patients with an abdominal strain are not able to reach overhand without pain, nor can they perform a pain-free Valsalva's maneuver. Indeed, those with a strain in this region cannot tense the abdominal muscles without pain, nor can they raise their head 6 to 8 inches off the ground when performing a bent-knee sit-up. Resting the affected muscles, applying cryotherapy to the area, and prescribing a thoracoabdominal support brace may decrease pain enough so the patient can be functional, allowing the person the ability to resume mild exercise such as walking, jogging, or biking fairly quickly. After 2 or 3 weeks of treatment most patients can slowly return to his or her chosen sport or activity, so long as the person strengthens and stretches the injured area until it is fully healed.[5]

Sports Hernia

Because body tissue does not actually protrude with this condition, a sports hernia, otherwise known as *athletic pubalgia*, is not a true hernia in the traditional sense. Rather, this condition refers to a spectrum of injuries involving the inguinal ligament, the internal and external oblique muscles, the lower portion of the rectus abdominis muscles, and the hip adductor muscles (discussed in Chapter 10). Almost exclusively seen in males, a sports hernia most commonly occurs in the area just superior to the pubis and results from overusing the muscles that attach to this bone, namely the hip adductors and the rectus abdominis. In these instances, the adductor muscles are stronger than the abdominals, causing a strength imbalance between these muscle groups. This places the weaker abdominal muscles at risk of becoming injured. Indeed, a sports hernia usually arises secondary to injury of the rectus abdominis. Unlike abdominal contusions and strains, a sports hernia can be very disabling, affecting a person's ability to move normally for extended periods.[9–13]

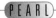

A sports hernia results from a strength imbalance between the hip adductor and abdominal muscles.

Though some patients can remember one specific activity that resulted in injury, most people with a sports hernia report an insidious onset of groin and inguinal canal pain that initially occurred immediately after or just before the termination of an exercise session. This pain usually occurs unilaterally, but it does occur bilaterally on occasion. At this beginning stage of injury, the pain continues to occur in this fashion, only to dissipate when the patient does not exercise. As the injury worsens, the person's pain starts occurring earlier and earlier during subsequent exercise sessions. Ultimately, pain inhibits the person's ability to cut when running, turn, bend, or stride and eventually affects their ability to run in a straight line. At this point, the patient reports pain radiating to the hip adductors and testicles, which is aggravated by sudden movements, coughing, and sneezing. Eventually, patients are forced to reduce or completely cease activities in which they participate.[10,12,13]

Though a sports hernia usually cannot be felt, patients with this condition have tenderness over the inguinal canal and the lower portion of the rectus abdominis at its attachment on the pubic bone. In males, these structures are easily palpated through the external inguinal ring (Fig. 14.3). Patients also experience pain when they perform a bent-knee sit-up, when they attempt Valsalva's maneuver, and, in some patients, with resisted hip adduction. This complex injury can be difficult to diagnose because it often occurs in conjunction with other conditions, such as a hip adductor strain (described in Chapter 10).[10,12,13]

Obtaining plain-film radiographs for patients with a suspected sports hernia helps to rule out bony involvement, though x-rays do not document the presence of this injury. Once bone injury has been ruled out, people with this injury are treated nonsurgically for up to 3 months, with rest and anti-inflammatory medication. Steroid injections have also been found to be helpful. Because sports hernias can be resistant to conservative management, surgery is the preferred course of action for patients who do not respond to 3 months of nonsurgical treatment. When surgery is performed, most patients can return to active sports within 3 to 6 weeks.[10,12,13]

Intra-abdominal Injury

Although any abdominal organ can be traumatized, in general solid organs, such as the spleen and liver, are more at risk of injury than hollow organs, such as the bladder and stomach. This is because when blunt-force trauma is applied to a hollow organ, it is able to dissipate the forces being delivered, whereas a solid organ is more likely to absorb these forces. Recognize that people who participate in collision and contact sports maintain the greatest injury risk, because blunt-force trauma is a common occurrence in these activities.

As previously mentioned, the presence of pain is the telltale sign that an abdominal injury has occurred, with intra-abdominal pain being more diffuse than the pain caused by an abdominal wall injury. The pain associated with abdominal organ injury can occur either immediately or some hours after the initial injury and increases with body movements such as walking, jumping, laughing, coughing, and bouncing. In addition, the patient with an intra-abdominal injury may experience pain radiating to one or more areas, another classic indicator of abdominal organ injury. The information provided in Table 14.2 identifies the possible source of a person's radiating pain. Other common signs and symptoms associated with intra-abdominal trauma are listed in Box 14.1.[3,7,12]

Examining someone with a suspected intra-abdominal injury is done with the patient laying supine, knees bent to 90°, because this relaxes the abdominal muscles, allowing better access to the underlying structures. Auscultation is performed first as doing so ensures peristalsis is not altered by the palpation portion of the examination. Auscultation begins in the abdominal area farthest away from the pain and slowly works toward the site of injury. Patients with an internal organ injury may present with hypoactive bowel sounds. As with auscultation, palpation begins in the area farthest away from the pain and is first performed with the patient's abdomen relaxed, and then contracted. Pain which decreases with the muscles contracted is

TABLE 14.2 Referred pain sites for abdominal organs

ORGAN	REFERRED PAIN SITE
Spleen	Left shoulder, ⅓ of way down left arm (Kehr's sign)
Liver	Right shoulder
Pancreas	Directly in front of or behind pancreas
Kidneys	Forward around flank into lower abdominal quadrant
Appendix	Initial: umbilical region; final: lower right quadrant
Bladder	Anterior upper thighs

BOX 14.1
SIGNS AND SYMPTOMS OF INTRA-ABDOMINAL INJURY

Nausea	Chills
Vomiting	Discomfort with inhaling and exhaling
Shock	Increased pulse rate
Change in stool pattern	Increased blood pressure
(constipation or diarrhea)	Increased respiratory rate
Fever	

Adapted from: Bergman RT. Assessing acute abdominal pain: a team physician's challenge. *Phys Sportsmed* 1996;24(4):72; Cody C, Standish WD. Emergencies in sports: the young athlete. *Clin Sports Med* 1988;7:625; Johnson R. Abdominal wall injuries: rectus abdominis strains, oblique strains, rectus sheath hematoma. *Curr Sports Med Rep* 2006;5:99.

indicative of intra-abdominal injury and a severe intra-abdominal condition is likely present if the patient cannot relax his or her muscles when palpated. An absence of rebound, as well as abdominal distention, are also signs of intra-abdominal injury.[3,5,8,9]

Once the presence of intra-abdominal damage is clinically confirmed, the patient should be referred to a specialist for additional testing, consultation, and possible surgical intervention. If an immediate referral cannot be made, the patient should be sent to an emergency department, because these injuries can be life-threatening.

Refer all patients with a suspected intra-abdominal injury to a specialist, because these injuries can be life-threatening.

Injury to the Spleen

The spleen is the most commonly damaged abdominal organ in people participating in sports. This organ bleeds easily if injured because it is extremely vascular. It is especially vulnerable to trauma when enlarged, otherwise known as splenomegaly. This most commonly occurs as a result of a viral disease, such as mononucleosis. Remember that mononucleosis is highly prevalent in the adolescent population, placing these patients at great risk for splenic injury from blunt-force trauma. It is for this reason people diagnosed with mononucleosis are disqualified from collision and contact sports until this condition has resolved and the enlarged spleen has returned to normal size. Because of the other symptoms associated with mononucleosis, such as extreme fatigue, patients with this condition will most likely not be able to successfully participate in any type of physical activity until the condition resolves.[1,3,7,14]

PEARL

Because mononucleosis causes splenomegaly, people with this condition should not participate in collision and contact sports until the organ has returned to normal size.

Because it is located in the LUQ, blunt-force trauma delivered to this region, to the lower left rib cage in the area of the 10th through 12th ribs, or to the upper region of the left back is the primary cause of splenic injury. As with injuries to most abdominal organs, the onset of symptoms when the spleen is traumatized may be rapid or delayed. In most instances, the patient initially reports LUQ pain, which progresses to the left shoulder and down the left arm. This is known as **Kehr's sign**. The patient has tenderness over the LUQ, left back, and left lower rib cage when these areas are palpated. As the condition progresses, pain from the spleen presents in the epigastric region, ultimately becoming more diffuse throughout the abdomen, resulting from the bleeding that accompanies this injury.[1,3,7]

Whereas a splenectomy was once the treatment of choice for an injured spleen, physicians now try to avoid removing the organ. This is particularly true in the pediatric population, because removing the spleen in this population has an adverse effect on the immune system and decreases the body's defenses to life-threatening conditions. Thus, if at all possible, a conservative treatment approach should be used by having the patient abstain from heavy work or sports participation for up to 6 weeks. A splenectomy is still the treatment of choice if the spleen has ruptured beyond repair.[3,7]

Injury to the Liver

Because of its healthy vascular supply, the liver, the second most commonly injured organ in the abdomen, also loses a lot of blood when traumatized. People who participate in collision, contact, and high-speed noncontact sports are at highest risk of liver injury. As with the spleen, a liver that is enlarged as a result of hepatitis is at an increased risk of injury, not only because of its size but also because the enlarged liver is softer than normal. Thus, athletes with **hepatomegaly** should not participate in collision and contact sports until the liver has returned to normal size.[1,3,7]

Blunt-force trauma to the RUQ or to the right lower chest is the most common way the liver is injured. Thus, patients with a damaged liver initially report RUQ tenderness that is sometimes referred to the right shoulder. Ultimately, the patient's abdominal pain becomes more diffuse as time goes on. A CT scan of the patient's abdomen can be used to gauge the amount of liver damage. If it is determined that the injury does not call for immediate surgery, the CT scan is repeated 5 to 7 days after the date of injury. If it is determined that the best course of treatment remains nonsurgical, the patient is treated conservatively, which includes instructing the patient to abstain from heavy work or sports participation for 6 weeks. Most people who injure their liver are encouraged to discontinue participation in collision and contact sports because of the extensive scaring the liver experiences during the healing process.[1,3,7]

Injury to the Kidney

For people who participate in collision sports such as football and rugby, the kidney is the most commonly injured organ. Though fairly well protected by the rib cage, surrounding musculature, and perirenal fat, this solid organ is frequently traumatized from one acute blow or from repeated blows to the right or left flank regions. These injury mechanisms usually cause the kidney to contuse, though the kidney can also be lacerated by a fractured rib. Indeed, contusions and lacerations account for 90% of all acute kidney injuries. The kidneys of younger people are at an increased risk for injury because, when compared with an adult's, a child's kidneys[1,3,7,15]

- have less perirenal fat,
- extend further below the rib cage,
- are more fragile to direct trauma,
- are large relative to their body size, and
- receive less protection from the ribs, because a child's ribs have yet to fully ossify, making them weak.

A child's kidney is at greater risk of injury from blunt-force trauma than an adult's.

Regardless of how a kidney is injured or the condition that results from the trauma (e.g., contusion, laceration), the signs and symptoms the patient presents with are similar. These include pain over the costovertebral angle, which can be reproduced with the blunt-percussion test or *kidney tap test* (Fig. 14.6). Pain may radiate around the flank into lower abdominal quadrant on the affected side and **Grey Turner's sign** may be present. Hematuria may also be present, because this condition usually results in microscopic or gross blood in the urine. When visible, blood makes urine assume a brownish tint. Clinically, the presence of hematuria is confirmed with a urinalysis dipstick. Though hematuria is considered the hallmark sign of renal trauma, the amount of blood in the urine does not necessarily indicate the degree of kidney injury. Indeed, visible hematuria does not have to be present for a kidney to be seriously damaged. Also, blood in the urine is a common response to people who participate in strenuous exercise, such as marathon running, and can occur as a by-product of an external irritation in the urethral area. Thus, findings of hematuria should coincide with a traumatic event before a diagnosis of kidney injury is made.[1,3,7,15]

Most people with an injured kidney are treated conservatively with rest, hydration, and analgesics for a few days. Realize it is common for a kidney that has stopped bleeding to experience clot resolution 2 to 3 weeks after the injury, causing

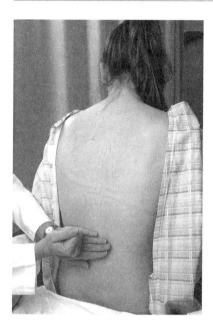

FIGURE 14.6 To perform the blunt-percussion, or kidney tap test, lay one hand flat over the patient's costovertebral angle and firmly tap it with the fist (ulnar side) of your other hand. Pain caused by this maneuver is indicative of kidney injury.
From Dillon: *Nursing Health Assessment: A Critical Thinking, Case Studies Approach*. 2003. Philadelphia: F.A. Davis Company, pg 504, with permission.

the kidney to rebleed. Thus, patients with an injured kidney must refrain from strenuous activity and from collision and contact sports for a minimum of 3 weeks, though some advocate instructing patients to abstain from heavy work or sports for 6 weeks.[7,15]

Injury to the Pancreas

Though the pancreas is not commonly injured, it presents an immediate life-threatening situation when traumatized. It is most commonly damaged from blunt-force trauma to the upper mid-abdomen, such as what occurs when a football helmet or bicycle handlebars strike this region. Patients with this injury report severe epigastric pain originating from directly in front of and behind the pancreas. When palpated, this area is extremely tender. As with most intra-abdominal injuries, the pain progresses to diffuse abdominal discomfort as time goes on. Immediate treatment includes surgical intervention.[7,8]

Injury to the Bladder

Because the bladder is a hollow organ, its incidence of injury to people participating in sports is fairly low. However, if it is not emptied prior to competition, the bladder acts more like a solid organ than a hollow one, making it less able to dissipate forces applied to it. It is for this reason that all who participate in collision and contact sports should empty the bladder before competition, because this helps to protect it from injury.[15]

Blunt-force trauma to the lower abdomen is the most common way the bladder is injured. When this occurs, the bladder usually ruptures, a condition that is more prevalent in adult males when compared with children and adolescents of the same gender. The incidence of bladder injury in females is much lower than it is in males, most likely because females do not participate in collision activities in great numbers. Patients with an injured bladder report lower abdominal pain and tenderness in the hypogastric region. They may also experience radiating pain to the anterior upper thighs. Hematuria may or may not accompany this injury. Treatment for a ruptured bladder is surgical repair, so patients with a bladder injury must immediately be referred for surgical consultation.[3,8,15]

Appendicitis

Though not usually injured as a result of sports participation, inflammation of the appendix is a fairly common occurrence, one that often presents in the primary care setting. This condition is characterized by generalized hypogastric and umbilical pain that eventually localizes to the RLQ. At times patients with appendicitis cannot jump without pain, owing to the fact that the inflamed appendix lies close to the iliopsoas complex (discussed in Chapter 10), a primary muscle group used for jumping. Nausea and vomiting may affect the patient's appetite, making the patient anorexic in appearance. In some instances nausea and vomiting are short lived, only appearing when the appendix ruptures. During the physical examination rebound tenderness is present over **McBurney's point**. A low-grade fever may also be present. Treatment includes appendix removal, so patients with appendicitis must immediately be referred for surgical consultation.[1,8]

Conditions of the Genitalia

Though sports-related trauma to the external genitalia is a rare occurrence for either gender, successful management requires prompt assessment and treatment. This should be coupled with sympathetic concern for the potential psychological impact of such an injury, particularly in younger patients.[16,17]

Mechanisms of Injury

The most common way to injure the external genitalia of both genders is from blunt-force trauma. In females, this usually results from a straddle injury mechanism, such as what happens when the genitals of a gymnast abruptly strike a balance beam. Though such an injury may occur from a macrotrauma event, female athletes may have difficulty recalling how they got hurt. The male genitals are usually traumatized by a direct blow to the scrotum, such as what happens when a person is kicked in the groin, but can also be injured by a straddle mechanism. Although it is exposed to trauma, the penis is rarely injured in sports.[2,3,16–18]

Conditions Involving the Male

Most injuries to the external male genitalia can be prevented by having the participant wear proper protective equipment. Indeed, those who partake in sports such as football, lacrosse, and ice hockey are required to wear a hard shelled "cup" over the external genitalia. This makes the testes the male's most protected organ during collision activities. However, even with this protection, and in other sports in which the genitals are exposed, trauma to this region does occur. Preexisting abnormalities, such as an undescended testicle, also predisposes a testicle to injury. Remember, too, that testicular cancer is the most common malignancy in males 16 through 35 years of age so any mass found in the testicle of those in this age group should be immediately referred for additional testing and evaluation.[3,16,19]

Males who experience blunt-force trauma to the external genitalia primarily complain of pain in the testicular region with the organs located in the scrotal sac being most at risk for injury. Indeed, any direct blow to the scrotum responsible for such pain can lead to significant injury.[16,19]

Conditions of the Scrotum

The most common traumatic condition occurring to this region is a testicular contusion. Patients with this injury typically report with pain, swelling, and discoloration of the scrotal sac. Such an injury may result in the testis retracting into the inguinal canal, otherwise known as *highball syndrome*. If the swelling associated with this injury keeps expanding after trauma or if the amount of pain the patient is in seems out of proportion with the severity of injury, the testicle may have been ruptured. Indeed, scrotal trauma great enough to rupture a testicle results in a painful, ecchymotic scrotal mass. These patients must be immediately referred to a urologist for treatment. All other patients with a testicular contusion usually respond well with ice, elevation, and, if needed, bed rest. The patient can return to activity once symptoms resolve.[1,2,3,16,17]

In addition to becoming contused, blunt-force trauma can also cause a testicle to rotate and the spermatic cord to twist upon itself in the scrotal sac. Known as *testicular torsion,* this condition, which can also occur spontaneously without trauma, is a true medical emergency. Patient's with testicular torsion report with acute testicular pain, a high-riding testicle, and an abnormal position of the epididymis. In order to have the best chance of salvaging the testicle, these patients must be treated surgically within 6 hours of the injury.[1,16,19]

Inguinal Hernia

A condition primarily seen in males, inguinal hernias are the most common form of abdominal wall hernias. This type of hernia occurs when a portion of intra-abdominal tissue, usually small intestines, protrudes into the lower portion of the abdominal wall or down the inguinal canal. When the intestines protrude through the abdominal muscles, it is known as a direct inguinal hernia, whereas an indirect inguinal hernia occurs when the intestines invade the canal by passing through the internal inguinal ring. Indirect hernias account for 75% of all inguinal hernias, are more common in children, and are congenital. In contrast, direct hernias are more common in adults and are an acquired condition because their occurrence is directly related to increases in abdominal pressure and weakness of the abdominal muscles.[19-21]

Initially, patients with an inguinal hernia do not feel pain. Rather, the person relates a feeling of heaviness or pressure in the groin region. Regardless of type, a person with an inguinal hernia usually presents with a lump in the affected area. This bulge can usually been seen with the patient standing but often disappears when the person sits or lies down. The hernia increases in size when the person strains, such as what happens when Valsalva's maneuver is performed. Eventually, the hernia becomes painful and tender to touch. The presence of an inguinal hernia can be verified by feeling inside the inguinal canal with the index finger as shown in Figure 14.3. If a hernia is present the abdominal contents bulge against the finger. Instructing the patient to cough during the examination exaggerates the presence of the bulge, which helps confirm the diagnosis. In some instances a hernia may become strangulated, resulting in a lack of blood supply to the affected abdominal contents. In these instances the tissue becomes necrotic, placing the entire abdominal contents at risk for infection. Clinically, the bulge associated with a strangulated inguinal hernia presents as a red, tender mass.[20,21]

Though some patients with an inguinal hernia are treated conservatively, most require surgical intervention. Thus, all patients with a suspected hernia should be referred to a surgeon for treatment. While waiting for this consultation, the patient should wear clothing, such as neoprene shorts (Fig. 14.7), that supports the area and decreases patient discomfort. Immediate surgical intervention is needed for all patients presenting with a strangulated hernia as this can be a life-threatening condition.[20,21]

Conditions Involving the Female

Because female genitalia are relatively well protected from trauma, they are not commonly injured during sports participation. This makes diagnosing conditions in this region challenging, particularly if the symptoms reported by the patient are not caused by trauma. Thus, non–sport-related genitourinary etiologies, such as pelvic inflammatory disease, ectopic pregnancy, and vaginal injury, should be included as part of the differential diagnosis when evaluating nontraumatic conditions to this region.[1,8,17,18]

Conditions of the Vulva

Vulvar injuries from blunt-force trauma almost always result in labial hematomas and tears, vaginal lacerations, and clitoral tears. These conditions are treated with cryotherapy and analgesics to reduce pain. Deep lacerations require primary repair under general anesthesia. Urinary retention may accompany any of these injuries, meaning that temporary drainage may be necessary. It most cases, normal activity can be pursued once pain subsides.[1,17]

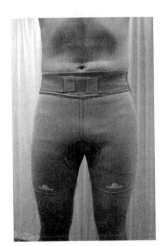

FIGURE 14.7 Neoprene shorts which can be used as a support device for those with an inguinal hernia or groin injury.
From Beam: *Orthopedic Taping, Wrapping, Bracing, and Padding.* 2006. Philadelphia: F.A. Davis Company, Fig. 7-16, pg 226, with permission.

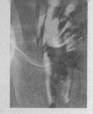

CASE STUDY:
Thorax, Abdomen, and Genitalia

SCENARIO
A 15-year-old high school ice hockey player is brought in by his father after sustaining an abdominal injury 3 days ago. The patient states being checked by another player into the ice hockey boards at the time of injury. The brunt of the force delivered to the body was absorbed by the patient's left lower abdominal quadrant and left mid-back region, causing him enough discomfort that he had to leave the ice immediately for a period of time. At the time, his father, who is also the coach, dismissed the condition as just a bruise. Though the injury occurred halfway through the game, the patient continued to play, albeit in increasing pain as time went on. The pain slightly subsided after the game but has remained consistent for the past few days.

PERTINENT HISTORY
Medications: Ibuprofen 400 mg QID since the injury incident. No other medications. No known drug allergies.

Family History: Older brother has diabetes. Otherwise unremarkable.

PERSONAL HEALTH HISTORY
Tobacco Use: Nonsmoker.

Alcohol Intake: None.

Recreational Drugs and Banned Substances: Denies use.

Caffeinated Beverages: Consumes 2 to 3 cola beverages per day.

Diet: To gain physical size and strength so he can successfully compete in high school ice hockey, the patient states he eats multiple times per day. Drinks a protein powder shake each morning and takes a daily multivitamin.

Past Medical History: Had chickenpox at age 7. Also had constant tonsillitis as a child but has not had an incident in many years.

History of Present Illness: The patient had an abdominal injury 3 days ago. He is currently experiencing extreme mid-back pain that radiates to the LLQ. The pain is intense enough that it limits his ability to move his torso. He states that he started feeling nauseous last night, which prevented him from eating breakfast. He has noticed that his urine has a slight brownish tint, though he is unsure of when this started.

PERTINENT PHYSICAL EXAMINATION*
The patient's back is tender around the area of ribs 11 and 12 on the left side. This region is starting to become ecchymotic. A blunt percussion test for the kidney is positive. Dipstick urine analysis confirms the presence of hematuria. The patient also has a low-grade fever.

*Focused examination limited to key points for this case.

RED FLAGS FOR THE PRIMARY HEALTH CARE PROFESSIONAL TO CONSIDER

- Any history of blunt-force trauma to the abdomen is indicative of intra-abdominal injury.
- The presence of hematuria and ecchymosis are indicative of a kidney injury.
- Because the father is the patient's ice hockey coach, there is the potential that the father will want to allow the son to resume playing quickly.

RECOMMENDED PLAN

- Refer the patient for urological consultation.
- Prescribe rest and an over-the-counter pain reliever, such as acetaminophen.
- Because the patient is still a minor, get signed permission from his father so you can communicate your findings and recommendations to the school's certified athletic trainer.
- This patient should be disqualified from participation for a minimum of 3 weeks.
- Explain to the father and the athlete about the risk involved if he returns to participation too early, including the potential that the kidney will rebleed if not fully healed.

REFERENCES

1. Amaral JF. Thoracoabdominal injuries in the athlete. *Clin Sports Med* 1997;16:739.
2. Wise CM, Semble EL, Dalton CB. Musculoskeletal chest wall syndromes in patients with noncardiac chest pain: a study of 100 patients. *Arch Phys Med Rehabil* 1992;73:147.
3. Coady C, Standish WD. Emergencies in sports: the young athlete. *Clin Sports Med* 1988;7:625.
4. Gregory PL, Biswas AC, Batt ME. Musculoskeletal problems of the chest wall in athletes. *Sports Med* 2002;32:235.
5. Lehman RC. Thoracoabdominal musculoskeletal injuries in racquet sports. *Clin Sports Med* 1988;7:267.
6. Karlson KA. Thoracic region pain in athletes. *Curr Sports Med Rep* 2004;3:53.
7. Diamond DL. Sports-related abdominal trauma. *Clin Sports Med* 1989;8:91.
8. Bergman RT. Assessing acute abdominal pain: a team physician's challenge. *Phys Sportsmed* 1996;24(4):72.
9. Johnson R. Abdominal wall injuries: rectus abdominis strains, oblique strains, rectus sheath hematoma. *Curr Sports Med Rep* 2006;5:99.
10. Diaco JF, Diaco DS, Lockhart L. Sports hernia. *Oper Tech Sports Med* 2005;13:68.
11. Hackney RG. The sports hernia. *Sports Med Arthroscopy Rev* 1997;5:320.
12. Johnson JD. Primary care of the sports hernia. *Phys Sportsmed* 2005;33(2):35.
13. LeBlanc KE, LeBlanc KA. Groin pain in athletes. *Hernia* 2003;7:68.
14. Maki DG, Reich RM. Infectious mononucleosis in the athlete. *Am J Sports Med* 1982;10:162.
15. York JP. Sports and the male genitourinary system: kidneys and bladder. *Phys Sportsmed* 1990;18(9):116.
16. York JP. Sports and the male genitourinary system: genital injuries and sexually transmitted diseases. *Phys Sportsmed* 1990;18(10):92.
17. Mandell J, Cromie WJ, Caldamone AA, et al. Sports-related genitourinary injuries in children. *Clin Sports Med* 1982;1:483.
18. Short JW, Pedowitz, RA, Strong JA, et al. The evaluation of pelvic injury in the female athlete. *Sports Med* 1995;20:422.
19. Junnila J, Lassen P. Testicular masses. *Am Fam Physician* 1998;57:685.
20. Bax T, Sheppard BC, Crass RA. Surgical options in the management of groin hernias. *Am Fam Physician* 1999;59:143.
21. Ruhl CE, Everhart JE. Risk factors for inguinal hernia among adults in the US population. *Am J Epidemiol* 2007;165:1154.

SUGGESTED READINGS

Congeni J, Miller SF, Bennett CL. Awareness of genital health in young male athletes. *Clin J Sport Med* 2005;15:22.
Coris EE, Higgins HW. First rib stress fractures in throwing athletes. *Am J Sports Med* 2005;33:1400.
LeBlanc KE, LeBlanc KA. Groin pain in athletes. *Hernia* 2003;7:68.

WEB LINKS

http://www.aic.cuhk.edu.hk/web8/abdominal_and_pelvic_injury.htm. Accessed 8/13/08.
Comprehensive website dedicated to abdominal and pelvic injury. Covers mechanisms of injury as well as history and examination for specific conditions.

http://www.emedicine.com/EMERG/topic1.htm. Accessed 8/13/08.
Provides background, differential diagnosis, treatment, and pathophysiology of blunt abdominal trauma.

15

Conditions Involving the Skin

● **Brian J. Toy, PhD, ATC, and Phyllis F. Healy, PhD, BC-FNP, CNL, RN** lthough not often considered in the broad spectrum of sports-related injuries, skin problems are among the most common conditions seen in people who are physically active. This is especially true for those who participate in competitive, team-orientated sports. In light of the inherent risks related to skin condition epidemics among athletic team members, primary health care providers must remain vigilant in recognizing and must properly manage the array of skin conditions that occur in those who participate in sports.[1]

Anatomy of the Skin

The skin consists of three layers: the epidermis, dermis, and subcutaneous tissue (Fig. 15.1). The most superficial layer, the epidermis, consists of four primary bands of stratum, the outermost most of which is called the *stratum corneum*. It is this band that acts as the primary protective barrier for the body. Pores, openings that connect to deeper situated sweat glands, are located within the stratum corneum. The dermis, the skin's middle layer, is comprised of thick connective tissue. It maintains the following skin appendages: hair follicles, sebaceous glands (which surround the hair

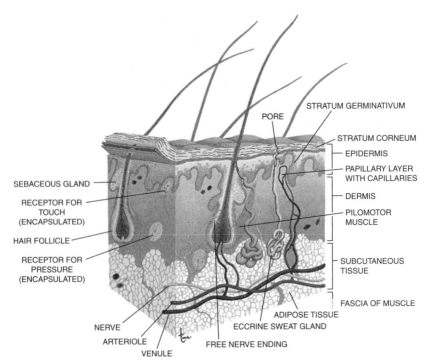

FIGURE 15.1 Anatomy of the skin.
From *Taber's Cyclopedic Medical Dictionary*, 20th ed. 2005. Philadelphia: F.A. Davis Company, pg 2009, with permission.

follicles), and sweat glands. The dermis, which maintains a rich supply of blood vessels, also has sensory (deep pressure, pain, light touch, thermo) and autonomic nerve endings. Subcutaneous tissue, the inner most skin layer, consists of fatty connective tissue. It connects skin to the underlying muscle fascia and insulates tissue below. Larger blood vessels and nerves are also located within this layer.

Functions of the Skin

The skin is a multifaceted organ that synthesizes vitamin D from sunlight and provides the body with sensory perception of external stimuli. It also helps to hold internal organs in place. However, its primary function is to act as a barrier to the external environment, protecting the body from harm (Box 15.1). Indeed, the importance of intact skin as the first line of defense in this regard cannot be overestimated, because any disruption of this largest body organ can have a marked impact on a patient's overall physical and mental health.[2]

The primary function of the skin is to act as a barrier to the external environment, protecting the body from harm.

Mechanisms of Injury

The skin of those who participate in sports faces many challenges when trying to do its job. This is especially true when the skin attempts to block pathogens from entering the body. Sweating, poor hygiene, exposure to environmental factors, a disruption in skin continuity, and skin-to-skin contact between participants are some of the more common reasons why skin infections occur in sports. Indeed, when skin-to-skin contact is an inherent part of a sport, such as in the case of wrestling, the potential for receiving and transmitting a contagious skin condition markedly increases. Others who maintain an increased risk of obtaining a skin infection are those who experience chaffing caused by equipment rubbing against the unprotected skin, such as in the case of football players, and those, like swimmers, who are exposed to **fomites.**[3,4]

Regardless of the sport a person plays, the risk of skin infection increases when someone participates with an open wound, because doing so provides pathogens easy access to the body. Though many types of wounds exist, those who participate with an abrasion are at highest risk of acquiring and spreading a contagious skin condition, because abrasions typically cover a wide body area. This makes the wound difficult to

BOX 15.1
THINGS FROM WHICH THE SKIN PROTECTS THE BODY

Pathogens	Ultraviolet light
Dehydration	Irritants
Temperature changes	Trauma

keep clean and protect during competition. Abrasions are caused by a shearing or friction injury mechanism, in which a body part is rubbed against a hard or immovable object or piece of equipment. For example, abrasions commonly occur in wrestling when an area of skin rubs against a wrestling mat and in football when a player's bare skin is exposed to artificial turf playing surfaces.[1,3,5,6]

People who participate with an open wound in sports requiring skin-to-skin contact between participants are at an increased risk of receiving and transmitting an infectious skin condition.

Preventing Skin Infections

In general, there are some easy, yet effective, measures that all people can take to prevent the occurrence and spread of skin infections (Box 15.2). Though these measures should be emphasized to all who participate in sports, it is especially important to do this for children and adolescents, because many in this age group have yet to fully understand the importance of practicing proper hygiene techniques.[1,3–8]

Part of preventing the spread of contagious skin conditions among athletes is evaluating all potential participants for the presence of a skin infection before the first day of practice. In fact, assessing the skin of a potential athlete should be a standard part of the pre-participation examination process (discussed in Chapter 2). However, those who maintain the highest risk of becoming infected should be evaluated periodically throughout the playing season. In recognition of this, certain sports, such as wrestling, require that participants receive skin assessments, otherwise referred to as *skin checks*, before certain competitions. These skin checks are usually performed by qualified medical personnel, such as physicians, nurse practitioners, and physician assistants.

BOX 15.2
MEASURES PEOPLE CAN TAKE TO PREVENT THE OCCURRENCE AND SPREAD OF SKIN INFECTIONS

Shower after all exercise sessions.	Regularly clean playing surfaces (e.g., wrestling mats).
Shower before activity if participating in a sport requiring skin-to-skin contact.	Avoid sharing washcloths, towels, clothing, razor blades, and equipment.
Wear protective footwear when showering in a communal setting.	Promptly clean and bandage all open wounds, especially abrasions.
Thoroughly dry all body parts after showering, paying particular attention to those areas where skin-to-skin contact occurs (e.g., groin, armpits, web spaces between toes).	Detect incidences of skin infections early.
Regularly wash all athletic clothing and equipment.	Remove those who are infected from skin-to-skin contact with others.

Typically, any lesion that cannot be completely occluded or that appears to be contagious necessitates that the participant be disqualified from competing. In most cases, the athlete is also removed from all skin-to-skin contact with teammates, being allowed to practice and compete only after completing a proper course of treatment and receiving clearance from a qualified medical professional.[5]

PEARL

In certain instances, qualified medical professionals, such as physicians, nurse practitioners, and physician assistants, are used to check wrestlers for contagious skin infections before competition.

Fungal Conditions

Of all infections that affect the skin, those of the tinea, or *fungal*, variety are among the most common. Otherwise referred to as *ringworm*, specific tinea infections are named in association with the body area affected, resulting in conditions such as **tinea corporis** (body), **tinea cruris** (groin), and **tinea pedis** (foot).

People who have skin fungal infections are typically treated with topical antifungal ointments, creams, powders, and solutions found in common over-the-counter products. When these prove to be ineffective for the patient with a single lesion, prescription-strength topical azole antifungals, containing agents such as fluconazole, itraconazole, or ketoconazole, are used. Oral therapy is prescribed when more than one lesion is present, when facial lesions are present, when lesions are resistant to topical therapy, and when infections are associated with widespread inflammation. Though for years griseofulvin was the oral antifungal of choice, the azoles and the newer allylamine antifungals, which maintain terbinafine, are now prescribed, because these agents, when compared with griseofulvin, are as effective and can be used for shorter periods of time. When intense itching accompanies the infection, the patient may need to be treated with topical corticosteroids, whereas topical or systemic steroids may be required in cases of widespread inflammation.[5,6,8]

Tinea Corporis

Tinea corporis is a fungal infection that affects the trunk and extremities (Fig. 15.2). Lesions typical of this condition present as distinct annular, red, scaly plaques that progress outward from a clearing center. The borders of these lesions are usually raised. Because of the close quarters that occur between participants during competition and the abrasions these athletes receive from the unyielding mats on which they participate, tinea corporis is extremely common in those who wrestle. Indeed, tinea corporis occurs so often in this sport that the term **tinea gladiatorum** is used when this condition occurs in a wrestler. Treatment consists of twice-daily topical applications of an antifungal ointment and should be continued for at least 2 weeks, or for at least 1 week after symptoms disappear.[5]

Tinea Cruris

Tinea cruris, commonly referred to as *jock itch*, is a condition mostly seen in males. This fungal infection affects the groin and surrounding area, though it usually does not

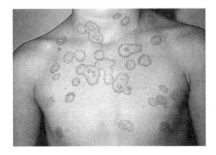

FIGURE 15.2 Tinea corporis.
From *Taber's Cyclopedic Medical Dictionary*, 20th ed.
2005. Philadelphia: F.A. Davis Company, pg 2192, with
permission.

involve the scrotum (Fig. 15.3). If severe enough, the infection may extend into the abdomen, perineum, and buttocks. Initially, this condition manifests itself by causing the patient to scratch the area because of an itching sensation. Raised, scaly plaques then develop, causing the region to appear red and inflamed. Treatment includes applying an antifungal ointment to the area twice per day for 2 to 4 weeks. Systemic treatment is reserved for unresponsive or very extensive cases.[9]

Tinea Pedis

Tinea pedis, otherwise known as *athlete's foot*, commonly appears as painful, red, macerated scales and fissures in the web spaces between the toes. It also presents in a moccasin distribution, with marked scaling and inflamed vesicles or bullae in the area of the foot's mid sole. Treatment includes applying antifungal ointment in the evening and a daytime antifungal powder to keep the foot dry. To further decrease moisture, absorbent cotton socks should be worn and changed frequently. Socks should be white, because moisture can cause the dye from colored socks to bleed into the infected area. At times, the underwear of those with tinea pedis becomes a fungus carrier, because these garments, when pulled from the feet to the waist, transport the fungus from the infected feet to the groin. This can result in the patient acquiring tinea cruris. To prevent this from happening, those with tinea

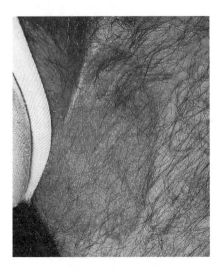

FIGURE 15.3 Tinea cruris.
From *Taber's Cyclopedic Medical Dictionary*, 20th ed.
2005. Philadelphia: F.A. Davis Company, pg 2192, with
permission.

pedis should put their socks on before their underwear when dressing. Only in rare instances does the person with tinea pedis require systemic treatment.[5,6,9]

Disqualification and Return-to-Play Decisions for Patients With Fungal Infections

In general, those with tinea pedis and cruris are rarely disqualified from participation, because the groin and feet are usually covered during competition, minimizing the risk of fungus transmission. However, at times these athletes must cease activity because of the pain and discomfort caused by chaffing during exercise. In contrast, unless a single lesion can be adequately covered, athletes with tinea corporis should be disqualified from participation. Even if a lesion can be covered, the policies of many athletic associations ban participants from competition if infectious lesions are present. In general, patients with multiple tinea corporis lesions or lesions that cannot be adequately covered are disqualified for a minimum of 72 hours after institution of topical therapy and for 2 weeks after the introduction of systemic therapy.[1,3,4]

Viral Conditions

Viral infections common in the athletic population include **herpes simplex virus (HSV)**, **molluscum contagiosum**, and **verruca plantaris**. When wrestlers are infected with herpes simplex, they are diagnosed as having **herpes gladiatorum**. Though it is clear that certain situations, such as skin-to-skin contact with an infected person, can transmit some viruses between people, there is some question as to the role that athletic equipment, such as the mats used in wrestling, has in transmitting common viral infections seen in athletes.[1,3,4,6,8]

Herpes Simplex Virus

An HSV infection, primarily caused by HSV-1, is a relatively common condition in sports such as wrestling and rugby, because those participating in activities requiring skin-to-skin contact, especially if they have an open wound, are at risk for such an infection (Fig. 15.4). Indeed, HSV-1 infections have been reported in wrestling in epidemic proportions. Though in the general population infections of this type typically occur on the lips, in herpes gladiatorum lesions are usually located on the head, neck, torso, and upper extremities. These lesions appear as grouped vessels on an erythematous base and eventually rupture, leaving crusted and eroded papules, making it easy to confuse HSV with tinea corporis, impetigo (discussed later in this chapter), or atopic dermatitis. Recognize that wrestlers use methods such as sandpapering and bleaching to avoid lesion detection so they can continue to participate. Other symptoms include localized pain and tingling, fever, chills, sore throat, and headache. A **Tzanck smear** can support the clinical diagnosis, but this should be confirmed through a viral culture.[1,3,4,6,10,11]

Those with an HSV infection are treated with an oral antiviral agent such as acyclovir, valacyclovir, or famciclovir. Realize, however, these drugs work only if administered during the first signs of lesion development and are minimally effective once the vesicles are formed, ruptured, or crusted. Applying warm compresses to the area can help with patient comfort. Most practitioners wait at least 4 to 7 days after the initiation of treatment before returning the person to practice and competition, though no data exist to support this guideline. Clinically, the lesions must be

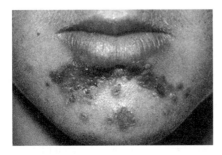

FIGURE 15.4 Herpes simplex.
From Dillon: *Nursing Health Assessment: A Critical Thinking, Case Studies Approach.* 2003. Philadelphia: F.A. Davis Company, pg 166, with permission.

scabbed and dried and the area must be properly covered before the patient can be allowed to have skin-to-skin contact with another peson.[1,3,5,6,8,11,12]

Molluscum Contagiosum

Molluscum contagiosum, an infection caused by a pox virus, has an unknown incidence (Fig. 15.5). Though commonly seen in those who participate in sports in which skin-to-skin contact occurs between people, this condition is also seen in swimmers, because these athletes contract the virus from contaminated water or from pool decks. Molluscum lesions are characterized by distinct white, 1- to 5-mm, centrally umbilicated, domed papules. In many instances, the person with this viral infection is symptom free, because the condition is usually self-limiting, typically resolving spontaneously in 6 or more months. When it is diagnosed, treatment is

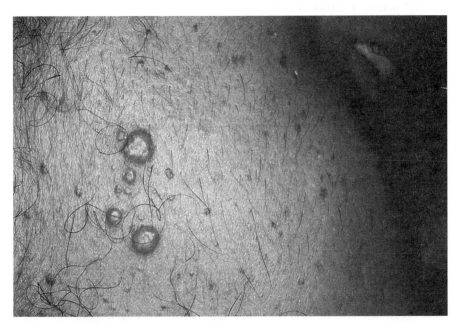

FIGURE 15.5 Molluscum contagiosum.
From Goldsmith, Lazarus, and Tharp: *Adult and Pediatric Dermatology: A Color Guide to Diagnosis and Treatment.* 1997. Philadelphia: F.A. Davis Company, pg 166, with permission.

usually limited to making sure the person does not have skin-to-skin contact with others and disqualifying him or her from competition. For those who do not respond to these conservative measures, invasive treatments such as laser therapy and cryotherapy are used, but people treated with these techniques may require longer recovery times.[1,4,6,10]

Verruca Plantaris

Verruca plantaris, otherwise known as a *plantar wart*, is caused by the human papilloma virus. Although this virus can infect any area of the body, in athletes it most commonly occurs on the plantar aspect of the foot. As with molluscum contagiosum, those who participate in water sports are at an increased risk of infection, because verruca is linked to fomites located on pool decks. Fomites are also located on the floors of showers, placing all who use communal showers without protecting the bottom of the foot at risk of getting a plantar wart. Clinically, the plantar wart appears as a hard, rough papule with a characteristic black dot in the center that is caused by capillary thrombosis. These warts are commonly covered by a callus, so it may be necessary to pare down the callus to see this diagnostic black dot. Though verrucae are not usually painful when they arise on other areas of the body, plantar warts typically cause patients great discomfort, particularly when they bear weight. In many instances, this impedes the person's ability to participate in sports.[1,3,4,9,10]

Treatment of a plantar wart includes surgical removal of the wart and/or the application of destructive techniques such as cryotherapy, curettage, and electrocautery. In some instances, a caustic agent such as salicylic acid, lactic acid, cantharidin acid, or trichloroacetic acid is used in combination with one of the above treatments. Typically, calluses must be pared down before a caustic agent is applied to the wart. Though effective, treatment methods that destroy tissue usually result in a longer recovery time, an outcome most athletes do not like. The recurrence of a plantar wart is common, making it important that the patient and health care provider stay vigilant with an established treatment plan.[1,3,9]

Bacterial Conditions

There is little debate that two organisms, **Staphylococcus aureus** (*S. aureus*) and **Streptococcus pyogenes** (*S. pyogenes*), are responsible for causing most of the bacterial skin infections in sports. These infections include **impetigo contagiosa, folliculitis, furunculosis**, and **community-acquired methicillin-resistant *S. aureus*** (CA-MSRA). Treatment of these conditions usually involves topical and/or oral antibiotic therapy and may or may not disqualify a person from participating in sports.[3,5,6,10]

Impetigo Contagiosa

Impetigo contagiosa, referred to simply as *impetigo*, is a highly contagious, superficial skin infection caused by either *S. aureus* or *S. pyogenes* (Fig. 15.6). People with this infection typically present with weeping, crusted, or pustular yellow honey-colored lesions on the face and/or extremities, which makes it difficult in the early stages of infection to differentiate impetigo from tina corporis and herpes simplex. As with all other skin infections, skin-to-skin contact is the most common way of transmitting impetigo from one person to another, though some believe the infection can also be

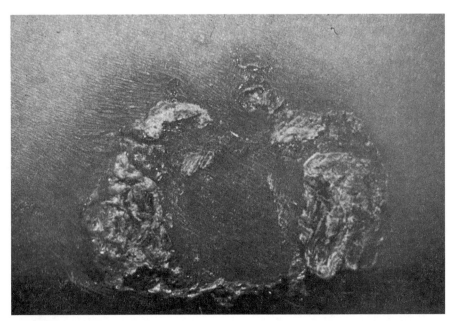

FIGURE 15.6 Impetigo.
From Goldsmith, Lazarus, and Tharp: *Adult and Pediatric Dermatology: A Color Guide to Diagnosis and Treatment*. 1997. Philadelphia: F.A. Davis Company, pg 331, with permission.

transmitted to a person from a piece of equipment that carries the bacterium. It is worth noting here that a strain of impetigo known as *bullous impetigo* produces toxins that can be very dangerous. This condition is characterized by erosions with flaccid bullae that split the epidermis. Traditionally, the diagnosis of impetigo has almost always been made clinically, making the need for a bacterial culture unnecessary in most cases. However, with the recent increased incidence of CA-MRSA (discussed later in this chapter), patients with impetigo may require a bacterial culture to determine antibiotic sensitivities.[1,3,5,6,10,13]

Treatment of patients with a single impetigo lesion includes applying mupirocin 2% ointment to the area. However, people with multiple lesions and those with bullous impetigo require oral antibiotic therapy with either dicloxacillin or cephalexin. Lesions should be cleaned two to three times per day with soap and water and should be completely covered the rest of the day and night. Because impetigo is very contagious, those with it must be disqualified from participation, preferably until all lesions have healed. However, some interscholastic and intercollegiate school policies and some practitioners require disqualification from participation for only 5 days after treatment is started, as long as the lesion has crusted. Because it is so contagious, many states do not allow an athlete to return to participation until a practitioner verifies that the patient is no longer contagious.[3–6,12,13]

PEARL

In many instances, impetigo, a highly contagious bacterial skin condition, must be treated with oral antibiotic therapy.

Folliculitis and Furunculosis

Folliculitis is a superficial infection of the hair follicles, whereas furunculosis, a condition derived from a furuncle, or *boil*, is a deeper skin infection. Folliculitis appears as pustules that are centered on hair-bearing areas, whereas furuncles present as large, distinct erythematous nodules over the extremities (Fig. 15.7). Both are caused by *S. aureus* and occur at a site of friction, making these conditions common in football, hockey, and lacrosse players in areas where equipment chafes the skin and where abrasions have occurred, particularly those that happen in response to playing on artificial turf. Folliculitis also appears on the face of males, resulting from the friction caused by daily shaving. As with most skin conditions, those who have an open lesion and skin-to-skin contact with an infected person maintain the highest risk of developing furunculosis.[1,6,10,12–14]

As with impetigo, the initial treatment of patients with folliculitis or an isolated furuncle includes daily cleaning with soap and water and applying mupirocin 2% ointment to the affected area. Those with multiple furuncles require oral antibiotic therapy with either dicloxacillin or cephalexin. Warm water compresses can also be of benefit to the patient. People with folliculitis can participate in athletics. However, those with furunculosis should be disqualified to avoid an epidemic outbreak among teammates.[1,3–6,14]

Community-Acquired Methicillin-Resistant
Staphylococcus aureus

Until fairly recently, methicillin-resistant *S. aureus*, a mutagenic, antibiotic-resistant variant of *S. aureus*, mostly occurred in traditional medical settings, such as hospitals

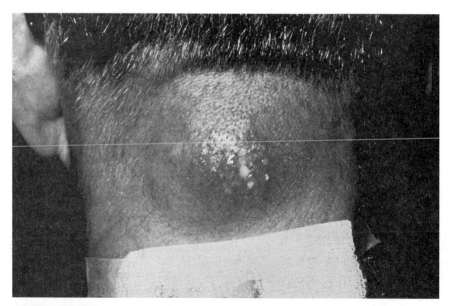

FIGURE 15.7 A furuncle associated with furunculosis.
From Goldsmith, Lazarus, and Tharp: *Adult and Pediatric Dermatology: A Color Guide to Diagnosis and Treatment.* 1997. Philadelphia: F.A. Davis Company, pg 364, with permission.

and nursing homes. Now, this bacterial infection is occurring with increasing frequency throughout many other settings. Indeed, within the past decade, the prevalence of CA-MRSA in the athletic setting has increased dramatically, with most cases affecting those who participate in team sports, such as football, wrestling, volleyball, and rugby. Though CA-MRSA occurs in people who are at an increased risk of becoming infected, such as those who have had contact with infected patients, realize that it also occurs in people who are not at an increased risk of infection.[7,15,16]

CA-MRSA occurs in otherwise healthy people who do not have risk factors commonly associated with the development of such an infection.

Patients with CA-MRSA typically present with a tender and erythematous abscess, though it is sometimes associated with furunculosis and impetigo. In some instances, multiple lesions are present. Common areas for abscess development include the axilla, buttocks, and thighs. A bacterial culture of the infection confirms a diagnosis of CA-MRSA and helps to determine the antibiotic treatment of choice. When CA-MRSA is confirmed, the abscesses are drained and treated with topical mupirocin 2% ointment. The region is bathed daily in an antibacterial agent, such as 10% povidone-iodine liquid soap. Mupirocin 2% ointment is also applied intranasally to treat possible bacterial colonization at that site. Oral antibiotics such as trimethoprim/sulfamethoxazole, clindamycin, and fluoroquinolone are prescribed for 10 to 14 days. In some instances, these are used in combination with rifampin. People not responding to this treatment and people presenting with systemic symptoms are hospitalized for intravenous antibiotic treatment.[5–7,13,16]

Inflammatory Conditions

Inflammatory skin conditions related to sports include allergic and irritant contact dermatitides, which typically result from exposure to an allergen located in items and on products listed in Box 15.3. Of note are items made of rubber, because these are a prime culprit in causing dermatitis. These conditions are characterized by distinct red vesicles with crusts or erosions and an eczematous rash that develops on the skin within 7 days after allergen exposure (Fig. 15.8). The area becomes itchy, causing many to scratch at the developing vesicles. Because they can produce similar signs and symptoms, it is easy to confuse contact dermatitis with an infection. For example, dermatitis caused by an allergic skin reaction to the soap used to launder athletic equipment can produce the same signs and symptoms as tinea cruris in a male who wears a jock strap during competition. Also, in certain instances, contact dermatitis produces hives on the skin, otherwise known as *urticaria*. Defined as a local anaphylactic reaction to an allergen, urticaria can also be precipitated by environmental factors, such as exposure to water, cold, heat, and the sun. A patch test is the best way to ultimately determine cause of the allergic reaction.[1,3,4,6,13,17]

The primary treatment of any contact or irritant dermatitis is for the patient to avoid the allergen that triggers the unwanted response. In some instances, this can easily be accomplished, such as by changing the laundry detergent used to clean a

BOX 15.3

ITEMS AND PRODUCTS THAT CONTAIN ALLERGENS RESPONSIBLE FOR CAUSING CONTACT DERMATITIS

Sports equipment (e.g., uniforms, shoes, undergarments, protective pads)	Cleaning products used to maintain indoor playing surfaces
Detergent used to launder athletic clothes	Athletic tape placed on body parts for prophylactic and treatment purposes
Lawn care products used to maintain outdoor playing fields	Topical medications used as a treatment modality

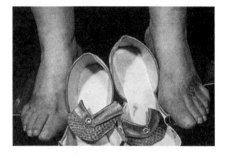

FIGURE 15.8 Contact dermatitis.
From Dillon: *Nursing Health Assessment: A Critical Thinking, Case Studies Approach.* 2003. Philadelphia: F.A. Davis Company, pg 167, with permission.

person's clothes. However, other allergens, such as those located in products used to maintain the safety of a playing surface on which the athlete participates, cannot be easily avoided. In these cases, topical corticosteroids and antihistamines may help control the patient's symptoms. Because a risk for anaphylaxis may exist for some highly sensitive individuals, these people should seriously consider disqualifying themselves from participating in any activity that exposes them to what they are allergic to. If these patients still insist on participating, appropriate immediate drug intervention, such as an epinephrine autoinjector, should be made available for use as needed.[1,3,4,6,13,17]

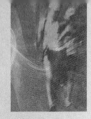

CASE STUDY
Conditions of the Skin

SCENARIO
A 21-year-old college wrestler presents in your office with a skin rash that started 1 week ago. Though official wrestling practice has yet to start, the patient has been preparing for the up-coming season by exercising and practicing with other members of the team. These unsupervised practice sessions are occurring at a local fitness club that rents out space for activities such as wrestling and martial arts.

PERTINENT HISTORY
Medications: No medications currently. No known drug allergies.

Family History: Unremarkable.

PERSONAL HEALTH HISTORY
Tobacco Use: Nonsmoker. Denies use of oral tobacco products.

Alcohol Intake: Regularly consumes 1 to 2 alcoholic drinks per day in the off-season. Abstains from alcohol intake during the wrestling season.

Recreational Drugs and Banned Substances: Denies use, but has used laxatives in the past to "make weight" during the season.

Caffeinated Beverages: Consumes 2 to 3 cups of coffee per day, sometimes more during the school year.

Diet: Has a regular, healthy diet when not wrestling. However, during the season, the patient reports modifying his diet so he can make and then stay at the weight he wrestles. This has included the need to "crash diet" on occasion, particularly when he was scheduled to wrestle at a lower weight than that at which he usually participates.

Past Medical History: While he was in high school, he experienced two incidences of herpes simplex outbreak around the lips and one case of tinea corporis. Absent of childhood diseases such as chicken pox and mumps. Has had numerous musculoskeletal injuries from wrestling, the most serious of which was a torn anterior cruciate ligament of the right knee when he was 18. This injury was repaired surgically.

History of Present Illness: *The* patient started noticing a rash on his neck 1 week ago. He tried treating the condition with an antifungal over-the-counter ointment, with no success. The rash has spread to his left cheek and ear and has become increasingly itchy.

PERTINENT PHYSICAL EXAMINATION*
Pustular yellow honey-colored lesions are present on the patient's neck, face, and ear. Some of the lesions are weeping, and a few are starting to crust over. Deep cervical, supraclavicular, and submaxillary lymph nodes are swollen and tender.

*Focused examination limited to key points for this case.

RED FLAGS FOR THE PRIMARY HEALTH CARE PROFESSIONAL TO CONSIDER

Skin-to-skin contact is the most common way of transmitting skin infections from one person to another, and any skin condition with weeping lesions is potentially contagious. Do not touch the area without protective gloves, and be sure to thoroughly wash your hands with soap and water after evaluating the region. Because the patient is wrestling in a communal setting, the cleanliness of the facility may be questionable.

RECOMMENDED PLAN

- Obtain a bacterial culture to confirm a diagnosis of impetigo.
- Prescribe oral antibiotic therapy (dicloxacillin or cephalexin).
- Instruct the patient to
  - stop using the topical antifungal,
  - clean the lesions two to three times per day with soap and water,
  - apply mupirocin 2% ointment to the affected areas daily,
  - not let others use his personal toiletries and items such as washcloths and towels,
  - keep lesions completely covered day and night, and
  - avoid bodily contact with others until all lesions have crusted.
- Recommend that the patient tell those with whom he has had skin-to-skin contact to report any sign of a skin rash to a qualified medical professional.
- Counsel the patient about the health dangers associated with using quick weight loss techniques.

REFERENCES

1. Adams BB. Sports dermatology. *Adolesc Med* 2001;12(2):305.
2. Finch M. Assessment of skin in older people. *Nurs Older People* 2003;15(2):29.
3. Adams BB. Dermatologic disorders of the athlete. *Sports Med* 2002;32:309.
4. Adams BB. Sports dermatology. *Derm Nurs* 2001;13(5):347.
5. Dienst WL, Dightman L, Dworkin MS, et al. Pinning down skin infections: diagnosis, treatment and prevention in wrestlers. *Phys Sportsmed* 1997;25(12):45.
6. Cordero KM, Ganz, JE. Training room management of medical conditions: sports dermatology. *Clin Sports Med* 2005;21:565.
7. Cohen PR. Cutaneous community-acquired methicillin-resistant *Staphylococcus aureus* infection in participants of athletic activities. *South Med Assoc* 2005;98:596.
8. Landry GL, Chang CJ, Harmon KG, et al. Herpes and tinea in wrestling. *Phys Sportsmed* 2004;32(10):34.
9. Burkhart CG. Skin disorders of the foot in active patients. *Phys Sportsmed* 1999;27(2):88.
10. Brenner IKM, Shek PN, Shephard RJ. Skin infection in athletes. *Sports Med* 1994;17:86.
11. Becker TM. Herpes gladiatorum: a growing problem in sports medicine. *Cutis* 1992;50:150.
12. Gorgos D. Skin care: proper treatment for skin infections. *Dermatol Nurs* 2006;18(3):283.
13. Kirkland R. Dermatological problems in the football player. *Int J Dermatol* 2006;45:927.
14. Sosin DM, Gunn RA, Ford WE, et al. An outbreak of furunculosis among high school athletes. *Am J Sports Med* 1989;17:828.
15. Beam JW, Buckley B. Community-acquired methicillin-resistant *Staphylococcus aureus*: prevalence and risk factors. *J Athl Train* 2006;41:337.
16. Lindenmayer JM, Schoenfeld S, O'Grady P, et al. Methicillin-resistant *Staphylococcus aureus* in a high school wrestling team and the surrounding community. *Arch Intern Med* 1998;158:895.
17. Fisher AA. Allergic contact dermatitis: practical solutions for the sports-related rashes. *Phys Sportsmed* 1993;21(3):65.

SUGGESTED READINGS

Adams ES, Dexter W. Identifying and controlling metabolic skin disorders. *Phys Sportsmed* 2004;32(8):29.
Romano R, Lu D, Holtom P. Outbreak of community-acquired methicillin-resistant *Staphylococcus aureus* skin infections among a collegiate football team. *J Athl Train* 2006;41:141.
Schnirring L. NFHS issues infectious skin disease policy. *Phys Sportsmed* 2005;33(10):18.

WEB LINKS

www.nlm.nih.gov/medlineplus/tineainfections.html. Accessed 8/30/08.
   Comprehensive information regarding the causes, signs and symptoms, treatment, and prevention of skin disorders.

www.kidshealth.org/parent/infections/bacterial_viral/impetigo.html. Accessed 8/30/08.
   Excellent resource related to contagiousness, treatment, and prevention of impetigo.

www.nlm.nih.gov/medlineplus/herpessimplex.html. Accessed 8/30/08.
   Comprehensive information and resource site for the herpes simplex virus.

Glossary

Accessory motions Small, nonmeasurable movements that occur when a diarthrodial joint moves through its full range.

Acclimatize To adapt to a new environment, such as what happens when the body becomes used to exercising in hot and humid weather.

Adhesion Fibrous connection between tissues that are normally separated, particularly soft tissues of the musculoskeletal system.

Adhesive capsulitis Inflammation of the shoulder's joint capsule, causing the region's soft tissues to adhere to one another. Also known as *frozen shoulder syndrome.*

Allograft Tissue harvested from one member of a species and transplanted into a different member of the same species.

Amino acids Organic compounds that serve as the building blocks of proteins.

Anatomic snuffbox Triangular area of the dorsum of the thumb formed by the thumb's extrinsic muscles. The scaphoid bone forms its floor.

Anorexia nervosa Eating disorder characterized by an unhealthy low body weight due to low self-esteem and a distorted body image.

Anterior drawer test Stress test used to determine the presence of either a lateral ankle sprain involving the anterior talofibular ligament or a knee sprain involving the anterior cruciate ligament.

Apley's compression test Special test used to evaluate the integrity of the knee menisci and collateral ligaments.

Apley's distraction test In light of a positive Apley's compression test, this is a special test used to differentiate between meniscal and collateral knee injury.

Apley's scratch tests Series of movements used to simultaneously assess multiple motions of the shoulder complex.

Articular cartilage Portion of hyaline cartilage located on a bone's joint surface.

Auricular hematoma Swelling between the ear's auricle external layer of skin and the underlying cartilage. Also known as *cauliflower ear.*

Autograft Tissue harvested and transplanted from one part of a patient's body to another.

Bennett's fracture Proximal end fracture of the first metacarpal associated with a dislocation of the carpometacarpal joint of the thumb.

Biceps tension test Special test used to evaluate the integrity of the glenoid labrum. Also known as the *SLAP test.*

Body composition Makeup of the body in terms of fat and lean body mass.

Body dysmorphic disorder Mental disorder characterized by a person having a distorted body image of himself or herself.

Bone scan Nuclear imaging technique where radioactive isotopes are injected into the body. In orthopedics, this test is primarily used to rule out the presence of a stress fracture.

Boutonnière deformity Flexion contracture of a finger's proximal interphalangeal joint. Also known as a *buttonhole deformity.*

Boxer's fracture Fracture to the shafts of the fourth and/or fifth metacarpals.

Bradykinin Plasma kinin that increases the permeability of blood vessels and irritates free nerve endings.

Bulimia nervosa Eating disorder characterized by binge eating followed by episodes of purging (e.g., vomiting, use of laxatives, enemas, diuretics, and medications) because of feelings of guilt and self-condemnation. Commonly associated with exercising for extended periods on a daily basis.

Bump test Special test used to determine the integrity of the fibula and tibia. Also known as the *heel tap test.*

Bursae Synovial fluid–filled sacs typically located near diarthrodial (synovial) joints. Bursae are responsible for decreasing friction between adjacent body tissues during movement.

Bursitis Inflammation of a bursa.

Calcaneal bursa Bursa located between the skin and the calcaneal tendon.

Calcaneal exostosis Bony growth arising from the calcaneus. Also known as a *heel spur.*

Calcaneal tendon Largest tendon of the body; formed by the muscles of the triceps surae. Also known as the *Achilles tendon.*

Cardiorespiratory endurance Ability of the heart, lungs, and blood vessels to supply oxygen to the working muscles over a prolonged period of time. Also known as *aerobic fitness.*

Carpal tunnel Tunnel that is formed by the carpal bones and transverse carpal ligament and passes vessels, nerves, and tendons from the forearm to the palmar aspect of the hand.

Carpal tunnel syndrome Entrapment of the median nerve in the carpal tunnel as it passes from the forearm to the hand.

Carrying angle The normal angle made by the elbow when standing in the anatomical position.

Cervical radiculopathy Any dysfunction of a cervical spine nerve root; typically caused by compression of the nerve root.

Chemotaxis Process by which leukocytes are brought to an area of inflammation.

Clunk test Special test used to evaluate the integrity of the glenoid labrum.

Cold erythema Nonallergic, erythematous rash response to the application of cold to the skin. Associated with pain, muscle spasms, and sweating. At times, it is congenital in nature.

Cold gel pack Form of cryotherapy where a commercially purchased pack is placed in a freezer, frozen to 10°F, and placed on the body. Because of the potential for frostbite to occur with this form of cryotherapy, a wet barrier, such as thin towel, should be placed between the pack and the skin.

Cold immersion Form of cryotherapy where an extremity is placed in a bucket filled with water chilled to 55°F.

Cold urticaria Anaphylactic reaction that occurs in the form of hives or welts in the immediate area where cold has been applied.

Collateral ligaments Ligaments that are positioned on either side of a diarthrodial joint. Most commonly associated with hinge and condyloid joints.

Community-acquired methicillin-resistant *Staphylococcus aureus* Strain of *S. aureus* resistant to methicillin.

Computed tomography Radiographic technique where a radiography tube emits x-ray beams in a 360° circle around the patient's body, producing three-dimensional image "slices" that are interpreted with computers.

Concussion Type of mild traumatic brain injury that causes an altered mental status.

Contrast therapy Alternating between hot and cold treatments during the same treatment session to decrease pain and to produce physiological effects beneficial to healing.

Contrecoup injury Injury that occurs at the site opposite to where the body is traumatized. This term is almost exclusively used to describe an injury to the brain.

Contusion Injury, to either hard or soft tissue, that is caused by blunt-force trauma and does not disrupt the continuity of the skin. Also known as a *bruise*.

Coracoacromial arch Structure that forms the roof of the subacromial space comprised of the coracoacromial ligament, coracoid process, and acromion process.

Corneal laceration Cut or scratch of the cornea. Also known as an *open globe injury*.

Coronary ligaments Structures that attach the peripheries of the medial and lateral menisci of the knee to the tibial plateaus.

Costochondritis Nonspecific idiopathic chest wall pain not associated with swelling.

Coup injury Injury that occurs at the site where the body is traumatized. This term is almost exclusively used to describe an injury to the brain.

Cross straight leg test Application of a straight leg test on the asymptomatic, contralateral extremity.

Crossover test Special test used to determine whether the acromioclavicular joint has been injured.

Cryotherapy Treatment modality that removes heat from the body to produce therapeutic effects.

Cubital recurvatum Hyperextension of the elbow not caused by trauma.

Cubital valgus Increase in the normal carrying angle.

Cubital varus Decrease in the normal carrying angle.

Cytotoxic Substances that are destructive to cells.

de Quervain's syndrome Paratenonitis (tenosynovitis) of the tendons that form the radial boarder of the anatomic snuffbox.

Dead arm syndrome Syndrome characterized by paresthesia and muscle weakness of the upper extremity; typically due to chronic instability of the glenohumeral joint.

Deltoid ligament Medial ankle ligament that protects the medial aspect of the foot and ankle by limiting the amount of foot eversion.

Detached retina Displacement of the retina from its normal position against the back of the eye.

Diapedesis Movement of leukocytes from capillaries to a site of inflammation.

Dislocation Displacement of a body part. Typically used to describe the disarticulation of a joint in musculoskeletal medicine.

Distraction test Special test used to determine whether the acromioclavicular joint has been injured.

Dorsiflexion Moving the foot toward its dorsal aspect by flexing the ankle.

Double straight leg test Special test used to differentiate sacroiliac joint pain from pain originating from the lumbar spine.

Drop foot Condition usually associated with anterior compartment syndrome, pathology to the common and/or deep peroneal nerves, or a herniated L4 lumbar disk resulting in a patient's inability to dorsiflex the ankle.

Drop arm test Special test used to determine the integrity of the rotator cuff muscle group.

Dual-energy x-ray absorptiometry (DEXA) scanning Test used to determine bone density and also to assess a person's body composition.

Empty can test Special test used primarily to determine the integrity of the supraspinatus; also may indicate the presence of subacromial impingement syndrome.

End-feel The amount and type of resistance provided by an injured soft tissue, as gauged by an examiner, during the application of a stress test.

Epidural hematoma Collection of blood between the dura mater and the skull.

Erythema Even reddening of the skin due to local histamine release and an increase of oxyhemoglobin in the area. Commonly associated with cryotherapy and thermotherapy modality treatments.

Esters Class of chemical compounds formed by combining an organic acid with an alcohol, which results in water loss.

Eversion Turning the foot outward by pointing the toes away from the midline of the body.

Eversion talar tilt test Stress test used to confirm the presence of a deltoid ligament sprain.

Exercise-induced bronchospasm Bronchospasm that occurs in response to exercise or strenuous activity. Also known as *exercise-induced asthma*.

External rotation test Special test to rule out the presence of a syndesmosis sprain. Also known as the *Kleiger test*.

FABERE test Special test used to rule out pathology of the sacroiliac and hip joint. Also known as *Patrick's test*.

False negative Diagnostic test finding that falsely states that a condition does not exist.

Fascia Supporting and connective tissue that forms a fibrous membrane.

Fasciotomy Surgical technique used to relive pressure in a compartment by cutting the fascia.

Female athlete triad Syndrome derived from the interrelated problems caused by disordered eating, amenorrhea, and osteoporosis.

Fibroplasia Formation of fibrous tissue.

Finkelstein's test Test used to determine the presence of de Quervain's syndrome.

Flexibility Capacity of a joint to move through its full range of motion.

Focal brain lesion Macroscopic bleeding in the brain. Also known as an *intracranial hemorrhage*.

Folliculitis Inflammation of the hair follicle.

Fomite An inanimate substance that carries infectious organisms.

Fracture Disruption in the continuity of a bone. Also known as a *broken bone*.

Freiberg's infraction Avascular necrosis of the epiphysis at the metatarsal head.

Full can test Special test used to determine the integrity of the supraspinatus.

Functional fitness The ability to perform activities of daily living, such as walking, bending, lifting, and climbing stairs, without pain, injury, or discomfort.

Furunculosis Deep, bacterial skin infection derived from a furuncle.

Gaenslen's test Special test used to rule out pathology of the sacroiliac joint.

Gamekeeper's thumb Sprain to the ulna collateral ligament of the thumb's metacarpophalangeal joint. Also known as *skier's thumb*.

Ganglia cyst Fluid-filled sac that forms on the dorsal aspect of the wrist.

Glenohumeral joint apprehension test Stress test used to determine the presence of anterior glenohumeral joint instability where the patient's joint is placed in a position that is vulnerable to dislocation.

Glenohumeral joint relocation test Stress test used to determine the presence of anterior glenohumeral joint instability where the examiner "relocates" a patient's joint that is on the verge of dislocating.

Glycerol Colorless, liquid, sugar alcohol found in fats.

Goniometer Tool used to measure a diarthrodial joint's range of motion.

Granulation Process that adds capillary beds to a fibrin clot.

Grey Turner's sign Discoloration of skin around the right or left flanks, commonly associated with an injured kidney.

Guyon's canal syndrome Compressive neuropathy of the ulnar nerve as it passes in Guyon's canal. Also known as *ulnar nerve palsy* and *cyclist's palsy*.

Haglund's deformity Thickened retrocalcaneal bursa on the lateral side of the heel with or without an underlying calcaneal exostosis. Also known as a *pump bump*.

Hawkins-Kennedy test Special test used to determine the presence of subacromial impingement syndrome involving the supraspinatus tendon.

Heart rate reserve Difference between a person's measured, or predicted, maximum heart rate and resting heart rate.

Hemarthrosis Bloody effusion usually associated with a severe ligament injury, particularly of the cruciate ligaments.

Hemothorax Collection of blood in the pleural cavity.

Hepatomegaly Enlargement of the liver commonly associated with hepatitis.

Herniated intervertebral lumbar disk Protrusion of a lumbar disk's nucleus pulposus into its annulus fibrosis. Also known as a *slipped disk*, the nucleus pulposus typically herniates in a posterolateral direction.

Herpes gladiatorum Term used to describe herpes simplex in the sport of wrestling.

Herpes simplex virus Virus that causes vesicular eruptions to mucosal areas.

Heterotopic ossification Abnormal formation of bone within skeletal muscle. Also known as *myositis ossificans.*

Hip pointer Contusion to the iliac crest.

Hip scouring test Special test used to evaluate the general health of the hip joint.

Histamine Chemical mediator that causes blood vessels to dilate and increases the permeability of vessel walls.

Hyaline cartilage Glassy, translucent cartilage that covers the surface of bone.

Hydrogenation Process of adding hydrogen to unsaturated organic compounds to form a solid saturated fat.

Hydrostatic weighing Method of determining body composition by measuring total body volume under water.

Hyperextension Extension of a joint beyond the anatomical position. Some joints have the ability to naturally hyperextend (e.g., shoulder), whereas others cannot (e.g., knee).

Hypertrophic cardiomyopathy Thickening of the heart muscle.

Hypertrophy Increase in size of a body organ, or tissue, not attributed to disease.

Hyphema Bleeding into the eye's anterior chamber in front of the iris.

Hypothenar eminence Area that is located on the lateral aspect of the hand's palmar aspect and contains the intrinsic muscles of the little finger.

Hypovascular Relating to an area of decreased blood supply.

Ice bag Form of cryotherapy where a plastic bag is filled with cube, disk, flake, or crushed ice and applied to the body with an elastic wrap. Also known as an *ice pack*.

Ice massage Form of cryotherapy where ice is rubbed on the body subsequent to allowing water to freeze in a paper cup.

Iliotibial band friction syndrome Irritation that occurs to the iliotibial band as it passes over the lateral condyle of the femur during knee flexion and extension.

Impetigo contagiosa Superficial skin infection caused by either *Staphylococcus aureus* or *Streptococcus pyogenes*.

Inguinal canal Passageway that passes the vas deferens and testicular artery and veins from the body to the scrotal sac in males.

Insoluble fiber Nondigestible substance that does not dissolve in water. Thus, it passes through the digestive track virtually intact to help increase bulk and soften stool.

Inversion Turning the foot inward by pointing the toes toward the midline of the body.

Inversion talar tilt test Stress test used to determine the presence of a lateral ankle sprain involving the anterior talofibular and calcaneal fibular ligaments. Also known as the *inversion stress test*.

Jersey finger Extension deformity of a finger's distal interphalangeal joint.

Jones fracture Fracture to the base of the fifth metatarsal.

Kehr's sign Pain that radiates to the left shoulder and one-third the way down the left arm. Commonly associated with an injured spleen.

Keloid Hypertrophied scar.

Kienböck's disease Avascular necrosis of the lunate.

Kyphosis Angulation of the posterior curve of the thoracic spine leading to decreases in the lordotic curve of the cervical and lumbar spines. Also known as *roundback* and *humpback*.

Lachman test Stress test used to assess the integrity of the anterior cruciate ligament.

Lateral epicondylitis Inflammation to the lateral epicondylitis of the humerus. Also known as *tennis elbow*.

Lazy bowel syndrome Condition where bowels become dependent on laxatives to function properly.

Lean body mass Everything in the body except for fat, including muscles, bones, ligaments, connective tissue, internal organs, and skin.

Legg-Calvé-Perthes disease Avascular necrosis of the femoral neck; usually congenital in nature.

Leucotaxin Chemical mediator responsible for aligning leukocytes delivered to an acutely inflamed region along the walls of surrounding intact blood vessels.

Lift-off test Special test used to evaluate the strength of the subscapularis muscle.

Ligaments Tissues that connect bone to bone. Extrinsic ligaments are discrete structures whereas intrinsic ligaments are thickened portions of a joint capsule.

Little league elbow Number of conditions, including apophysitis, avulsion fracture, and articular changes involving the medial epicondyle of the humerus in the adolescent.

Ludington's test Special test used to confirm a rupture of the long head of the biceps tendon.

Lysosomes Cells that contain enzymes that contribute to the digestion of pathogens taken into a cell by phagocytosis.

Macronutrients Nutrients that supply the body with energy and help body tissues develop.

Macrophages Phagocytes that develop from monocytes and play a major role in phagocytosis.

Magnetic resonance imaging Technique that produces body images from the interaction of a magnetic field with a radiofrequency signal.

Mallet finger Flexion deformity of a finger's distal interphalangeal joint. Also known as *baseball finger* and *drop finger*.

Manual muscle testing Clinical technique used to qualitatively assess the strength of a muscle group.

March fractures Stress fractures to the shafts of the second and third metatarsals.

Marfan's syndrome Congenital connective tissue disorder that dilates and weakens the aorta, predisposing it to dissection or rupture during intense physical activity.

Margination Accumulation and adhesion of leukocytes to the epithelial cells of blood vessel walls at the site of injury in the early stages of inflammation.

Mast cells Histamine- and heparin-rich cells that are present in connective tissue and play an essential role in the inflammatory process. Also known as *mastocytes*.

McBurney's point Area located one-third of the way between the anterior superior iliac spine and umbilicus. Pain at this point is commonly associated with appendicitis.

McMurray's test Special test used to evaluate the integrity of the knee menisci.

Mechanism of injury Manner in which forces are applied to the body that result in musculoskeletal pathology.

Medial epicondylitis Inflammation to the medial epicondylitis of the humerus. Also known as *golfer's elbow*.

Medial tibial stress syndrome Term used to describe atraumatic pain along the medial aspect of the tibia. Also known as *shin splints*.

Menorrhagia Unusually heavy menstrual flow.

Metatarsalgia Generic term used to describe any pain in the plantar aspect of the metatarsal heads.

Micronutrients Nutrients that regulate cell function.

Mild traumatic brain injury Injury to the brain arising from blunt-force trauma and/or acceleration or deceleration forces.

Minerals Inorganic compounds that are found in foods and are necessary for proper bodily function.

Molluscum contagiosum Skin infection caused by a pox virus.

Mottling Condition where the skin appears blotchy with red and white patches caused by blood vessel changes in the underlying tissue. A common response to intense heating of the skin, indicating unequal distribution of heat in the underlying tissue.

Murphy's sign Indicative of a dislocated lunate where the third metacarpophalangeal joint appears equal in height with the other metacarpophalangeal joints when the patient makes a fist.

Muscular endurance Ability of a muscle or muscle group to repeatedly contract or to sustain a contraction over a period of time.

Muscular strength Capability of a muscle or muscle group to exert force against resistance.

Myocardial contusion Bruising of the heart due to blunt-force trauma. Also known as a *cardiac bruise*.

Necrosin Toxic substance in injured tissue that attracts leukocytes to an injured area and mediates the phagocytic process.

Neer's impingement test Special test used to determine the presence of subacromial impingement syndrome involving the supraspinatus and/or long head of the biceps tendon.

Nerves Part of the peripheral nervous system, nerves are tissues comprised of neuron bundles that transmit information to and from the central nervous system.

Noble's compression test Special test used to confirm the presence of iliotibial band friction syndrome.

Nutrients Elements that supply the body with chemicals needed for metabolism.

Ober's test Special test used to determine whether the iliotibial band is shortened.

Organomegaly Enlargement of a visceral organ.

Osgood–Schlatter disease Traction apophysitis condition occurring when the patellar ligament pulls excessively on the tibial tubercle. Also known as *tibial tubercle apophysitis*.

Osteolysis Destruction and reabsorption of bone into the body. Commonly occurs at the distal end of the clavicle in response to heavy resistance training exercise.

Osteopenia Decrease in bone mineral density that, if left unchecked, leads to osteoporosis.

Osteophyte Bony outgrowth that typically forms near freely moveable joints. Also known as a *bone spur*.

Osteoporosis Loss of bone mass due to factors such as aging, poor nutritional status, and, in women, a lack of estrogen production.

Otitis externa Bacterial infection of the ear canal that alters the canal's normal pH balance. Commonly known as *swimmer's ear*.

Painful arc Pain that occurs between 60° and 120° glenohumeral joint abduction.

Paratenonitis Umbrella term used to refer to the inflammation and degeneration of the outer layer of a tendon's sheath.

Patellar apprehension test Stress test that assesses the stability of the patella within the femoral groove.

Patellar grind test Special test used to determine the presence of chondromalacia patella. Also known as *Clarke's sign*.

Patellar ligament Structure that attaches the distal pole of the patella to the tibial tubercle. Also known as the *patella tendon*.

Patellar tendon rupture Complete tearing of the patellar tendon (ligament); typically occurs at the tendon's patella attachment.

Patellar tendonitis Irritation that occurs at the patellar tendon's (ligament) attachment site on the patella. Also known as *jumper's knee*.

Patellofemoral joint Joint formed by the articulation between the patella and the patellar, or femoral, groove.

Peritendinitis Paratenonitis condition referring to inflammation of a tendon's sheath. Also known as *tenosynovitis* and *tenovaginitis*.

Phagocytosis Ingestion and digestion of debris and bacteria by phagocytes.

Phalen's test Definitive clinical diagnostic test for carpal tunnel syndrome.

Plain-film radiography Most common form of x-ray examination. Also known as *standard radiography*.

Plantar fascia Tough, fibrous tissue supporting the foot's plantar aspect. Also known as the *plantar aponeurosis*.

Plantar fasciitis Inflammation of the plantar fascia.

Plantar flexion Moving the foot toward its plantar aspect by extending the ankle.

Plasma exudate Protein-rich substance normally found in blood.

Pneumothorax Collection of air in the pleural cavity.

Polypeptide Chain of two or more amino acids.

Position of function Normal position assumed by the hand and wrist with the patient standing and the upper extremity relaxed.

Postconcussion syndrome Diagnosis used when concussion symptoms are experienced by a patient for weeks or months after a mild traumatic brain injury.

Posterior drawer test Stress test used to determine the presence of either a lateral ankle sprain involving the posterior talofibular ligament or a knee sprain involving the posterior cruciate ligament.

Pre-participation examination Comprehensive medical examination provided to those desiring to participate in sports and exercise.

Primary motions Major motions that are allowed by a diarthrodial joint and can typically be measured in degrees of motion.

Prostaglandin Chemical mediator that stimulates free nerve endings in response to injury.

Pseudoboutonnière deformity Finger deformity defined by hyperextension of the distal interphalangeal joint and flexion of the proximal interphalangeal joint.

Pulmonary contusion Bruising of a lung, usually by a deceleration injury mechanism.

Radiculopathy Generalized term used to describe any irritation of a nerve root.

Range of motion Amount of movement, measured in degrees of motion, allowed by a diarthrodial joint.

Raynaud's phenomenon Constriction of arteries and arterioles in a body part due to exposure to cold.

Resting metabolic rate Rate at which calories are burned when at rest.

Retinacula Membranes that hold body tissue and organs in place.

Retrocalcaneal bursa Bursa located between the calcaneal tendon and the calcaneus.

Reye's syndrome Acute encephalopathy and fatty infiltration of the liver, sometimes involving the kidneys, pancreas, spleen, heart, and lymph nodes. Prevalent in children aged 15 years and younger. Its development is associated with the use of salicylates, notably aspirin.

Rotator cuff Muscle group comprised of the supraspinatus, infraspinatus, subscapularis, and teres minor muscles.

Sacroiliac joint compression test Special test used to rule out pathology of the sacroiliac joint where the examiner compresses the joint.

Sacroiliac joint distraction test Special test used to rule out pathology of the sacroiliac joint where the examiner distracts the joint.

Sag test Stress test used to assess the integrity of the posterior cruciate ligament.

Salter-Harris fracture classification System of categorizing growth plate fractures based on injury mechanism and the relationship of the fracture line(s) with the epiphysis. Salter-Harris fractures are also known as *physeal fractures.*

Scapula winging Inability of the scapula's vertebral border to sit flush against the rib cage.

Sciatica Generalized term used to describe radiating pain that follows the course of the sciatic nerve.

Second impact syndrome Occurs when the brain of a patient still experiencing symptoms from a mild traumatic brain injury is traumatized, resulting in respiratory failure and death.

Secondary amenorrhea Condition defined clinically by a history of three missed menstrual periods in a row or the lack of menstrual period for 6 months in the absence of pregnancy.

Secondary hypoxia Hypoxia that occurs secondary to acute trauma due to a decreased supply of oxygen to the injured area.

Sesamoid bone Bone embedded in a tendon or joint capsule.

Sever's disease Apophysitis of the calcaneus.

Shear test Special test used to determine whether the acromioclavicular joint has been injured. Also known as the *compression test*.

Sinding-Larsen-Johansson disease Traction apophysitis condition that occurs when the patellar ligament pulls excessively on the inferior pole of the patella.

Skeletal muscles Ttissue composed of contractile elements that move the joints of the appendicular and axial skeleton. Also known as *striated muscles*.

Slipped capital femoral epiphysis Posterior slippage of the femoral epiphysis in relation to the femoral head.

Slipping rib syndrome Hypermobility of the anterior end of a false rib, causing it to slip under the adjacent superior rib. Also known as *painful rib syndrome*.

Snapping hip syndrome Audible snapping sound originating from the hip region caused by the proximal portion of the iliotibial band and/or tendon of the gluteus maximus muscle passing over the femur's greater trochanter.

Soluble fiber Nondigestible chemical substance that dissolves in water. When ingested, it undergoes metabolic processes that aid in digestion, though it is not absorbed into the bloodstream.

Spondylolisthesis Forward slippage of one vertebral body over another.

Spondylolysis Defect of the pars interarticularis of a vertebra; typically seen in the fourth and fifth lumbar vertebrae.

Sports hernia Term used to describe a spectrum of injuries resulting from overusing the rectus abdominis and hip adductor muscles at their attachment to the pubic bone. Also known as *athletic pubalgia*.

Sprain Stretching or tearing of a ligament or joint capsule.

Sprengel's deformity Condition characterized by scapulae that sit higher than normal on the rib cage.

Spurling's test Special test used to determine the presence of cervical radiculopathy, especially if the radiculopathy is caused by compression of the nerve root. Also known as the *foramen compression test*.

Squeeze test Special test used to assess the integrity of the fibula.

Staphylococcus aureus (S. aureus) Resident flora bacterium of the skin and of the nasal and oral cavities.

Step deformity Elevation of the distal portion of the clavicle due to a sprain to the acromioclavicular joint.

Step-off deformity Condition where the spinous process of a vertebra cannot be palpated because of a forward slippage of the vertebra.

Sternal compression test Test that differentiates between a thorax contusion and a rib fracture.

Sterols Fatty compound subgroup of steroids that provide important metabolic communications and prevent the absorption of cholesterol in the intestines.

Stimson's maneuver Method that uses traction to allow for a gentle reduction of an active glenohumeral joint dislocation.

Straight leg test Special test used to confirm the presence of pressure, typically caused by a herniated intervertebral lumbar disk, on one or more of the nerve roots comprising the sciatic nerve.

Strain Stretching or tearing of a muscle or tendon. Also known as a *pulled muscle*.

Streptococcus pyogenes (S. pyogenes) Resident flora bacterium of the respiratory tract.

Stress fracture Fracture caused by repetitive microtrauma to a bone. Also known as a *fatigue fracture.*

Stress radiograph Plain-film radiograph taken while an examiner applies a stress test to an injured joint.

Subacromial impingement syndrome Compression of the structures (supraspinatus, long head of the biceps, subacromial bursa) occupying the subacromial space.

Subconjunctival hemorrhage Bleeding that occurs beneath the conjunctiva.

Subdural hematoma Collection of blood between the dura mater and brain.

Subtalar joint Intertarsal joint located between the talus and calcaneus.

Sudden cardiac death Unexpected death occurring in a short time frame resulting from cardiac disease from known or unknown origin.

Sulcus sign Stress test used to determine the presence of inferior glenohumeral joint instability.

Syndesmosis sprain Sprain involving the anterior inferior tibiofibular ligament. In certain instances, the interosseous membrane and posterior inferior tibiofibular ligament are also involved. Also known as a *high ankle sprain.*

Syndesmotic complex Complex comprised of the distal tibiofibular joint, anterior and posterior inferior tibiofibular ligaments, and interosseous membrane.

Tendinosis Focal area of tendon degeneration that does not exhibit either clinical or histological signs of inflammation.

Tendonitis Inflammation of a tendon, though it is questionable whether a tendon undergoes the normal inflammatory process when injured.

Tendons Structures that connect muscle to bone.

Tendinopathies Pathologic conditions involving a tendon.

Tennis elbow test Definitive clinical diagnostic test for lateral epicondylitis.

Tenosynovitis Paratenonitis condition referring to inflammation of a tendon's sheath. Also known as *peritendinitis* and *tenovaginitis.*

Tenovaginitis Paratenonitis condition referring to inflammation of a tendon's sheath. Also known as *peritendinitis* and *tenosynovitis.*

Theater sign Patellofemoral pain resulting from placing the knee in a continuous flexed position for an extended period. Most commonly associated with chondromalacia patella.

Thenar eminence Area that is located on the medial aspect of the hand's palmar aspect and contains the intrinsic muscles of the thumb.

Thermogenesis Energy expenditure not accounted for by resting metabolic rate or activity.

Thermotherapy Treatment modality that adds heat to the body to produce therapeutic effects.

Thomas test Clinical test signifying tightness of the hip flexors.

Thompson test Special test used to determine the integrity of the calcaneal (Achilles) tendon.

Thumb abduction stress test Definitive clinical diagnostic test for a sprain to the ulnar collateral ligament of the thumb's metacarpophalangeal joint.

Tibiofemoral joint Joint formed by the articulation between the tibia and femur. Also known as the *knee joint.*

Tietze's syndrome Idiopathic anterior chest wall pain associated with swelling.

Tinea corporis Fungal skin disease of the body and extremities. Also known as *ringworm.*

Tinea cruris Fungal skin disease of the groin that can involve the genitals and anus. Also known as *jock itch*.

Tinea gladiatorum Term used to describe tinea corporis in the sport of wrestling.

Tinea pedis Fungal skin disease of the foot. Also known as *athlete's foot*.

Tinel's test Determines the health of a nerve by tapping over a superficial portion of the nerve. Also known as *Tinel's sign*.

Torsion Rotation of a body part around its long axis.

Transient paresthesia Paresthesia that disappears gradually over time.

Trendelenburg sign Clinical sign indicating weakness of the hip abductor weakness.

Triceps surae Muscle complex formed by the gastrocnemius, soleus, and plantaris muscles.

Turf toe Sprain to the metatarsophalangeal joint of the great, or first, toe.

Tzanck smear Microscopic test used to diagnose infections caused by the herpes virus.

Ulnar collateral insufficiency Stretching of the elbow's ulnar collateral ligament.

Ulnar nerve neuropathy Any nerve condition involving the ulnar nerve.

Valgus Angulation of an extremity where the extremity's distal segment is angulated away from the body's midline.

Valgus stress test Stress test used to assess the integrity of a medial collateral ligament.

Varus Angulation of an extremity where the extremity's distal segment is angulated toward the body's midline.

Varus stress test Stress test used to assess the integrity of a lateral collateral ligament.

Verruca plantaris Plantar wart.

Vitamins Organic compounds that are found in foods and are necessary for proper bodily function.

Volkmann's contracture Permanent claw-like deformity of the hand and fingers caused by a disruption to the neurovascular supply to the region.

Yergason's test Special test used to determine the presence of tendonitis and/or subluxation of the long head of the biceps tendon.

Index

Note: Page numbers followed by *b* refer to boxed material; page numbers followed by *f* refer to illustrations; and page numbers followed by *t* refer to tables.